Gastrointestinal Endoscopy 3rd Edition

Gastrointestinal Endoscopy **3rd Edition**

Fred E Silverstein MD

Clinical Professor of Medicine
University of Washington
Seattle, Washington

Partner, Frazier & Company
Seattle, Washington

Guido NJ Tytgat MD PhD

Chief, Division of
Gastroenterology–Hepatology
University of Amsterdam
Academic Medical Center

Professor of Medicine and Gastroenterology

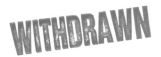

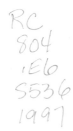 **Mosby**

London   Philadelphia   St. Louis   Sydney   Tokyo

Copyright © 1997 Times Mirror International Publishers Limited.
Published in 1997 by Mosby-Wolfe, an imprint of Times Mirror International Publishers Limited.

Typeset on Apple Macintosh.
Body text set in Sabon roman 9.5 pt/12 pt; legends set in Gill Sans italic 9 pt/11 pt.

Colour reproduction and final film by Spectrum Colour, Needham Market, Ipswich, UK.
Printed and bound by Grafos SA, Arte sobre papel, Barcelona, Spain.

Reprinted in 1998 by Mosby International Limited

10 9 8 7 6 5 4 3 2

ISBN 0 7234 2195 1

For full details of all Mosby International Limited titles, please write to Mosby International Limited, Lynton House, 7–12 Tavistock Square, London WC1H 9LB, UK.

A CIP catalogue record for this book is available from the British Library and the US Library of Congress.

Project Manager Nigel Wetters

Development Editors Gina Almond and Jennifer Prast

Design and Layout Louise Bond

Illustrators Sandie Hill, Diane Kinton, and Daniel Pyne

Production Controller Jane Tozer

Copyeditor John Halliday

Index Angela Cottingham

Proofreader Alison Creedy

Publisher Richard Furn

Contents

Preface

Endoscopy is one of the most exciting and expanding fields of clinical medicine. It provides accurate diagnostic information and is being used increasingly to provide therapy for intestinal disorders. Furthermore, it is less invasive and safer than many other therapeutic approaches, and often can be accomplished on an outpatient basis to achieve a favorable cost–benefit ratio.

The success of endoscopy creates several dilemmas. How is one to learn these techniques? How can one learn to interpret the images? How can one learn about the appearances of newly recognized diseases? Many of us who teach endoscopy know that the mechanical performance of the procedure is only the beginning. Accurate interpretation of images is at least as important, and learning this skill requires the highest quality endoscopic images.

The purpose of writing this book is to provide an organized series of photographs documenting the appearance of gastrointestinal organs in health and disease.

Endoscopic photography is not simple. Many of us have taken thousands of photographs for teaching and for documenting a patient's abnormality. Unfortunately, most of these photographs turn out to be of poor quality. The unique aspect of this book is the high quality of the photographs and the vast clinical experience from which they are drawn. Dr Tytgat has mastered the art of endoscopic photography. When his interest and skill are combined with his large clinical facility, the large number of patients, and the wide variety of gastrointestinal problems encountered, the result is an exceptional set of photographs. The majority of images in this book are reproduced from Dr Tytgat's collection. Carefully labeled line drawings and schematic diagrams were added to clarify the critical diagnostic information.

In this third edition of *Gastrointestinal Endoscopy*, we have made a number of improvements. We have added images of several diseases not previously covered and we have included additional and better images of diseases that were discussed in the earlier editions. We have continued to emphasize diseases associated with AIDS because this is a problem of increasing importance in gastroenterology. We have also expanded the sections on early diagnosis of tumors. It is vital that clinicians attempt diagnosis at a sufficiently early stage so that endoscopic or surgical resection can be effective.

We were faced with a challenge in this third edition. Should we add images of a variety of types to the book, or stay focused on endoscopy? Although the temptation was to add more ERCP, CT, histological images, etc., we chose to keep the emphasis of the book on the endoscopic appearance of disease. Each other imaging discipline has developed a core set of images of its own and to try and represent each field with inclusion of only a few such core images is unfair to these disciplines. We continue to present some endoscopic ultrasound images, histology and ERCP radiographs, but for details of these and other approaches, the reader is referred to books specifically written about these techniques.

A new aspect of endoscopy is the availability of video images of high quality. Most of our images are obtained via a fiber-optic endoscope as these are from Dr Tytgat's extensive collection. However, many excellent images are now available with video imaging both in still and motion formats. The fiber-optic images in this book should be equally applicable to interpretation of video images.

Fred E Silverstein MD
Guido NJ Tytgat MD PhD

Acknowledgements

We have many people to thank for helping us prepare this book. Dr Tytgat would like to thank his colleagues at the Academic Medical Center and his ex-fellows in training who referred patients with uncommon abnormalities. In particular, he would like to thank Drs Kees Huibregtse, Joep Bartelsman, Lisbeth Mathus-Vliegen, Lok Tio, Paul Fockens, Eric Rauws, Willem Dekker, Max Schrijver, and the staff of the Department of Medical Photography. He would also like to thank the Board of Directors of the Academic Medical Center for their support and appreciation.

Dr Silverstein would like to thank Mary Hill who helped edit the text and organize the slide set, and his colleagues who provided thoughtful comments and some excellent examples of unusual diseases. He would like to thank in particular Drs David Saunders, Charles Pope, Charles Rohrmann, Rodger Haggitt, Cyrus Rubin, Michael Kimmey, Lok Tio, George MacDonald, and Brian Reid.

Dr Silverstein would also like to thank his partners at Frazier & Company – Alan D Frazier, Charles H Blanchard, Jon N Gilbert, Robert Kupor, and Nader J Naini – who remained patient and supportive during the preparation of this third edition.

Dr Douglas Levine, Associate Professor of Medicine at the University of Washington, Division of Gastrointestinal Endoscopy, provided clinical guidance and thorough comments as we prepared both the second edition and this new third edition.

Finally, we would like to thank Ellie Silverstein and Christiane Tytgat who assisted us with this project. Our famililes encouraged us, provided critical comments, and allowed us to devote the time necessary to complete this book.

junction is called the ora serrata or 'Z' line (Fig. 1.9). The normal junction may appear irregular (Fig. 1.10). Note that this line may appear to straighten if the area is distended with air during endoscopy.

The esophageal lumen is usually free of debris, and normally has longitudinal mucosal folds that are pliable and flatten with distension. These folds can be easily distinguished from esophageal varices, which appear beaded and may have a bluish color. Four or five longitudinal folds usually form a symmetrical, rosette-like structure at the esophagogastric junction. This junction is normally closed but can be easily opened with gentle air insufflation. No resistance is usually encountered at this junction as the endoscope passes into the stomach. In addition to longitudinal folds, transverse ridges may occasionally be seen, especially before vomiting or during retching (Fig. 1.11.).

The longitudinal folds gradually taper over a 2–3 cm section of distal esophagus and extend to the Z line. The squamocolumnar junction is usually located at the distal end of the lower esophageal sphincter, 0.5 cm below the diaphragmatic hiatus, though it may be observed 1 cm above the hiatus as a result of variations that occur with respiration and air insufflation. Gastric folds extend up from below and end just below the squamocolumnar junction.

The submucosal vasculature of the esophagus can be seen at endoscopy as fine, small, delicate blood vessels. In the distal esophagus it may be possible to see delicate vessels that are straight and parallel. These correspond to the 'palisade' zone. These vessels are only visible on the esophageal side of the ora serrata (Figs. 1.8, 1.12 and 1.14).

In older individuals, one may commonly see glycogen-rich nodular or granular structures in the esophageal squamous mucosa, a condition referred to as glycogenic acanthosis (Fig. 1.13). The presence of these granules is of no clinical relevance. Such areas may also be seen in the distal esophagus (Fig. 1.14).

Motility in the esophagus is difficult to appreciate at endoscopy. Occasionally, contractions will be seen, especially tertiary contractions. Likewise, in certain diseases that involve the esophageal muscle, the lack of motility can be observed by endoscopy (e.g. a nonperistaltic esophagus in a patient with scleroderma).

A variety of normal and abnormal conditions cause narrowing of the esophageal lumen. These include intrinsic structures such as rings, webs, tumors, or strictures, and extrinsic structures such as normal and abnormal vascular structures adjacent to the esophagus, mediastinal tumors, etc. The intrinsic lesions are dealt with in the following chapters on esophageal pathology.

The importance of extrinsic compression on the esophagus is best understood when one remembers that the esophagus is positioned in a central location within the thorax: immediately posterior to the heart, between the lungs, and adjacent to the vertebral column, the inferior vena cava, and the aorta. It is attached at its upper end to the cricopharyngeus muscle and at its lower end to the diaphragm. Normal (Fig. 1.15) and abnormal (Fig. 1.16) structures may impinge on the esophagus and can be seen during

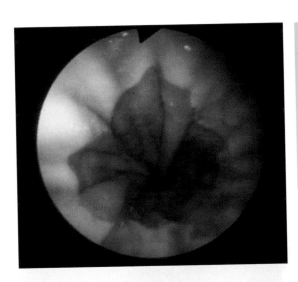

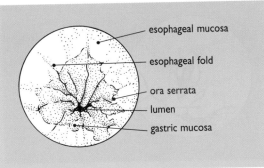

Figure 1.9 Normal squamocolumnar junction is well seen. Note esophageal folds that can be seen at the esophagogastric junction. These folds are pliable and can usually be distinguished from esophageal varices.

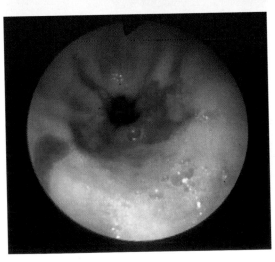

Figure 1.10 Normal squamocolumnar junction may appear irregular.

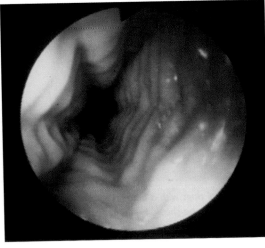

Figure 1.11 Transverse ridging of the esophagus with retching.

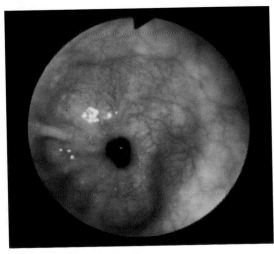

Figure 1.12 View of normal distal esophageal mucosa with a delicate vascular pattern.

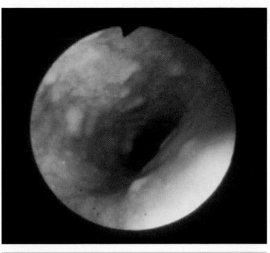

Figure 1.13 *Glycogenic acanthosis of the esophagus.*

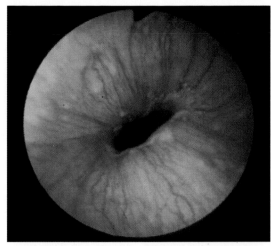

Figure 1.14 *This endoscopic view of the distal esophagus demonstrates normal blood vessels and glycogenic acanthosis of the mucosa.*

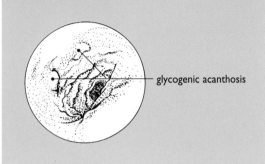

glycogenic acanthosis

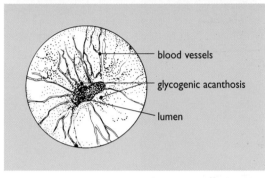

blood vessels

glycogenic acanthosis

lumen

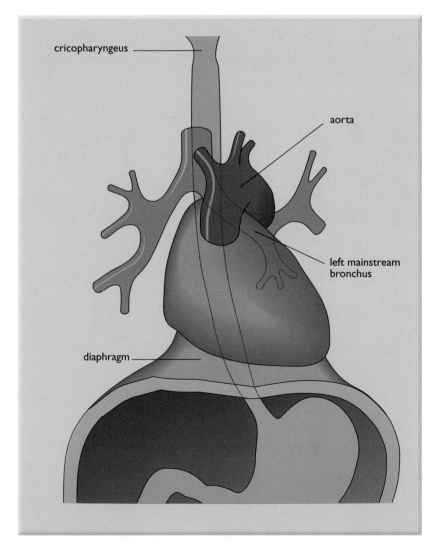

cricopharyngeus

aorta

left mainstream bronchus

diaphragm

Figure 1.15 *The normal areas of narrowing of the esophagus.*

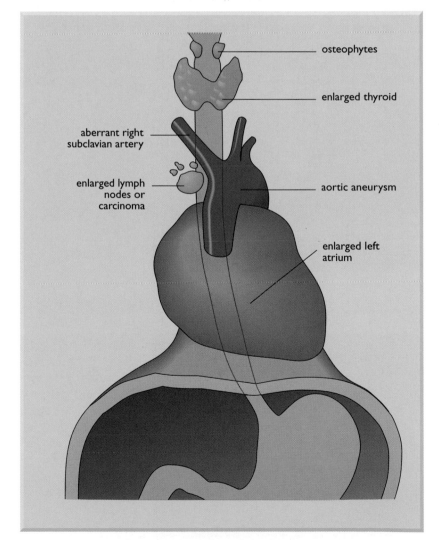

osteophytes

enlarged thyroid

aberrant right subclavian artery

aortic aneurysm

enlarged lymph nodes or carcinoma

enlarged left atrium

Figure 1.16 *The abnormal areas of narrowing of the esophagus.*

esophagoscopy. The normal structures include the aorta, approximately 25–30 cm from the incisor teeth (Fig. 1.17), and the left mainstem bronchus, slightly below the aorta. Both of these structures cause a smooth indentation of the esophageal wall. The abnormal structures include osteophytes from the cervical spine, an enlarged thyroid gland, an enlarged aorta, and enlarged left atrium, bronchogenic tumors, lymph nodes, and abnormal vascular structures. An anomalous origin of the right subclavian artery from the descending aorta may cross behind the esophagus and compress it anteriorly against the trachea, causing difficulty in swallowing. This condition is referred to as dysphagia lusoria. In each case, the esophageal mucosa is indented but otherwise appears normal.

The esophagus terminates at the ora serrata and at the lower esophageal sphincter. Anatomically, the lower esophageal sphincter appears as a slight thickening of the smooth muscle of the esophageal wall. It is normally closed at rest, and functions to keep gastric contents out of the esophagus.

▼ A

▼ B

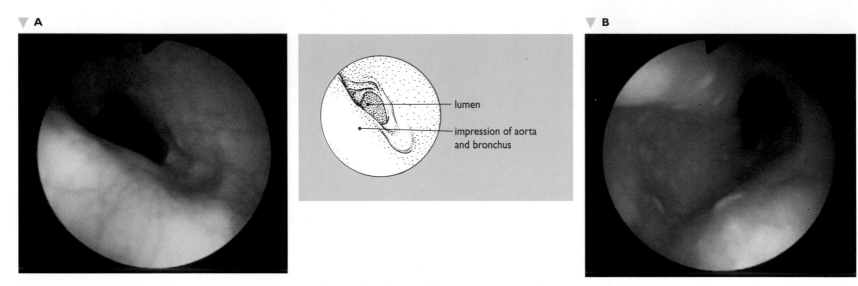

Figure 1.17 (A and B) *Two different patients, each demonstrating normal esophagus with an impression caused by the adjacent aorta and left mainstem bronchus. The covering mucosa is normal.*

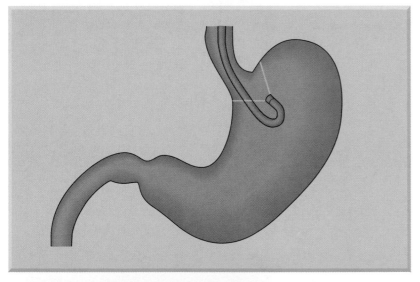

Figure 1.18 *Diagram demonstrates retroflexion to inspect the gastric cardia, fundus, and lesser curvature.*

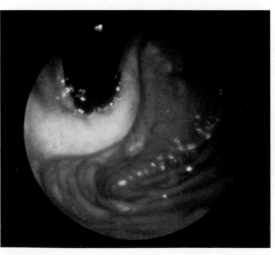

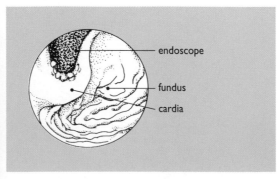

Figure 1.19 *Normal cardia seen with the endoscope retroflexed. The cardial tissue is snug around the endoscope. The fundus is partially seen.*

POSITIONING AND ENDOSCOPIC EXAMINATION

The endoscope is passed under direct vision from the esophagus into the stomach. When using a forward-viewing endoscope, advancemeent should be accomplished with the lumen constantly in view; blind passage is not desirable. This passage often requires a turn to the left and anteriorly to track the esophagus as it enters the stomach. The lumen can usually be easily and gently followed into the stomach. The area of the stomach just below the

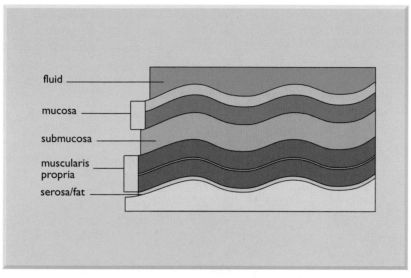

Figure 1.20 *Basic intestinal wall structure. The two layers of muscle in the muscularis propria separated by connective tissue. Exact configuration varies in different intestinal organs.*

esophagogastric junction is the cardia. Endoscopic examination of the esophagus should include careful inspection of the cardia, which can only be partially accomplished during insertion of the instrument into the stomach. For complete and accurate examination, the instrument must be placed into the stomach and the tip bent back on itself, or retroflexed, to see the gastric tissue of the cardia as it surrounds the endoscope (Figs. 1.18 and 1.19). This is the only reliable method of viewing ulcers, mucosal tears, or tumors in the cardia. When a hiatal hernia is present a large, incompetent cardia will be observed in the retroflexed view, with a space surrounding the endoscope as it enters the stomach.

The retroflexion maneuver is also essential to permit adequate inspection of the gastric fundus and the lesser curve of the stomach. This is achieved by retroflexing the endoscope and then moving it in and out with rotation clockwise and counterclockwise. If one limits an endoscopic examination to direct endoscopy without performing careful retroflexion, significant lesions in the stomach can be missed. Because of the risk of impaction, the retroflexed endoscope should not be pulled up into a hiatal hernia or the distal esophagus. The instrument should always be straightened first in the more distal part of the stomach.

ENDOSONOGRAPHY OF THE NORMAL ESOPHAGUS

In the normal esophagus the typical five-layer intestinal wall structure can be recognized (Fig. 1.20). The interface with the mucosa is echogenic or white, the deep mucosa is echo poor, and the submucosa, again, is echogenic. The muscularis propria is echo poor and the periesophageal fat is echogenic (Figs. 1.21 and 1.22).

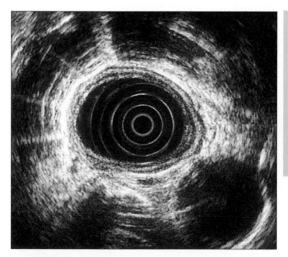

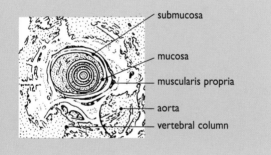

Figure 1.21 *The five normal esophageal wall layers are seen, as in the aorta. The wall layers are thin. The ultrasound endoscope and balloon are seen in the center of the image. (Courtesy of Dr T.L. Tio)*

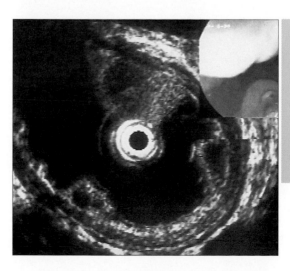

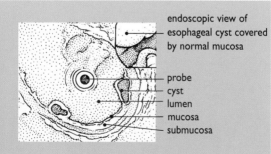

Figure 1.22 *This image was made of esophageal wall using a rotating ultrasound probe passed via the channel of a video endoscope. The insert in the upper right is the endoscopic image. The ultrasound image shows several submucosal esophageal cysts and the normal layers of the esophageal wall. (Courtesy of Dr Mitsahiko Kubo)*

THE NORMAL STOMACH

ANATOMY

The stomach is divided into several anatomical areas (Fig. 1.23): the fundus (Fig. 1.24), the cardia (seen in Fig. 1.19), the body or corpus (Figs. 1.25 and 1.26), and the antrum (Fig. 1.27). There is a lesser curve and a greater curve. Endoscopically, the incisura angularis usually marks the entrance into the antrum on the lesser curvature. This anatomic division is different from the histologic or physiologic boundary because of the distribution of the antral and fundal mucosa. Histologically the antral mucosa may extend high up on the lesser curvature to within a few centimeters of the cardia. This is higher than the incisura angularis, the anatomic boundary for the beginning of the antrum. For the endoscopist, this mucosal boundary is important because benign gastric ulcers often occur at the margin of the antral and fundal mucosa. As this boundary can occur high on the lesser curvature, especially in elderly patients, this is an area where gastric ulcers may be encountered. For this reason the lesser curvature must be carefully inspected during endoscopy, both directly and with the tip retroflexed.

POSITIONING AND ENDOSCOPIC EXAMINATION

Stomachs have a variety of normal shapes. Some are long and vertical whereas others are transverse. Most of the these distinctions are not important to the endoscopist. The general principles for inspection are the same for all configurations.

The tip of the endoscope is passed through the distal esophagus and cardia into the upper body of the stomach. At this point, gentle inflation with air is necessary to inspect the stomach wall. The gastric pool is inspected and observations made as to the amount of fluid and the presence of blood, bile, and food (Fig. 1.28). Recently ingested antacid or barium may compromise the endoscopic examination (Fig. 1.29), whereas other debris may suggest abnormal gastric emptying. A bezoar consisting of retained food residue or other material may be seen. After inspecting the gastric pool, it is usually wise to aspirate as much fluid as possible in order to prevent reflux and aspiration during the procedure and to facilitate the further inspection of the stomach.

The gastric mucosal surface is briefly inspected for color, surface appearance, blood vessels, and fold thickness. The complete gastric examination

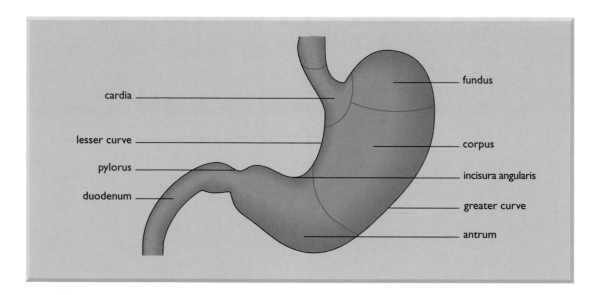

Figure 1.23 *The anatomy of the stomach.*

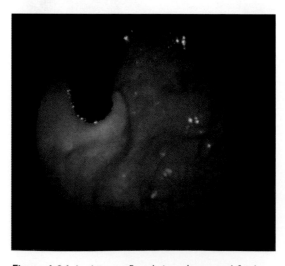

Figure 1.24 *In this retroflexed view, the normal fundus of the stomach is seen in addition to the cardia.*

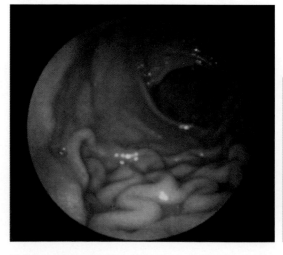
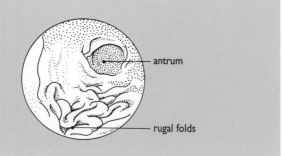

Figure 1.25 *In this view of the stomach with the endoscope straight, one can appreciate the normal rugal folds in the body of the stomach and observe that these folds do not extend into the antrum in the distance.*

is usually performed after the duodenum has been intubated and inspected. One exception is when an abnormality is encountered during the initial examination of the stomach in which case the area is carefully inspected immediately. In this way the endoscopist knows that erythema or bleeding was present before passing the endoscope through that area and was not caused by the shaft of the endoscope during inspection of the duodenum.

Although it seems that the area just below the cardia should be easy to inspect endoscopically, this is often not the case. In the high lesser curvature position, even large gastric ulcers can be missed with a forward-viewing endoscope. A similar problem occurs with other lesions of the cardia such as tears and tumors. Therefore, it is essential that these areas be observed on retroflexed view (Figs. 1.19 and 1.24).

When fiberoptic endoscopes were first developed, complicated maneuvers were necessary to achieve retroflexion in order to inspect the cardia and fundus. This is no longer the case. The new flexible fiberoptic or video endoscopes can mechanically turn 180° with motion on the control handles. In fact, most can turn 210°, allowing simple retroflexion for inspection of the cardia and fundus. With experience, the retroflexion maneuver can be easily performed, allowing complete inspection of the lesser curvature, cardia, and fundus.

Normally, the gastric mucosa is a uniform salmon color (Fig. 1.26). With careful inspection one can observe the areae gastricae, the macroscopic patterns of gastric glandular architecture (Fig. 1.30). This pattern is irregular and occasionally absent in patients with atrophic gastritis, and accentuated in patients with hypersecretion and duodenal ulcers. Blood vessels are not usually seen through the mucosa. The folds, or rugae, begin in the upper body of the stomach near the entrance to the esophagus and course distally, in a parallel longitudinal fashion, to the antrum. They may be seen in the fundus but are often not longitudinally oriented in this area. These folds are normally soft and pliable, and in most cases will flatten almost completely with moderate but not excessive distension of the stomach.

The antrum is usually smooth and free of folds, although a prepyloric semicircular fold may be seen (Fig. 1.27). Gastric peristalsis begins in the midbody and progresses down into the antrum. Contractions, at a frequency of three per minute, continue to the gastric outlet or pylorus where they stop (Fig. 1.31). The pylorus is usually open (Fig. 1.32) but closes when the contraction wave reaches it. This probably allows for mixing of food, and for

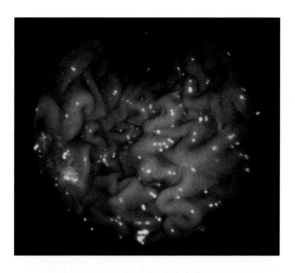

Figure 1.26 The normal mucosa of the stomach is glistening and moist, and normal rugae are also seen. The white spots are highlights of the endoscope lights reflecting off the mucosa.

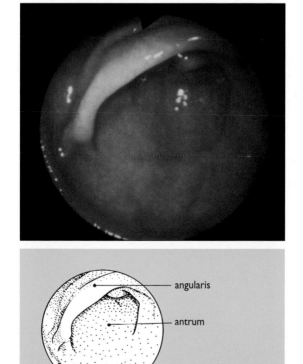

Figure 1.27 Normal antrum and angularis. The pylorus is located under the incisura angularis and is therefore not seen in this view. There are no rugal folds.

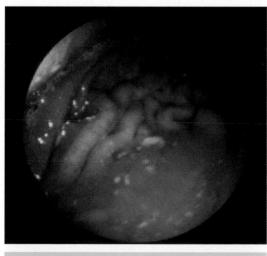
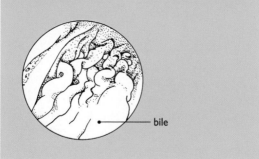

Figure 1.28 Normal stomach, with bile present in the gastric pool.

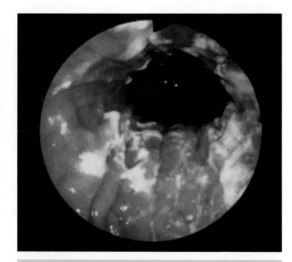
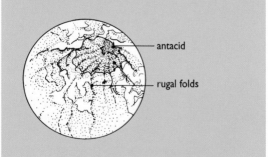

Figure 1.29 Normal stomach. The normal mucosa of the midbody is covered with antacid taken by mistake just before endoscopy. The rugal folds are normal.

liquid contents to pass into the duodenum while the stomach continues to liquefy solids. It is often useful endoscopically to watch a contraction wave move from the body to the antrum to determine whether there is an area that is asymmetrical, stiff, and not moving well. If such as area is observed, it should be carefully inspected for signs of an abnormality. An ulcer or tumor may first be noted as an abnormal area observed during an antral contraction wave. This is especially important with infiltrating carcinomas, which may be covered by relatively normal looking mucosa.

There are several organs adjacent to the stomach that can cause extrinsic impressions of the gastric lumen. The most commonly seen is the spleen, which may cause an impression in the posterior greater curvature area. Abnormalities of other structures, such as aneurysms of the splenic artery or pancreatic pseudocysts, may also appear as areas of extrinsic compression. When using a forward-viewing endoscope, the gastric configuration is usually easily understood. This is not the case, however, when side-viewing endoscopes are used. With the latter instrument, one may get somewhat lost

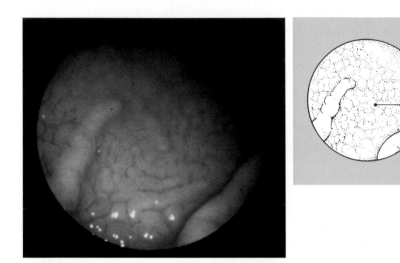

Figure 1.30 Normal areae gastricae are seen. The gastric pits empty into these glandular structures.

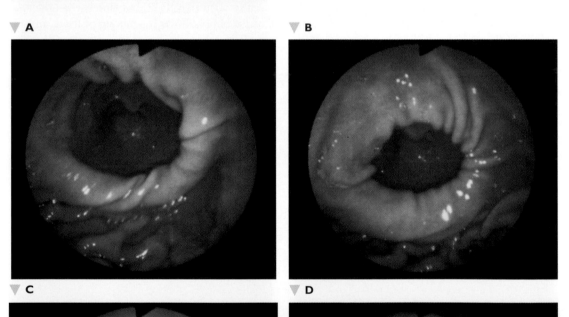

Figure 1.31 (A–D) This sequence demonstrates a normal antrum with a contraction wave moving towards the pylorus. If one watches this wave as it progresses, areas of decreased contractility can be identified and studied. The final view shows the wave ending at the pylorus.

in the proximal stomach and have difficulty finding the antrum and pylorus. This may be problem during endoscopic retrograde cholangiopancreatography (ERCP), which requires that a side-viewing endoscope be passed via the esophagus and stomach into the duodenum to locate and cannulate the papilla of Vater. This problem is especially noted in the 'cup-and-pour' or 'cascade' stomach, in which a pouch of fundus lies directly below the cardia. The tip of the endoscope may enter this pouch, and the endoscopist is then unable to locate the route to the gastric body, antrum, and pylorus. The endoscope may continue to turn around in the pouch presenting a retroflexed view, but the anatomy is confusing (Fig. 1.33).

Although the 'cup-and-pour' stomach is mainly a problem for side-viewing endoscopes, it is also occasionally a problem with forward-viewing endoscopes. The instrument may be damaged because of extreme angulations and, more important, a complication such as a perforation can result because of the confusing anatomy, especially if excessive force is used. This problem may be solved by pulling the endoscope back to just below the esophagogastric junction and then looking to the left. One often sees a ridge that separates the fundic pouch from the rest of the stomach (Fig. 1.34). A turn to the left will then allow the endoscope to pass easily into the gastric body and down into the antrum.

The incisura angularis is a useful marker for locating the lesser curvature, as well as the pylorus. The latter is found several centimeters distal to the angularis. Although it is usually not difficult to find the pylorus, it may be a problem with a side-viewing endoscope, or with any endoscope if the area is distorted by current or past peptic ulcer disease or surgery.

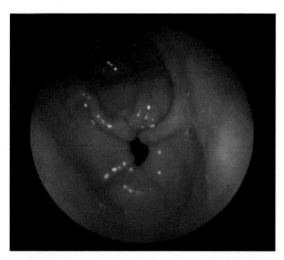

Figure 1.32 *The pylorus often appears open as does in this photograph.*

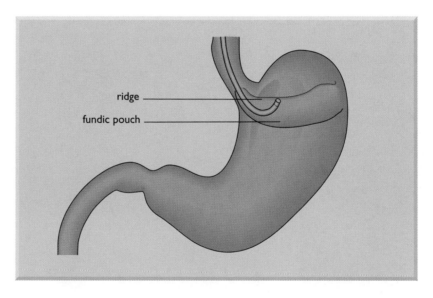

Figure 1.33 *Diagram of a 'cup-and-pour' stomach demonstrating the problem this can create for the endoscopist.*

ridge

fundic pouch

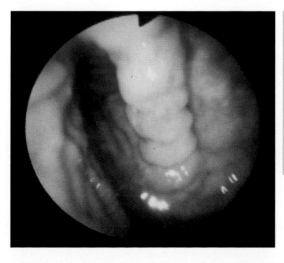

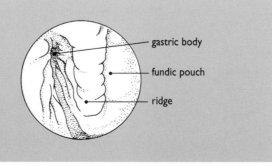

gastric body

fundic pouch

ridge

Figure 1.34 *Cup-and-pour stomach. The fundic pouch, which may confuse the endoscopist, is seen to the right. In the center is the ridge separating the pouch from the main body of the stomach to the left.*

ENDOSONOGRAPHY OF THE NORMAL STOMACH

The endoscopic application of ultrasound to the stomach allows examination of the stomach wall as well as structures such as the lymph nodes, pancreas, liver, blood vessels, and so on, which lie adjacent to it. The five layers of the normal stomach wall can clearly be seen when the transducer orientation is correct (Fig. 1.35).

THE NORMAL DUODENUM

ANATOMY

The duodenum, measuring 25–30 cm in length, marks the beginning of the small bowel. It is composed of four portions (Fig. 1.36). The first is the duodenal bulb, which is approximately 4–5 cm long and begins at the pylorus and runs to the right and posteriorly. The bulb is in the peritoneal cavity; the other portions are retroperitoneal. The second portion is approximately 7–8 cm in length and runs caudally. The third portion is approximately 10 cm long and runs to the left across the spine and great vessels. The fourth portion is 4–5 cm long and runs cephalad and to the left where it turns and joins the jejunum at the ligament of Treitz.

The mucosa of the duodenal bulb is usually free of folds, but the other portions demonstrate characteristic folds of Kerckring. The mucosal villi are similar to those found in the jejunum and ileum. Peculiar to the duodenum are Brunner's glands, which occur mainly in the submucosa of the first one-half or two-thirds.

The papilla of Vater, located on the medial wall of the descending duodenum 3–6 cm distal to the apex of the bulb, is the main papilla that drains the bile duct and the pancreatic duct in most patients. An accessory papilla (papilla of Santorini) may be located 2–4 cm proximal to the papilla of Vater on the medial duodenal wall. It is important to understand the anatomy of the duodenum around the papilla of Vater if one is to be able to find the papilla and cannulate it with a side-viewing endoscope. The papilla is often located at the distal end of a bulge in the medial duodenal wall. This bulge is the intramural portion of the distal common bile duct. Just distal to the papilla there is a characteristic longitudinal fold, the plica duodeni longitudinalis. Likewise, there may be several folds that converge proximally at the papilla. The experienced endoscopist focuses on the area at the distal end of the bulging intramural common bile duct and the proximal end of the longitudinal fold to locate the papilla. This anatomy may be appreciated on barium contrast x-ray studies of the duodenum, especially during hypotonic duodenography with air contrast (Figs. 1.37 and 1.38).

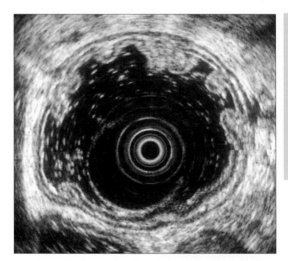

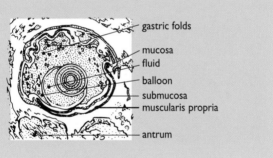

Figure 1.35 *Endosonogram of the normal stomach. The stomach is fluid filled and the ultrasound endoscope is in the center. A balloon over the tip is visible. The normal layers of the stomach wall can be seen. (Courtesy of Dr T.L. Tio)*

Figure 1.36 *Anatomy of the duodenum.*

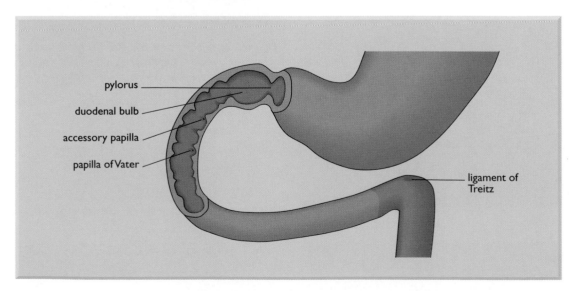

POSITIONING THE ENDOSCOPE

Once the pylorus is located, the tip of the endoscope is advanced into the duodenal bulb. In most instances the tip passes easily, but occasionally persistence is required. Touching the pylorus, backing away, and then touching it again will sometimes assist passage. Force should never be used, as there may be an organic cause for an obstruction to passage and excessive force could result in a tear or perforation. In a vertically oriented or J-shaped stomach, the endoscopist may have to create a long, greater curvature gastric loop before the tip of the instrument can be advanced up to and through the pylorus into the duodenal bulb.

In some cases, the duodenal bulb is first inspected with the endoscope tip at the pylorus. This is referred to as the transpyloric view. This view may be useful if there is difficulty passing the pylorus or if, as the tip of the endoscope is passed into the bulb, it slips immediately down into the second or descending portion of the duodenum. This latter problem may occur in a patient with a J-shaped stomach, because once the tip of the endoscope passes the pylorus, pressure from the gastric loop pushes the tip beyond the duodenal bulb, interfering with adequate inspection of the bulb. As the endoscope is withdrawn in an attempt to see the bulb, the reverse problem occurs. First the gastric loop is removed. Then, when the instrument is straight, the tip begins to move back up the duodenum and comes out through the bulb very rapidly into the stomach, again not allowing adequate inspection of the bulb. One can repeat this in–out sequence several times and never adequately inspect the bulb. The solution is to stop the forward advance at the pylorus, inspect the bulb transpylorically, and then very slowly advance into the bulb. Similarly, when the tip is in the descending duodenum, pulling out very slowly will often allow the tip to come back into the bulb for adequate inspection of the area.

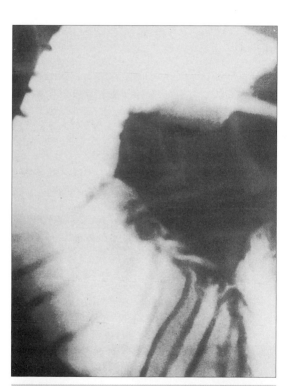

Figure 1.37 In this hypotonic duodenogram, barium outlines the papilla on the medial portion of the descending duodenal wall. The intramural common bile duct (CBD) and the plica duodeni longitudinalis can be seen along with a gathering of folds just distal to the papilla. (Courtesy of Dr Charles Rohrmann)

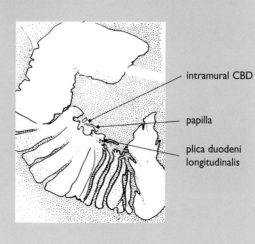

intramural CBD

papilla

plica duodeni longitudinalis

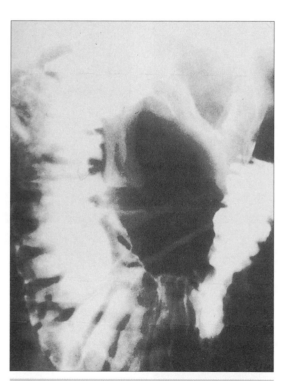

Figure 1.38 In this duodenal x-ray study, the papilla and the longitudinal fold distal to it are easily seen. This anatomy, as might be seen on a prior upper gastrointerinal contrast x-ray, can orient the endoscopist and help locate the papilla. (Courtesy of Dr Charles Rohrmann)

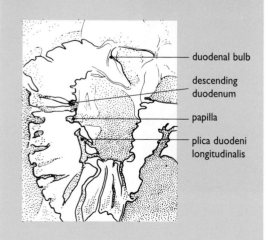

duodenal bulb

descending duodenum

papilla

plica duodeni longitudinalis

ENDOSCOPIC EXAMINATION

Nearly the entire surface of the duodenal bulb can usually be well visualized with a small-caliber endoscope. The most difficult areas to inspect are the fornices, just distal to the pylorus. The mucosa of the bulb often has a slightly reticulated appearance when contrasted with the stomach, though the color may be similar (Fig. 1.39). There are usually few if any folds (Fig. 1.40). Bile is often present (Fig. 1.41) and may cause a bubbly foam that can interfere with duodenal inspection. Using a wash fluid with simethicone or other surfactant will immediately break up these bubbles and permit excellent inspection of the mucosa. Active peristalis may also make endoscopy of the duodenum difficult. Here, a hypotonic agent such as glucagon or buscopan will rapidly cause duodenal hypotonia and allow endoscopic inspection of the duodenal bulb and descending duodenum.

If a red, reticulated area of mucosa is noted, careful inspection is essential because it may be adjacent to a duodenal ulcer that might otherwise be missed. This is especially problematic if heavy folds and scarring from previous peptic ulcer disease are present. Blood vessels are not visible in the duodenal bulb, nor are they visible further down in the descending duodenum. In addition to inspection for ulcers and erosions, surgical anastomoses such as a choledochoduodenostomy may be located. Using an end-viewing instrument, this orifice can be inspected and, if appropriate, cannulated for contrast x-ray studies of the common bile duct.

The endoscope is then routinely passed by the apex of the bulb and the superior duodenal angle into the descending duodenum. This portion of the duodenum is posterior and retroperitoneal, therefore a turn to the right and down is usually required. In most cases this can be accomplished under direct vision, with the lumen maintained in view at all times. Occasionally, it may be necessary to turn the tip to the right and down without advancing the instrument to see if one can enter the descending duodenum blindly. This maneuver may pass the tip gently into the descending duodenum. As soon as the descending duodenum is intubated, the lumen can again be imaged and the rest of the examination performed with the lumen clearly in view.

The descending duodenum can be recognized by the folds of Kerckring, which run transversely around the lumen (Fig. 1.42). There is considerable variability in the fold pattern, and in some patients longitudinally oriented folds connect the transverse folds (Fig. 1.43). The mucosal surface is smooth, and blood vessels are not seen. In close up, it may be possible to see duodenal villi. Bile is often present and may help locate the papilla of Vater.

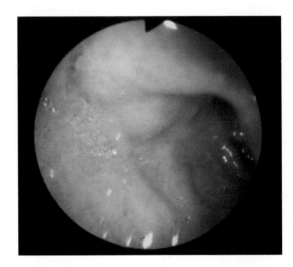

Figure 1.39 *Normal duodenal bulb. The mucosa is slightly reticulated, and no blood vessels are seen. The apex of the bulb and the entrance into the descending duodenum are seen to the right.*

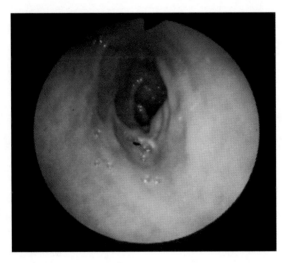

Figure 1.40 *Normal duodenal bulb. Folds of Kerckring can be seen in the distance just beyond the apex of the bulb.*

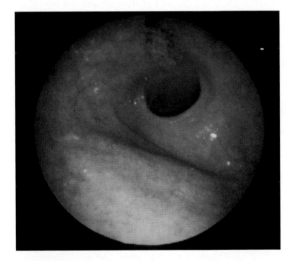

Figure 1.41 *The apex of a normal duodenal bulb is seen; bile is present.*

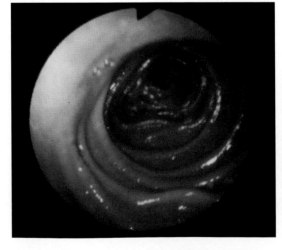

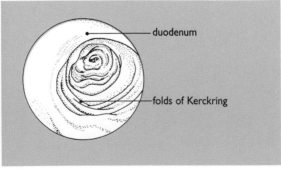

Figure 1.42 *Normal descending duodenum, with the transverse folds of Kerckring clearly evident.*

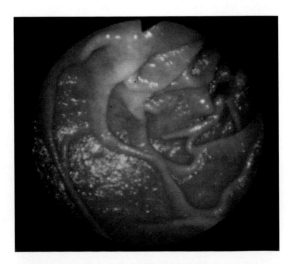

Figure 1.43 *Normal descending duodenum, with a reticulated or velvet mucosal surface. In this case, some of the folds are longitudinally oriented.*

Inspection of the descending duodenum is usually performed to determine the presence of a postbulbar ulcer, as may be seen in gastric hypersecretory states, or to examine the papilla of Vater. Other indications include possible inflammatory disease in the postapical portion of the duodenum (Crohn's disease), inspection to detect telangiectasias that may be responsible for gastrointestinal bleeding, or evaluation of masses noted on barium upper-gastrointestinal x-ray studies. Examination of the postbulbar duodenum is usually brief, and is part of routine upper endoscopy. Duodenoscopy may also be performed to obtain mucosal biopsies for the diagnosis of infections such as cytomegalovirus in immunocompromised hosts or gluten-sensitive enteropathy.

Location and inspection of the papilla of Vater is not as easily accomplished with a forward-viewing endoscope as with a side-viewing endoscope. With a forward-viewing endoscope, the intramural portion of the common bile duct may be seen bulging into the duodenal lumen. One may also see the papilla of Vater protruding into the lumen (Fig. 1.44), as well as the vertical fold below the papilla, the plica duodeni longitudinalis. It is not usually possible to cannulate the papilla with a forward-viewing endoscope. On occasion, one will see the accessory papilla in the duodenum (Fig. 1.44). This structure is usually on the same side of the duodenum as the main papilla but is located several centimeters closer to the pylorus. The accessory papilla is smaller, less red, and is usually not reticulated as is the main papilla.

The papilla of Vater may have several shapes, varying from a prominent papillary projection to relatively flat. The surface of the papilla has a characteristic red, reticulated appearance which clearly distinguishes it from surrounding duodenal mucosa (Fig. 1.45). In some cases, yellow or golden bile is seen flowing from the papilla or is noted on the mucosa adjacent to the papilla, especially after a migrating motor complex passes through the duodenum and upper small bowel.

The endoscope is slowly withdrawn from the descending duodenum, inspecting the descending duodenal surface, the apex of the bulb, the duodenal bulb, the pylorus, and the stomach along the way. The detailed gastric examination is usually performed at this point. Once the stomach examination, including retroflexion, is completed, gentle suction is used to remove air, reducing the patient's discomfort after the procedure. The endoscope is then pulled back into the esophagus, and the observations that were made as the endoscope was first passed are confirmed. If one moves slowly and gently as the tip of the endoscope passes up through the cricopharyngeus muscle, the anatomy of the hypopharynx and vocal cords can be observed. The patient can be asked to phonate so that vocal cord appearance and movement can be evaluated. The instrument is then removed from the mouth and the endoscopy is complete.

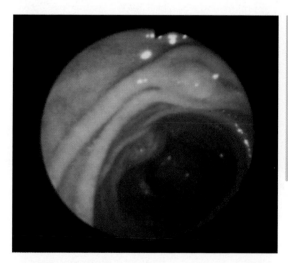
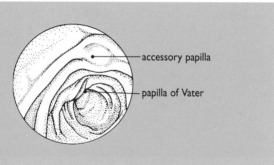

Figure 1.44 *Descending duodenum with the main papilla of Vater seen in the distance. The smaller accessory papilla is seen proximal to the main papilla.*

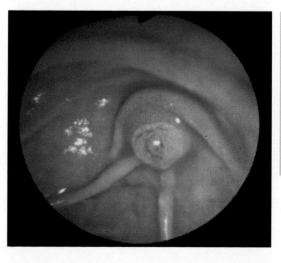
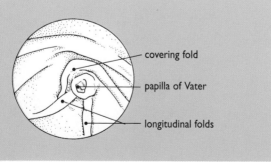

Figure 1.45 *Normal papilla of Vater, with its characteristic red, reticulated surface. Two longitudinal folds distal to the papilla can be appreciated.*

THE TERMINAL ILEUM

ANATOMY

The terminal ileum, the end of the small bowel, attaches to the colon at the ileocecal valve. The colonoscopist may place the tip of the colonoscope in the cecum and then enter the terminal ileum for a variable distance. This distal segment of ileum is not as mobile as the rest of the ileum because it is attached to the cecum, which is usually not mobile. The circular folds characteristic of the duodenum and jejunum are often absent in the terminal ileum, whereas lymphoid aggregates may be seen.

POSITIONING THE ENDOSCOPE

The tip of the colonoscope is routinely passed retrograde into the cecum, the most proximal portion of the colon. In most cases the ileocecal valve can be identified.

Endoscopy of the terminal ileum may occasionally be difficult and is often not indicated in routine colonoscopy. In some diseases, such as inflammatory bowel disease, it may be useful to inspect the terminal ileum, though it may not be possible to pass the valve because of narrowing.

The most commonly used technique is to pass the tip of the colonoscope just beyond the proximal lip of the ileocecal valve and then turn into the valve, often medially and posteriorly, to lift the lip of the valve and permit entry of the tip of the colonoscope into the terminal ileum (Fig. 1.46). In some cases one can then gently withdraw the colonoscope in this hooked position causing the colonoscope tip to advance slightly into the ileum. It may then be possible to insert more colonoscope length gently and further intubate the terminal ileum. The optimal position of the patient for ileal intubation may vary from left lateral to dorsal and even right lateral. Rarely can one pass the ileocecal valve 'en face'.

Entry into the terminal ileum is readily suspected when a villus pattern is observed endoscopically. On occasion, a biopsy may be used to identify villi in the mucosa of the terminal ileum (Fig. 1.47). The technique should be gentle, with minimal force and intermittent removal of air to help the tip advance into the ileum.

ENDOSCOPIC EXAMINATION

Colonoscopy of the terminal ileum is useful in the differential diagnosis of radiographic abnormalities and in patients presenting with suspected Crohn's

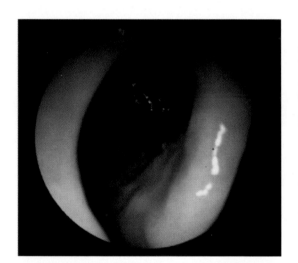

Figure 1.46 *Opening of lips of normal ileocecal valve, permitting entry of colonoscope tip into the terminal ileum.*

A

B

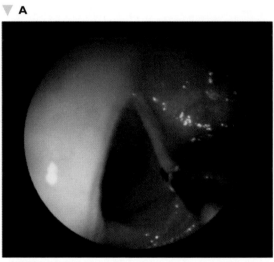

Figure 1.47 *(A) A biopsy forceps is used to take a sample of terminal ileal mucosa. (B) Minimal bleeding is noted at the biopsy site.*

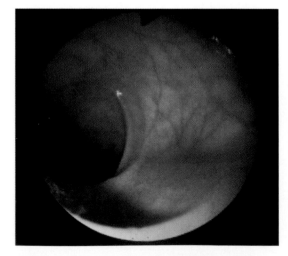

Figure 1.48 *View of a normal terminal ileum. A fine vascular pattern can be seen with inflation of the lumen. Folds are subtle and the mucosa less glistening than in the colon.*

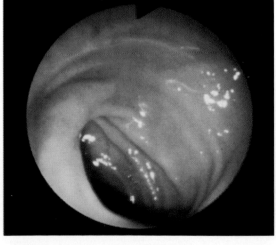

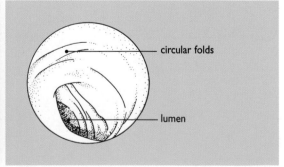

Figure 1.49 *Normal terminal ileum with less inflation. Folds are seen although they are less prominent than in the duodenum. The lumen tends to collapse readily with suction.*

disease. Normally, the terminal ileum mucosa is smooth, and blood vessels may be seen, especially with air insufflation (Fig. 1.48); Kerckring folds are less marked in the terminal ileum than in the duodenum and jejunum (Fig 1.49; compare with Figs. 1.42 and 1.43). The appearance of the mucosa is not glistening as in the colon but more villous and dull as in the duodenum (Fig. 1.50). There is usually vigorous (contractility) motor activity. The lumen tends to collapse more readily than in the colon and is usually of smaller caliber than is the ascending colon or cecum. All of these factors can be clues to the fact that the tip of the instrument is, in fact, in the terminal ileum.

Occasionally, lymphoid nodules covered with normal mucosa are seen. These nodules can vary in size from one to several millimetres and may cause a nodular surface. The appearance of active peristalsis also helps to distinguish the terminal ileum from the colon. Mucosal changes may indicate the presence of Crohn's disease or other inflammations of the terminal ileum, including tuberculosis and infection with *Yersinia*.

THE NORMAL COLON

ANATOMY
The colon is a tubular organ that runs from the cecum in the right lower quadrant to the rectum (Fig. 1.51). It is widest in the cecum and ascending colon and gradually narrows as it approaches the rectum. The colon is divided into the following sections: the cecum; the ascending colon, which runs cephalad from the cecum to the hepatic flexure; the transverse colon, which runs from the hepatic flexure in the right upper quadrant to the splenic flexure in the left upper quadrant; the descending colon, which runs caudad from the splenic flexure to the left lower quadrant; the sigmoid colon, which runs from the left lower quadrant to the rectosigmoid junction; and the rectum, which extends down to the anal canal.

The inner layer of circular muscle is present throughout the colon. The outer longitudinal muscle in the wall of the colon is fused into three bands, the teniae coli. These bands start at the base of the appendix and run in the wall of the colon down to the rectum where they diffuse into the muscular coat. The three teniae cause the colon to have a triangular appearance endoscopically; this is especially prominent in the ascending and transverse colon. The haustra are outpouchings of the colon, separated by folds. In the descending colon the endoscopic appearance is often tubular.

POSITIONING THE COLONOSCOPE
The patient's perianal area is inspected and a digital examination performed. The colonoscope is then placed into the patient's rectum. Colonic cleansing is required. For upper endoscopy, simply having the patient fast for 8–12 hours is sufficient for an adequate examination. However, for colonoscopy, a preparative program is essential. There are two approaches. The first is to give the patient clear liquids for 1–2 days and a purge with oral magnesium and enemas the day of the examination. The second, increasingly widespread, technique is to purge the gut with a nonabsorbable electrolyte solution. This can be accomplished the night before or the morning of the examination. The solution can be administered orally or via a nasogastric tube. Some endoscopists favor a combination of these techniques. Either prep, or the combined prep, if followed correctly, removes both fecal material and potentially explosive hydrogen and methane gases.

Most experienced colonoscopists use similar intubation techniques. As little air as possible is introduced to prevent overdistension. The pressure on the device is gentle to avoid stretching the colonic wall or mesentery, which can cause pain, a vagal reaction or a perforation. The lumen is kept in view at all times; little or none of the examination is performed blindly. A variety of in and out maneuvers are used to 'accordion' the colon on the colonoscope, keeping the colonoscope as free of loops as possible. In the difficult colon, special maneuvers such as creating an alpha loop in the sigmoid colon are used to pass the sharply angulated sigmoid/descending colon junction. This maneuver requires fluoroscopic guidance and training in the technique.

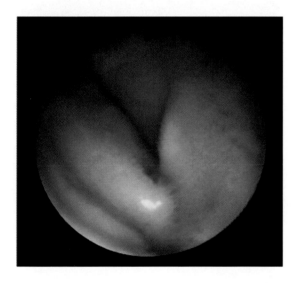

Figure 1.50 *Normal terminal ileum. The velvet mucosal appearance is caused by the presence of villi.*

Figure 1.51 *Anatomy of the colon.*

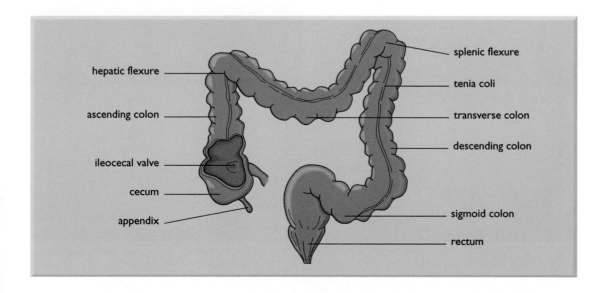

hepatic flexure
ascending colon
ileocecal valve
cecum
appendix
splenic flexure
tenia coli
transverse colon
descending colon
sigmoid colon
rectum

The colonoscope is advanced to the cecum under direct vision. The detailed examination of the mucosa is usually performed as the colonoscope is slowly removed from the cecum. If the colonoscope has been kept free of loops, the tip responds well to steering maneuvers and the examination is facilitated. This is especially true if a therapeutic procedure such as polypectomy is to be undertaken, because large, redundant loops of colonoscope can make control of the tip difficult.

Understanding the colonic anatomy is important for several reasons; first, to determine where the tip of the colonoscope is located and to determine the location of an abnormality if one is encountered; second, to determine whether a structure encountered is normal or not; and third, to determine whether the colonoscope tip has reached the cecum and whether the entire surface has therefore been inspected. The latter point is critical, for in most indications for colonoscopy the endoscopist should examine the entire length of the colon. For example, if a patient presents with blood in the stool, the entire length of the colon must be examined for a bleeding source. If one encounters a polyp in the descending colon, it is necessary to look higher for a possible synchronous polyp or cancer. There are, however, circumstances under which total colonoscopy is not possible; for example, when it is impossible to advance the colonoscope tip safely beyond an area of diverticular disease, anatomic variation, or scarring from previous operations.

It is imperative to determine whether the tip of the colonoscope has arrived in the cecum or whether it is trapped at a difficult bend or flexure. Several clues can be used. Light from the tip of the colonoscope may transilluminate the patient's right lower quadrant when the tip is in the cecum. This may be more easily observed if the lights in the room are turned down and if the patient is not greatly obese. Note, however, that this may also occasionally occur when the tip is in the sigmoid colon or transverse colon, especially if a redundant transverse colonic loop is present. Transillumination is more difficult when using videoendoscopic equipment. When in doubt, observe with x-ray fluoroscopy. The best method of assuring a complete examination is to recognize the cecum anatomy (ileocecal valve, appendiceal orifice, etc.).

ENDOSCOPIC EXAMINATION

The first characteristic aspect of the cecum is the presence of the appendiceal orifice, a slit-like or crescent-shaped opening located near the coalescence of the three teniae coli (Figs. 1.52 and 1.53). The appendiceal orifice may assume one of two general forms: flat, or protruded in which the base protrudes into the cecum (Fig. 1.54). Occasionally, small bits of food residue such as seeds or pits may be seen at the orifice (Fig. 1.55), as may a fecalith (Fig. 1.56).

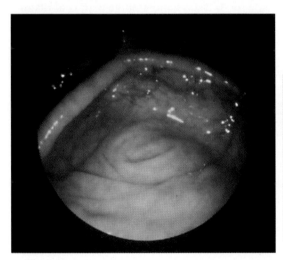
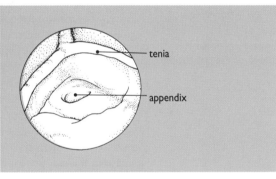
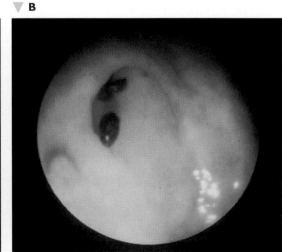

Figure 1.52 *Crescent-shaped orifice of a normal appendix, seen in the base of the cecum.*

Figure 1.53 *Crescent-shaped opening of the appendix on the wall of the cecum. The normal colonic vasculature can be appreciated.*

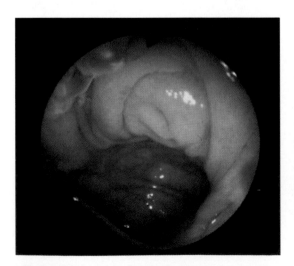
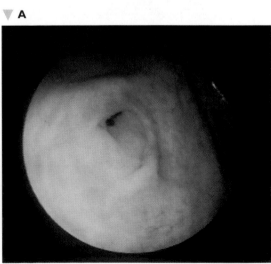

Figure 1.54 *Opening of the appendix in the protruded type of configuration. The orifice appears closed.*

Figure 1.55 *(A) Normal, crescent-shaped appendiceal orifice with seeds noted. (B) A close-up view.*

The cecum, located just beyond the ileocecal valve, may be difficult to evaluate radiographically during barium enema examination. Likewise, polyps and cancers can be missed colonoscopically. Therefore, careful inspection of this area is essential.

The ileocecal valve may provide another clue to the location of the colonoscope tip. The valve has several appearances, varying from a subtle flattening of a colonic fold (Fig. 1.57), to a prominent lip-like structure bulging into the lumen (Fig. 1.58), to the most prominent papillary or multilobed appearance (Figs. 1.59, 1.60 and 1.61). The ileocecal valve may also have a fatty,

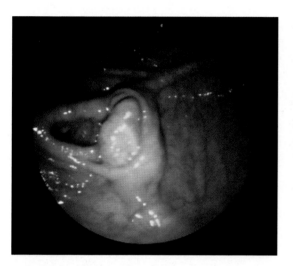

Figure 1.56 *Normal appendix with a fecalith in the orifice. Convergence of the teniae can be seen at the orifice.*

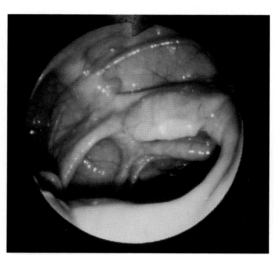
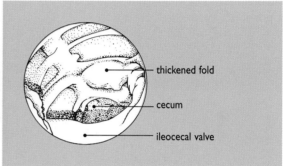

Figure 1.57 *Normal ileocecal valve. The cecum can be seen distal to the valve. This area should be carefully inspected endoscopically, as the fold marking the valve is subtle.*

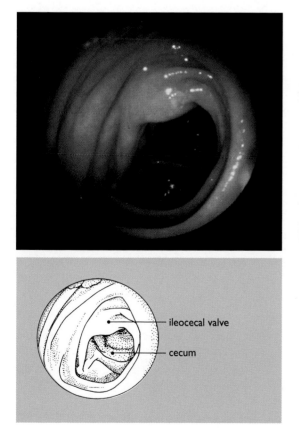

Figure 1.58 *A slightly more prominent ileocecal valve.*

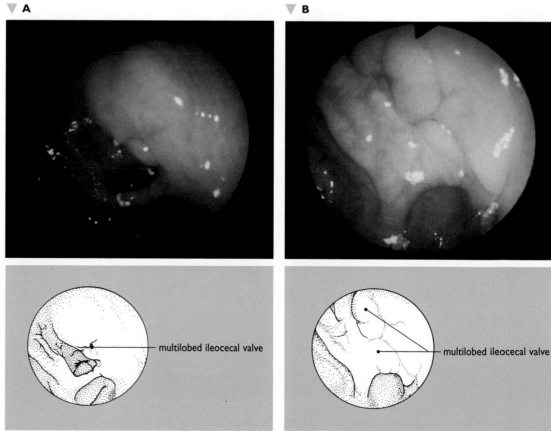

Figure 1.59 *(A)* A very prominent ileocecal valve with a papillary or multilobed appearance. *(B)* A close-up view. Valves in this configuration may be difficult to enter with the colonoscope.

or lipomatous, appearance (Fig. 1.62). In some cases, green ileal fluid (succus entericus) may be seen entering the colon through the ileocecal valve. Occasionally, air in the small intestine from colonoscopy insufflation can distend an adjacent loop of small bowel and cause an impression on the cecal wall that may appear similar to the ileocecal valve (Fig. 1.63).

As the colonoscope is pulled out, it is advanced up the ascending colon. In this area, the typical colonic appearance is noted. The mucosa is smooth; normal, fine, delicate blood vessels are apparent (Fig. 1.64). The vessels may appear in a double pattern with a vein accompanying each artery (Fig. 1.65). Occasionally, bluish submucosal veins are seen (Fig. 1.66). The teniae coli

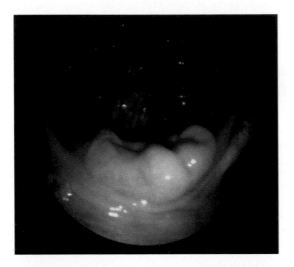

Figure 1.60 Prominent papillary ileocecal valve.

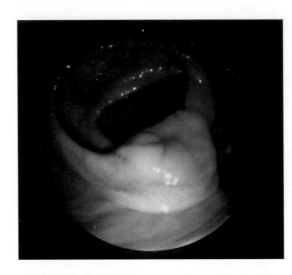

Figure 1.61 Papillary ileocecal valve.

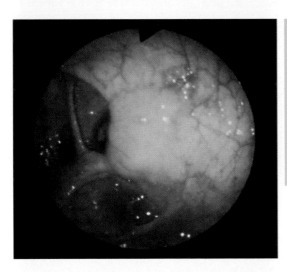

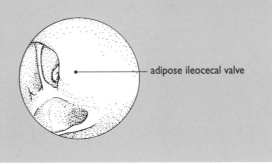

Figure 1.62 Normal ileocecal valve containing slightly yellow adipose tissue (often referred to as lipomatous transformation of the ileocecal valve).

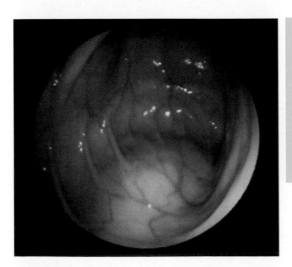

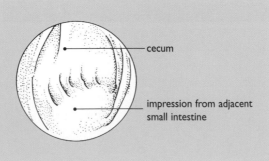

Figure 1.63 Impression of adjacent air-filled loops of small bowel on the wall of the cecum. This could be confused with the ileocecal valve but no orifice is seen.

cause sacculations or haustra to occur in the colon. It may be necessary to look carefully beyond each haustral fold to detect the presence of a small lesion such as a polyp or cancer. The lumen in the cecum and ascending colon is often wide and clearly more capacious than the terminal ileum or the transverse, descending, or sigmoid colon. In the ascending and transverse colon the appearance is characteristically triangular because of the three teniae coli.

The folds in the cecum and ascending colon (Fig. 1.67) are thicker than the folds in the tranverse colon. The contents of the right colon are often slightly different in color than the rest of the colon because of the succus entericus, which imparts a dark green color, except after saline lavage. This change is only seen in the cecum and ascending colon.

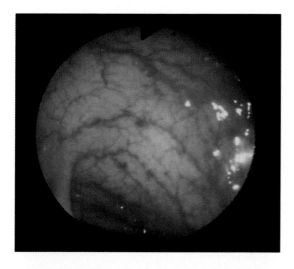

Figure 1.64 *View of the normal, delicate vascular pattern of the colonic mucosa.*

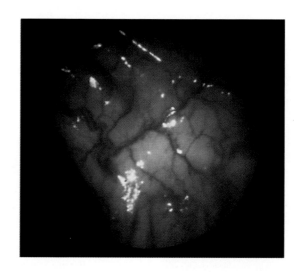

Figure 1.65 *Normal colonic vessels in a double pattern. An artery is seen running parallel to each vein.*

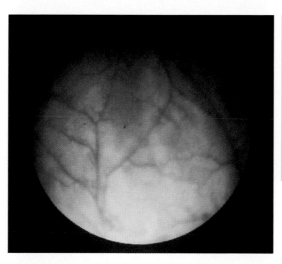

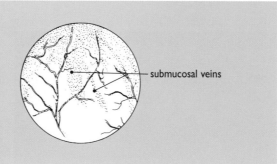

Figure 1.66 *Normal submucosal veins of the colon can be seen adjacent to small arterial structures.*

— submucosal veins

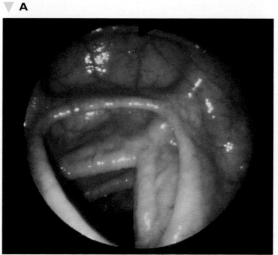

▼ A

Figure 1.67 *(A and B)* *Views of the folds in the normal ascending colon. The folds are slightly thicker than in the transverse colon. The triangular configuration is evident, as in the normal colonic vascular pattern.*

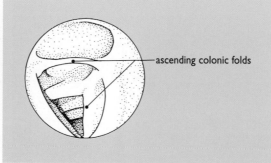

— ascending colonic folds

▼ B

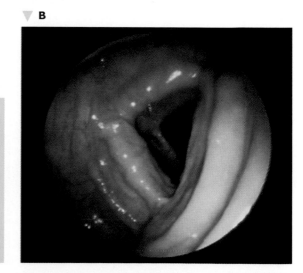

Contractions of the colon may be noted, and in some patients with muscular colonic walls one may encounter a series of contracted haustrations with luminal orifices that must be intubated as the instrument is advanced proximally to the cecum. As the colonoscope is advanced up the colon, these haustral folds can usually be gently passed if attention is directed to keep the lumen in the center of the endoscopic visual field. Each area must then be carefully inspected as the instrument is withdrawn (Fig. 1.68). Rarely, antispasmodics such as glucagon are required. The tip may have to be passed through the area several times, and the colonoscopist must carefully inspect behind each fold to examine these relatively blind areas and avoid missing a lesion.

The hepatic flexure is occasionally identifiable by a slightly bluish discoloration from the adjacent liver and/or gall bladder. The transverse colon has a typical triangular appearance with finer or thinner folds (Fig. 1.69), and may be seen to move readily with respiration. Here, as in the rest of the colon, the vessels are fine and delicate, and the mucosa is smooth. The splenic flexure is difficult to identify endoscopically, except as a bend located between the obviously triangular transverse colon and the more circular, tubular descending colon. The spleen may be noted through the colonic wall as a bluish discoloration at the splenic flexure (Fig. 1.70).

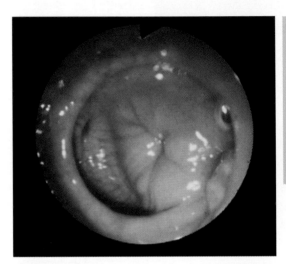
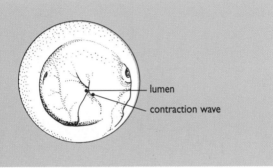

Figure 1.68 *Normal colon with a contraction wave. With patience the orifice will open and allow intubation. The colon just beyond the orifice may represent a relative blind spot and must be carefully inspected.*

▼ **A**

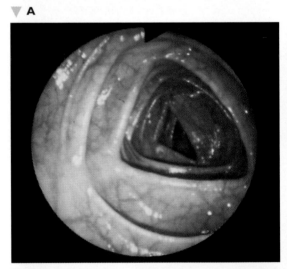

▼ **B**

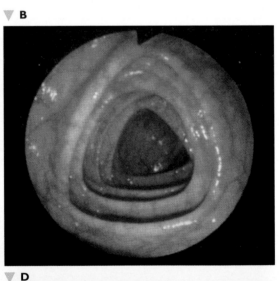

Figure 1.69 (A–D) *Views of a normal transverse colon demonstrate its typical configuration, caused by the three teniae.*

▼ **C**

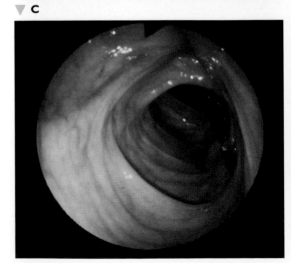

▼ **D**

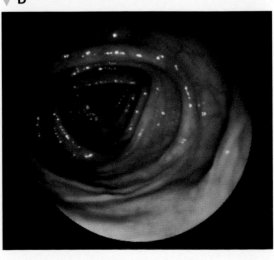

The descending colon usually has less marked haustra and is not as triangular (Fig. 1.71). The colonoscope is pulled down the descending colon, past the sigmoid/descending colon junction, into the sigmoid colon. The sigmoid/descending colon junction is often a sharp angle with a potential blind spot, as are the hepatic and splenic flexures. These areas must be carefully examined to avoid missing a lesion. The sigmoid colon is often circular and may be of highly variable length from patient to patient (Fig. 1.72). The technique of withdrawal should allow inspection of the entire mucosal surface. If a sharp bend or fold is encountered, the colonoscope may have to be passed up through the area again to inspect the segment thoroughly.

At 16–18 cm from the anus one encounters the rectosigmoid junction. This is an acute bend that must also be carefully inspected to avoid missing a lesion.

THE RECTUM

The colonoscope is now back in the rectum. The lumen here is wider than in the sigmoid, descending, and transverse colon. Blood vessels are easily observed and are more prominent than in other areas of the colon (Fig. 1.73). The mucosa is usually smooth and glistening.

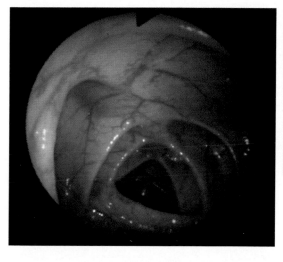
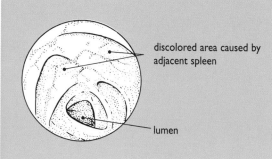

Figure 1.70 The spleen is seen as a bluish discoloration through the colonic wall at the splenic flexure.

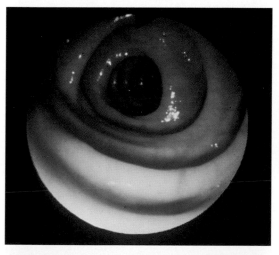
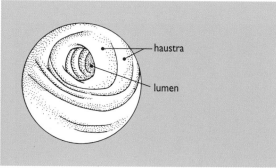

Figure 1.71 Normal descending colon. The haustra are less marked and the lumen is more tubular and less typically triangular.

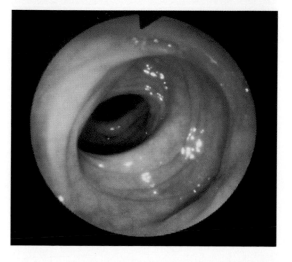

Figure 1.72 Normal sigmoid colon. The lumen has several bends and is tubular or circular.

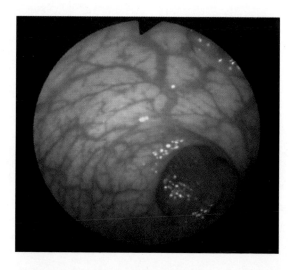

Figure 1.73 Normal prominent veins in the rectum.

Three rectal valves are seen (Fig. 1.74). A complete examination often requires that the endoscopist look behind each valve to be certain that a lesion is not missed. It is possible in many patients to retroflex the instrument in the rectum and, by rotating the shaft, look back at the distal rectal mucosa surrounding the endoscope as it passes through the anal canal (Fig. 1.75). This technique allows one to detect lesions that might go unnoticed by direct inspection with a straight tip. Lesions such as internal hemorrhoids, condylomata, and tumors can be seen with this maneuver. After retroflexion, the tip of the device is straightened and gas is gently suctioned from the colon. This makes the patient more comfortable at the conclusion of the procedure. The colonoscope is then slowly removed from the patient; the anal canal can be inspected directly during removal, although this can often be better accomplished by using an anoscope.

ENDOSONOGRAPHY OF THE NORMAL RECTUM

An ultrasound probe can be passed into the rectum to visualize the layers of the rectal wall and surrounding structures (Figs. 1.76 and 1.77). Any of the three types of ultrasound device – a blind probe, an imaging endoscope probe or an echo endoscope – can be used.

THE PERIANAL EXAMINATION

Examination of the rectum and colon is not complete without a careful inspection of the perianal area, a digital examination of the anal canal, and a stress test. The inspection and digital examination are usually performed before colonoscopy. Inspection of the perianal area may reveal a bluish discoloration or lateral ridging, typical findings in Crohn's disease. The opening of fistulas or fissures may also be noted. The digital examination is essential before the introduction of the colonoscope detect the presence of any low-lying rectal masses as well as areas of tenderness that might represent a fissure or abscess.

TECHNICAL CONSIDERATIONS

Some general comments that relate to the endoscopic imaging of the gastrointestinal tract are now appropriate. It is essential to ascertain that the endoscope is functioning properly before the procedure is started. If the

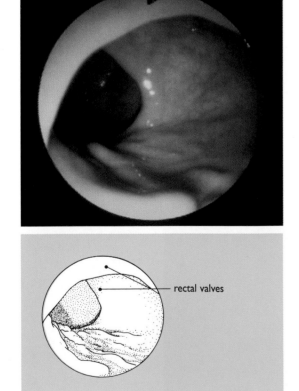

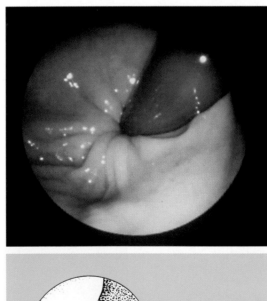

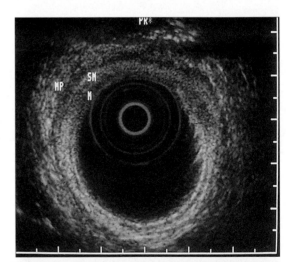

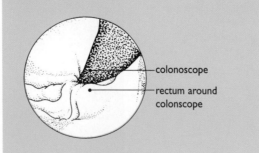

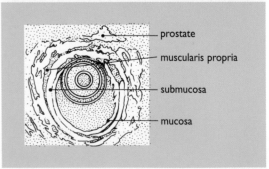

Figure 1.74 *Rectum distended with air. Two of the three normal rectal valves are seen.*

Figure 1.75 *The rectum just above the anal canal, as seen from the inside with the colonoscope retroflexed. This enables the endoscopist to see lesions just inside of the anal canal that can be easily missed otherwise.*

Figure 1.76 *Ultrasound image of normal rectal wall. The layers of the wall can be seen, as can the prostate, which is adjacent to the wall. (Courtesy of Dr T.L. Tio)*

endoscope is not working properly, the examination can be severely compromised, yield little or no information, and actually pose a higher risk of complication to the patient. Air insufflation is essential to expose the luminal organ being examined gently, thus allowing the endoscopist to see. If the water wash is not working and the endoscopist is unable to clean the lens, the field may be partially obscured with blood or mucus, markedly interfering with the endoscopy. If the suction channel is plugged, secretions or excessive insufflated air cannot be removed, and this may interfere with the

examination and increase the patient's discomfort. The mechanisms of the bending sections must be working so that retroflexion is possible to inspect the cardia, lesser curve, and fundus during upper endoscopy. Obviously, the optics must function correctly. If any of these problems exist, the endoscope should not be used until the problem is corrected.

Some additional comments are required regarding the use of the suction channel. As mentioned earlier, when used properly this channel is very helpful in reducing patient discomfort by preventing gas distension, and in the

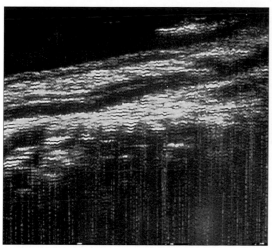

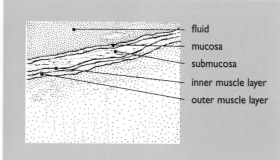

fluid
mucosa
submucosa
inner muscle layer
outer muscle layer

Figure 1.77 *Ultrasound probe image of the normal rectum. Fluid separates the transducer on the tip of the probe from the rectal wall. The probe was passed via the biopsy channel of a colonoscope. The mucosa, submucosa, and muscularis propria can be seen, as can surrounding fat. The muscularis propria has two layers, the inner, circular, and the outer, longitudinal, separated by the area of the myenteric plexus.*
(Courtesy of Dr Michael Kimmey)

▼ **A**

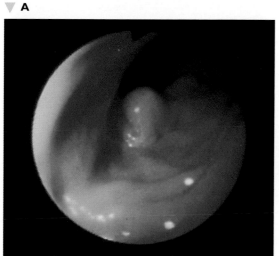

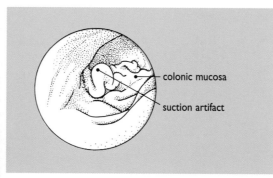

colonic mucosa

suction artifact

Figure 1.78 (A) *Iatrogenic 'polyp' caused by pulling the mucosa of the colon into the biopsy channel in the tip of the endoscope and then releasing the suction.* **(B)** *After several seconds the polyp begins to fade.* **(C)** *After 1 or 2 minutes the suction artifact is gone.*

▼ **B**

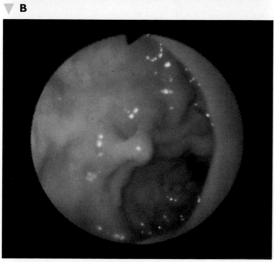

▼ **C**

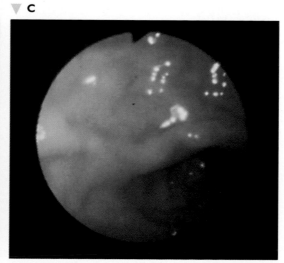

removal of secretions and blood that can cover lesions. In addition, the channel is essential for passing accessories during diagnostic procedures such as biopsy and cytology, or therapeutic procedures such as polypectomy, laser therapy, electrocoagulation, foreign body removal, etc. If a piece of stool is pulled against the tip of the endoscope, it may be difficult to dislodge, and on occasion may necessitate removal of the endoscope for cleaning. As the device must then be passed again, it causes significant inconvenience for both the patient and the examiner.

Another problem occurs if mucosa is suctioned into the tip of the endoscope's instrumentation channel. The experienced endoscopist often knows this has happened when he or she observes a crescent of red in the visual field and the suction stops working. The tip also moves less well. If this is recognized immediately, the tip can be maneuvered to release the mucosa, or the suction channel can be temporarily disconnected from the suction system and the channel opened to room air, which will also immediately release the mucosa. If this problem is not recognized and the mucosa remains in the channel, a pseudopolyp or iatrogenic polyp may develop. If it has been recognized early, one can see this polyp gradually fade (Fig. 1.78). However, if not recognized early, the polyp may appear red and 'adenomatous' or may cause a small amount of bleeding (Fig. 1.79). This iatrogenic problem creates confusion and slows the endoscopic procedure. The endoscopist should be aware of this problem and try to avoid it, and should release the mucosa immediately if it is pulled into the tip of the instrument. These considerations are essential to make endoscopy as complete, gentle, safe, rapid, and informative as possible.

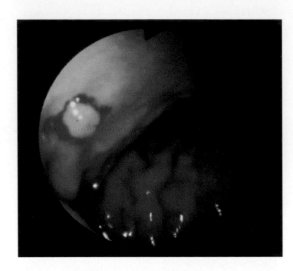

Figure 1.79 Bleeding suction artifact in the stomach. This can be very confusing for the endoscopist, especially in the patient being examined because of gastrointestinal bleeding.

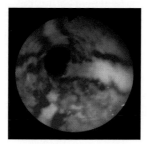

Esophagus I: Diverticula, Hiatal Hernias, Webs, Rings, Reflux, and Barrett's Metaplasia

This chapter is the first of three that presents diseases of the esophagus. In this chapter we consider structural abnormalities such as diverticula, hiatal hernias, and esophageal webs and rings, as well as reflux, reflux-associated complications, and Barrett's metaplasia.

DIVERTICULA

Esophageal diverticula may be symptomatic or asymptomatic. Endoscopy does not play a primary role in their diagnosis or management; however, these entities are important to the endoscopist because a diverticulum can complicate endoscopy. For example, an unsuspected diverticulum can be traumatized or perforated during intubation of the esophagus. Such a perforation can occur with end-viewing and side-viewing endoscopes. A diverticulum of the upper esophagus can be perforated with the routine passage of an end-viewing endoscope because passage of the endoscope through the upper sphincter and upper part of the esophagus is often performed blindly. The routine passage of a side-viewing endoscope could perforate a

▼ A

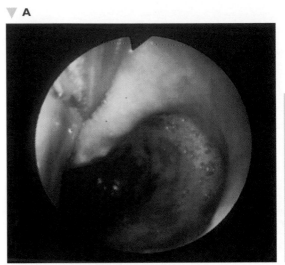

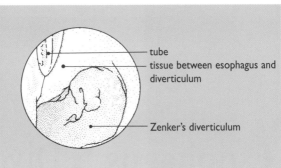

▼ B

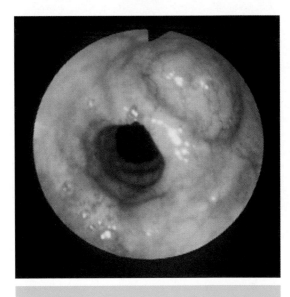

Figure 2.1 (**A** and **B**) Two views of Zenker's diverticulum. A tube has been passed into the esophagus. The orifice into the esophagus is difficult to see.

Figure 2.2 Barium esophagram demonstrating a large Zenker's diverticulum. A radio-opaque tube has been placed in the esophagus, bypassing the diverticulum.

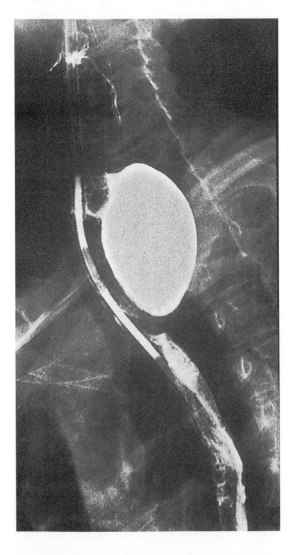

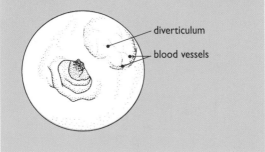

Figure 2.3 Midesophageal diverticulum. Small blood vessels are seen in the base of the diverticulum.

diverticulum anywhere along the esophagus because it is difficult, if not impossible, to inspect the esophageal lumen as the instrument is being passed. It is important to remember that if the endoscope is not passing easily or is causing discomfort, one should stop the procedure, remove the endoscope and establish whether an organic obstruction or a proximal diverticulum is present (Figs. 2.1 and 2.2). This may be accomplished by obtaining and carefully examining a barium x-ray esophagram of the area. An alternative is to pass a small-caliber, end-viewing endoscope through the hypopharynx and on through the cricopharyngeus muscle using a constant inspection technique by which the lumen is always in view. Both radiologic and otolaryngologic evaluation may be necessary to study the hypopharyngeal area and the very proximal portion of the upper esophagus.

Diverticula may be observed in three possible configurations: (1) in which the diverticulum empties into the esophagus in a downstream direction parallel to the esophagus; (2) in which the diverticulum is located at a 90° angle to the esophagus (Fig. 2.3); and (3) in which the diverticulum is dependent, meaning that the entrance to the lumen of the diverticulum points towards the stomach (Fig. 2.4). Of these three configurations, the dependent causes the most problems, as food and/or gastrointestinal instruments tend to enter the diverticulum rather than stay in the lumen (Fig. 2.5). These configurations can be applied to the three types of esophageal diverticula: upper esophageal (Zenker's), midesophageal, and epiphrenic (just above the diaphragm). Each is now be discussed in detail.

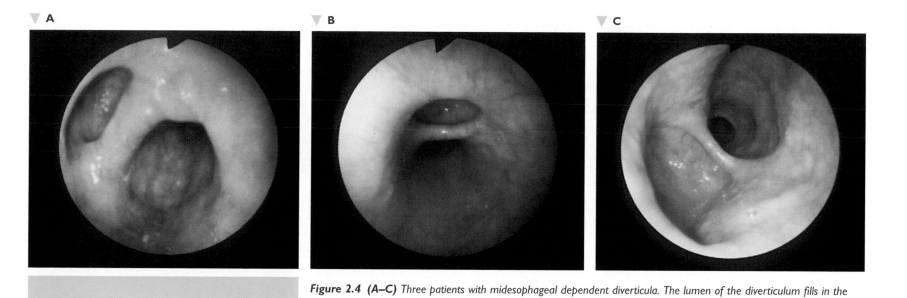

Figure 2.4 (A–C) *Three patients with midesophageal dependent diverticula. The lumen of the diverticulum fills in the direction of food moving down the esophagus.*

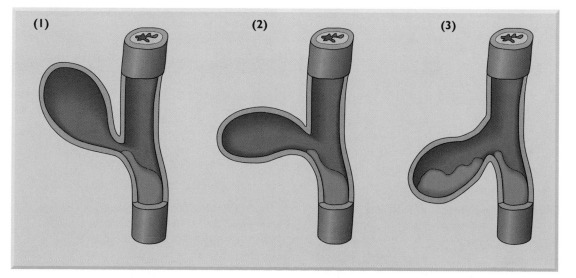

Figure 2.5 *Configurations of esophageal diverticula. (1) The diverticulum empties caudad in a direction parallel to the esophagus; (2) the diverticulum fills at 90° to the esophageal long axis; (3) the diverticulum fills in the same direction as food passing down the esophagus. One can clearly see how food or instruments can be diverted into the lumen of the dependent diverticulum.*

ZENKER'S DIVERTICULUM

Zenker's diverticulum is an outpouching of the esophagus typically occurring just above or at the level of the cricopharyngeus sphincter (see Figs. 2.1 and 2.2). It is usually found in adults. The etiology of the diverticulum is not known, although motor dysfunction with incoordination of the cricopharyngeus muscle may be the cause. The initial presenting symptom is usually dysphagia, which may gradually increase with time. If the diverticulum is large, symptoms associated with fluid retention such as sudden regurgitation of liquid with choking or aspiration may be noted. Gurgling sounds may be heard in the neck.

Although diagnosis is usually made by barium esophagram (Fig. 2.2), a Zenker's diverticulum can be missed unless careful attention is paid to the cricopharyngeal area. If this diverticulum is suspected, endoscopy should be performed with utmost care and gentleness. The orifice of a diverticulum is usually difficult to visualize and, as one advances an end-viewing instrument, one may inadvertently enter the Zenker's diverticulum. Because further advancement could result in a perforation, the instrument should be withdrawn until the esophageal lumen is visualized. The endoscope can then be advanced with the lumen constantly in view. Alternatively, the endoscope can be passed over a guidewire that is introduced through the lumen of a sump tube placed in the stomach. The sump tube is removed, leaving the guidewire in place.

MIDESOPHAGEAL DIVERTICULA

Midesophageal diverticula are mostly asymptomatic, and their cause is unclear. These diverticula are usually single but may be multiple. They are often associated with motor abnormalities of the esophagus.

EPIPHRENIC DIVERTICULA

Epiphrenic diverticula are frequently associated with motor abnormalities such as diffuse esophageal spasm and achalasia. Symptoms are more common with this type of diverticulum than with the midesophageal type. Diagnosis is usually made radiographically or by endoscopy. These diverticula may be multiple or single (Fig. 2.6), and often occur in association with esophagitis with stricture or ulceration. An epiphrenic diverticulum may create difficulty in passing an endoscope into the stomach, even under direct vision. The opening into the esophagogastric junction may appear cervix-like adjacent to the wide mouth of the diverticulum, making it easier to enter the diverticulum than the stomach. Therefore, there is a risk of perforation, especially with dependent diverticula. One also may note pseudodiverticula of the distal esophagus, with bands creating outpouchings of the esophageal lumen (Fig. 2.7).

INTRAMURAL DIVERTICULOSIS

Intramural diverticulosis is an unusual condition in which many small diverticula of the esophagus are seen. Patients often present with dysphagia. Diagnosis is usually made by barium esophagram, which demonstrates numerous small outpouchings or irregularities of the esophageal wall, each approximately 1–2 mm in diameter. They are thought to represent dilated submucosal esophageal glands. Endoscopically, the mucosa may appear granular and friable, with tiny orifices of the diverticula visible (Fig. 2.8). In many cases these diverticula are associated with esophageal candidiasis (Fig. 2.9), including the mucocutaneous type, and may be associated with motor disorders.

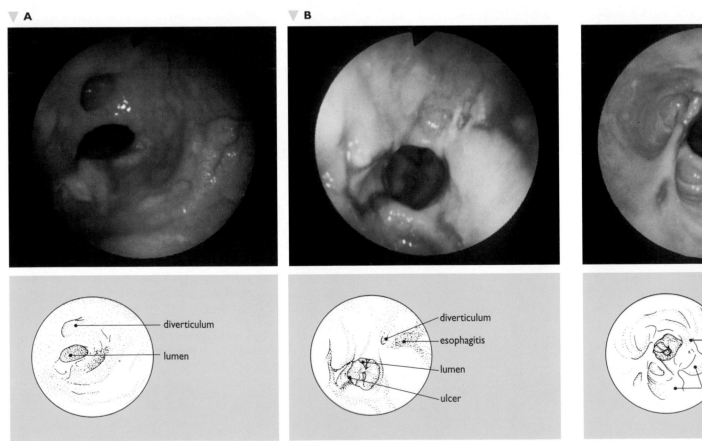

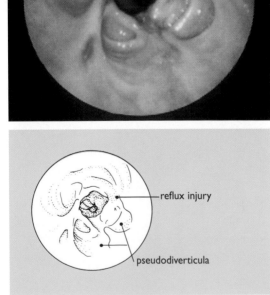

Figure 2.6 (A) Epiphrenic diverticulum in a patient with a motor disorder. After pneumatic dilation of the esophagus, the lower esophageal sphincter became incompetent, and reflux and a reflux-associated ulcer occurred. **(B)** A closeup view demonstrates the ulcer, but the diverticulum is less well seen.

Figure 2.7 Bands in the distal esophagus creating pseudodiverticula. There is minimal associated reflux injury, with red streaks on the tops of the folds.

HIATAL HERNIA

There are two types of hiatal hernia: axial and paraesophageal. Each is identified and discussed below.

AXIAL HIATAL HERNIA

An axial (sliding) hiatal hernia is the more common type of hernia encountered in clinical medicine. There are two issues in the diagnosis: first, how to

define what appears to be a small hiatal hernia; second, how to relate the presence of an axial hiatal hernia to symptomatic gastroesophageal reflux.

Radiologically, diagnosis of an axial hiatal hernia is usually made when a barium esophagram demonstrates a portion of the stomach above the diaphragm (Fig. 2.10). Endoscopically, diagnosis requires recognition of the squamocolumnar junction and the level of the diaphragmatic hiatus. If, during quiet respiration and without excessive air insufflation, the squamocolumnar junction is located more than 2 or 3 cm above the diaphragmatic

▼ **A**

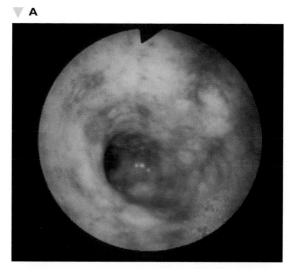

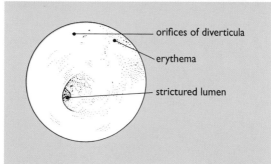

▼ **B**

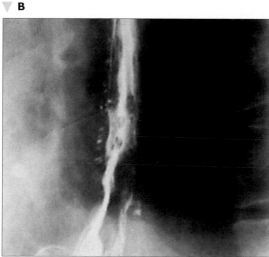

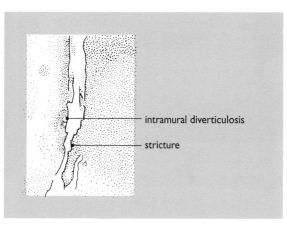

Figure 2.8 (**A**) Intramural diverticulosis. The mucosa appears pale, friable, and granular. Tiny orifices of the diverticula or outpouchings are seen. (**B**) A barium esophagram confirms the diagnosis.

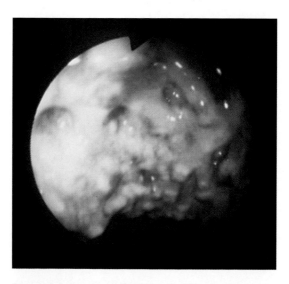

Figure 2.9 Intramural diverticulosis. The mucosa appears irregular with multiple small diverticula, or outpouchings. The white exudate is caused by candida associated with this condition.

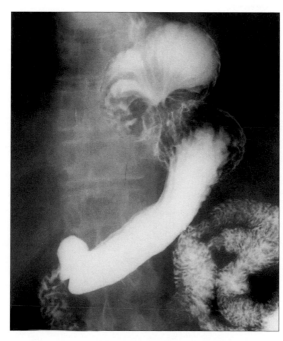

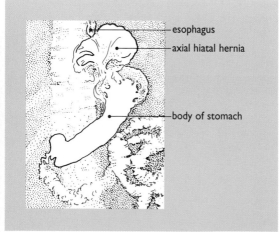

Figure 2.10 Barium esophagram demonstrates a large axial hiatal hernia. The proximal stomach has herniated through the diaphragm into the thorax.
(Courtesy of Dr Charles Rohrmann)

impression, some will diagnose an axial hiatal hernia. Often, the hernia appears as a pouch-like area just below the mucosal junction and above the diaphragm. The squamocolumnar junction may be patulous, allowing the endoscopist to look through into the hiatal hernia pouch (Figs. 2.11 and 2.12).

To inspect the cardia, the endoscope is passed into the stomach and retroflexed. Normally, the tissue of the cardia appears snug around the endoscope. With an axial hiatal hernia, a space is evident around the instrument as it passes through the cardia (Fig. 2.13). Small ulcers may be seen in the

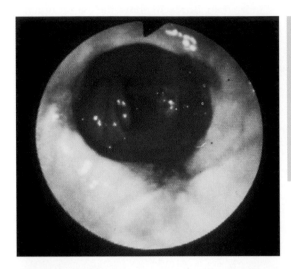

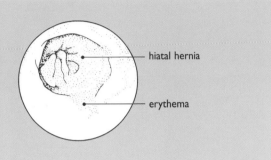

Figure 2.11 *An axial hiatal hernia is seen just beyond the squamocolumnar junction, with minimal erythema on one rim of the junction. Gastric mucosa is seen in the pouch. (Courtesy of Dr Eric Harder)*

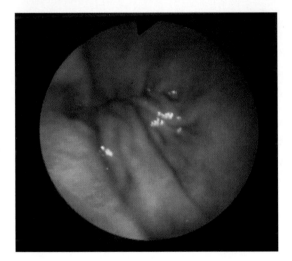

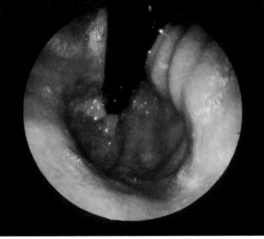

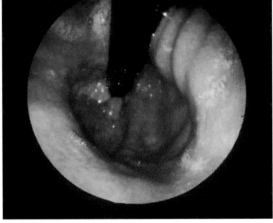

Figure 2.12 *View of hiatal hernia from endoscope inserted to just beyond the squamocolumnar junction.*

Figure 2.13 *An axial hiatal hernia, seen with the endoscope retroflexed. The tissue of the gastric cardia is not snug around the endoscope, and one can see into the hernia.*

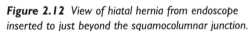

Figure 2.14 *(A and B) Two small, relatively flat 'riding' ulcers as seen in hiatal hernias, in separate patients.*

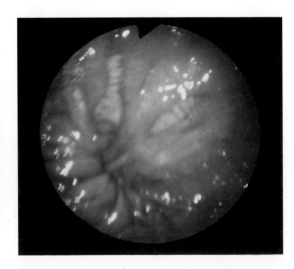

Figure 2.15 *Multiple 'riding' ulcers in a hiatal hernia.*

hernia. These are referred to as 'riding' ulcers if they occur on the gastric tissue separating the hiatal hernia from the remainder of the stomach (Fig. 2.14). The ulcers may bleed and be multiple (Fig. 2.15).

The symptoms of gastroesophageal reflux are often associated with the diagnosis of hiatal hernia. Reflux can occur without a hernia, and patients with a hernia may be free of reflux, but frequently these diagnoses occur together.

PARAESOPHAGEAL HIATAL HERNIA

A paraesophageal hiatal hernia is much less common than an axial hiatal hernia and may present a significant clinical problem. This hernia is defined as a pouch of stomach that has herniated up into the chest and is in a position adjacent to the esophagus. The esophagus does not necessarily empty into the most cephalad margin of the hernia. Patients present with a fullness in the chest after eating; they may also present with dysphagia, bleeding, and chest discomfort. Patients usually do not have gastroesophageal reflux. Paraesophageal hernias have been reported to cause obstruction, ulceration,

and strangulation with infarction. Diagnosis is usually made radiographically (Fig. 2.16). Endoscopy may be problematic, as one may get lost inside the hernia pouch and have considerable trouble locating the main gastric lumen. However, the endoscope may be valuable in discovering the presence of an ulcer in the hernia, which may be the cause of bleeding.

WEBS AND RINGS

Webs and rings are infrequently encountered in the esophagus but are of significance because they may cause symptoms that require therapy, and because they can cause difficulty during endoscopy.

WEBS

A web is usually defined as a thin, membrane-like structure containing mucosa and submucosa but without muscle layers (Figs. 2.17 and 2.18).

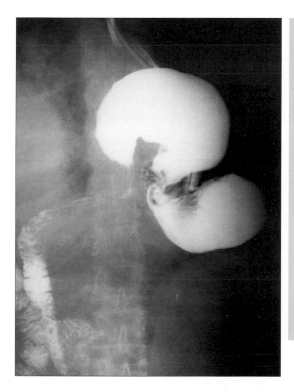

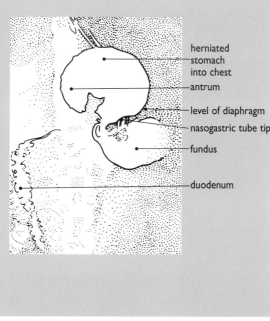

herniated stomach into chest
antrum
level of diaphragm
nasogastric tube tip
fundus
duodenum

Figure 2.16 Barium esophagram reveals a large paraesophageal hernia. A nasogastric tube is seen with its tip below the diaphragm in the cardia of the stomach. The fundus is below the diaphragm, and the body and antrum are herniated into the chest. (Courtesy of Dr Charles Rohrmann)

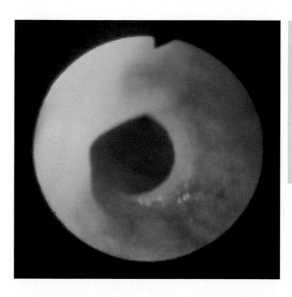

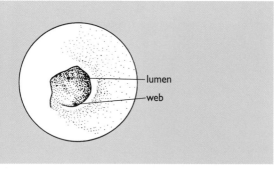

lumen
web

Figure 2.17 This thin esophageal web does not extend around the circumference of the esophagus. (Courtesy of Group Health Hospital)

Webs can occur anywhere in the esophagus and may be single or multiple. Patients may present with dysphagia if the diameter of the lumen through the web is less than 12 mm. Etiology is unknown, though they may occur in chronic graft-versus-host disease.

Webs may be noted incidentally on barium esophagrams (Fig. 2.19) or during endoscopy. Distension of the esophagus is necessary to see a thin web radiographically. A water-soluble bolus, such as a marshmallow, is usually swallowed with barium to determine whether there is obstruction to passage. Endoscopically, the web can usually be seen if the esophagus is gently distended with air (Fig. 2.17). Occasionally, the web may be difficult to see. This will be the case if the endoscope gets caught in a web that is out of the field of view (Fig. 2.20). As the endoscope is advanced, the web may be inadvertently ruptured (Fig. 2.21). This may cure the problem, as treatment for these webs is disruption using dilation with an esophageal dilator or with an endoscope.

Plummer-Vinson syndrome is an unusual condition in which a web occurs in the proximal 4 or 5 cm of the esophagus (Fig. 2.22). The syndrome may be associated with dysphagia, aspiration, and iron-deficiency anemia, and is associated with an increased incidence of hypopharyngeal carcinoma. The web is often eccentric. Such webs may be difficult to see endoscopically if they are located in the upper esophagus just beyond the cricopharyngeus muscle. In this position the web may be ruptured as the endoscope is passed through the cricopharyngeus muscle into the upper esophagus. In addition to receiving iron therapy, these patients with Plummer-Vinson syndrome must be screened periodically for hypopharyngeal cancer.

Webs in the midesophagus and distal esophagus may be asymptomatic or may be associated with dysphagia; they are usually not associated with reflux.

Diagnosis is by careful radiology or endoscopy. Endoscopically, these webs appear the same as those in the upper esophagus. Some investigators have suggested treatment using endoscopic biopsy forceps to biopsy the margin of the web or diathermy electrosurgical current to incise the structure radially, but most prefer routine dilation.

RINGS

Esophageal rings are often thicker than webs and are most frequently seen in the distal esophagus. There are two types of lower esophageal ring: the A ring and the B ring. The A ring occurs in the distal esophagus at the proximal margin of the lower esophageal sphincter (LES). It is covered with squamous mucosa and is usually located 2 or 3 cm proximal to the squamocolumnar junction. This ring does not cause symptoms except in rare instances.

The B, or Schatzki, ring is more common than the A ring. It is located at the squamocolumnar junction, with squamous mucosa on the upper side of the ring and columnar mucosa on the lower side (Fig. 2.23). The thickness of a B ring is usually 2 or 3 mm, rarely thicker; it tends to be symmetrical. The B ring is seen endoscopically only if the LES is located in the chest above the diaphragmatic hiatus. This may be accomplished by gently insufflating the distal esophagus, causing the LES to move upwards into the chest. Having the patient sniff may also accentuate a B ring. In addition, the B ring is usually seen when a hiatal hernia is present because the hernia displaces the LES above the diaphragm. Therefore, the B ring is a dynamic structure that changes configuration with a variety of factors. If the diameter of the lumen through the ring is less than 12 or 13 mm, dysphagia may be present.

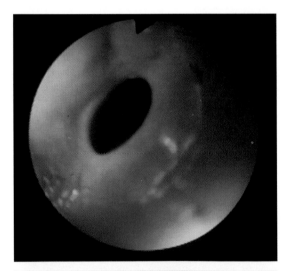
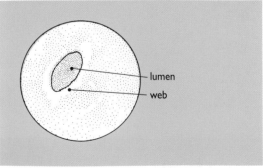

Figure 2.18 Web in the proximal esophagus.

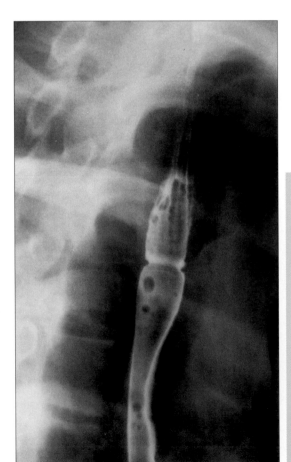

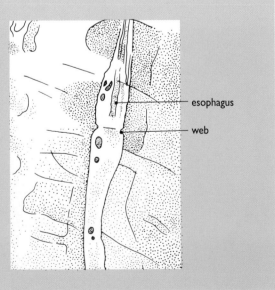

Figure 2.19 In this air-contrast view of the esophagus, a relatively thin web is seen in the proximal third. This patient presented with dysphagia.
(Courtesy of Dr Charles Rohrmann)

Only rarely is a ring seen with reflux esophagitis. The B ring is not seen after a Nissen fundoplication because the LES is intra-abdominal (below the diaphragm), nor with Barrett's metaplasia when the squamocolumnar junction is displaced proximally.

The most common symptom of a ring is dysphagia, but a somewhat unique form of dysphagia; the patient frequently complains of intermittent dysphagia that may occur with the first swallow of solid food in a meal, but then does

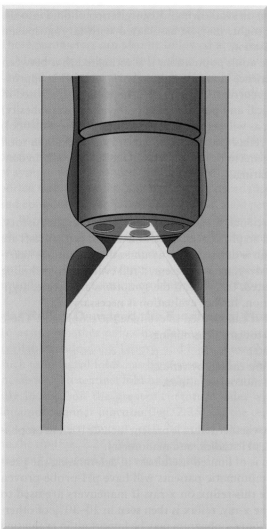

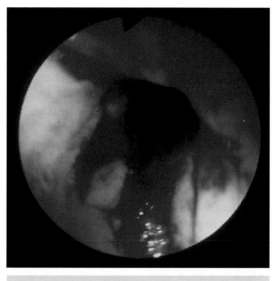

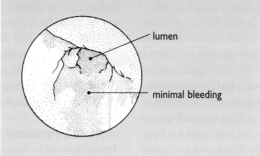

Figure 2.21 Web after rupture with Savary dilator. Mild bleeding is noted.

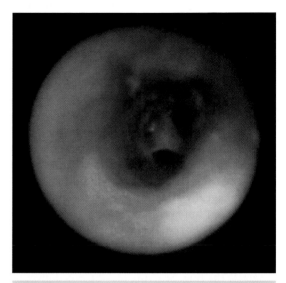

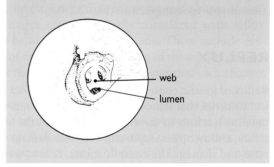

Figure 2.22 Web in the proximal esophagus of a patient with Plummer-Vinson syndrome. This is a complicated web with small lumen on either side. (Courtesy of Dr George McDonald)

Figure 2.20 In this diagram, the web is preventing the passage of the endoscope while remaining out of view. If the endoscope is advanced, the web may be ruptured.

▼ **A**

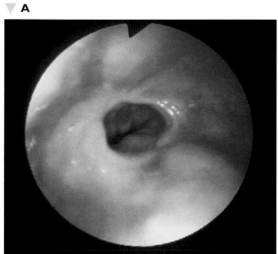

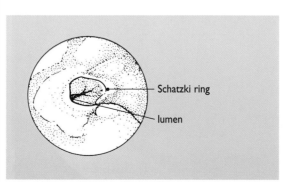

▼ **B**

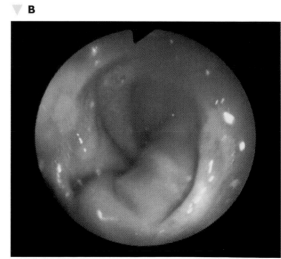

Figure 2.23 (A and B) Early incomplete Schatzki B ring.

In stage I, nonconfluent red patches or streaks are noted at and just proximal to the squamocolumnar junction. The shape of these patches may be longitudinal, triangular, or oval. They often occur along a fold and may be covered with a white exudate. Patches may occur singly or in multiple nonconfluent areas (Figs. 2.28–2.30).

As the damage progresses, the injury becomes confluent but still does not extend around the entire esophageal circumference. This marks stage II mucosal damage (Figs. 2.31–2.33). The typical appearance involves finger-like lesions, with a white exudate in the center of the lesion surrounded by erythematous mucosa, extending cephalad up the esophagus. They may be

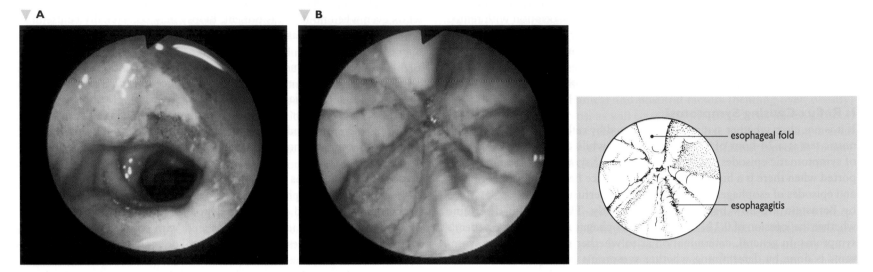

Figure 2.27 This patient presented with a duodenal bulb ulcer **(A)** in conjunction with stage II reflux esophagitis **(B)**. This is a common manifestation associated with increased gastric acid production.

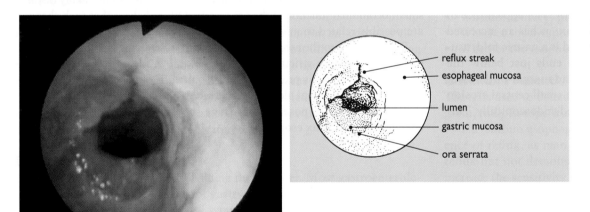

Figure 2.28 Stage I (mild) reflux esophagitis in a patient with an incompetent LES. The ora serrata is seen, and there is a single erosion extending up the esophagus.

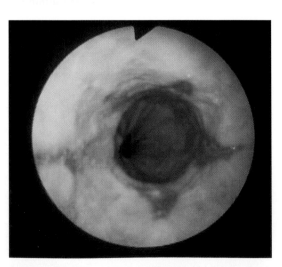

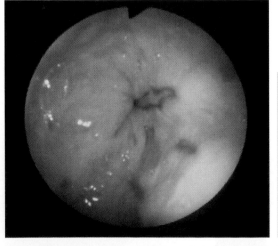

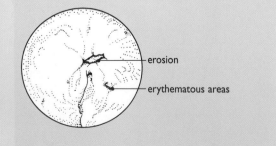

Figure 2.29 Stage I reflux esophagitis. Here, the reflux is slightly more extensive, with several linear, nonconfluent red streaks extending up the esophagus.

Figure 2.30 Stage I reflux esophagitis. A single erosion with a red perimeter and a white exudative base is seen, as are several small erythematous areas.

friable and bleed. If there is no exudate on the area of esophagitis, it may be difficult to distinguish this lesion from patches of columnar epithelium. Reflux changes characteristically involve the distal esophagus at the squamo-columnar junction and extend proximally. If the esophageal mucosa just above the squamocolumnar junction is normal but inflammation is noted proximally in the esophagus, this favors a diagnosis of candida infection, herpetic infection, drug injury, etc. rather than reflux.

In stage III, the inflammatory lesion extends to the entire circumference of the esophagus and is accompanied by more edema, hyperemia, friability, and bleeding; however, no stricture is present (Figs. 2.34–2.37).

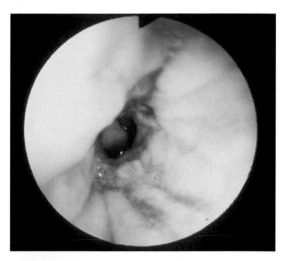

Figure 2.31 *Stage II reflux esophagitis. Confluent erythematous areas are seen extending up the esophagus.*

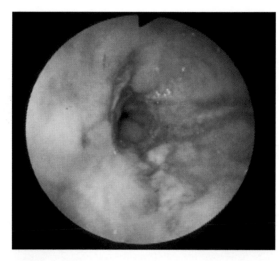

Figure 2.32 *Stage II reflux esophagitis. These early confluent erosions have a white base and erythematous surrounding mucosa.*

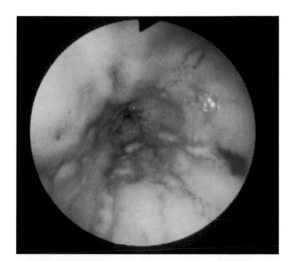

Figure 2.33 *Stage II reflux esophagitis. White-based erosions extend up the esophagus. Confluence but noninvolvement of the entire circumference is noted.*

Figure 2.34 *Severe reflux esophagitis stage III with erosions involving the entire circumference of the distal esophagus. Friability and a small amount of bleeding are evident.*

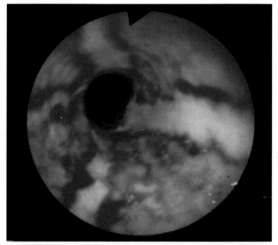

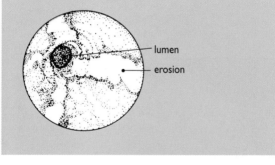

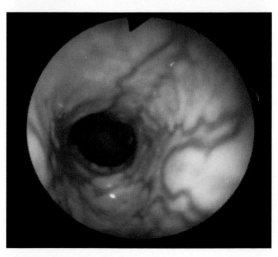

Figure 2.35 *Stage III reflux esophagitis with confluent erosions involving the entire circumference of the distal esophagus.*

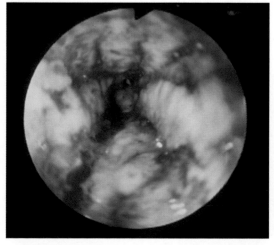

Figure 2.36 *Stage III reflux esophagitis. Denudation and friability are observed.*

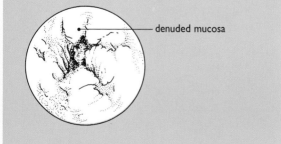

Stage IV is divided into IVa and IVb. In IVa there are one or several esophageal ulcers that may be associated with circumferential stricturing, esophageal shortening, or Barrett's metaplasia (Figs. 2.38–2.41). In IVb a peptic stricture is noted, with or without evidence of erosion or ulceration in the strictured area (Fig. 2.42).

There are several systems for grading esophagitis (Fig 2.43).

Therapy

In most patients with reflux, medical therapy relieves symptoms. In a small number of patients, surgery is necessary because of severe reflux or complications of reflux that do not respond to medical therapy. One procedure considered to be effective is the Nissen fundoplication. In this operation, the fundus is wrapped around the distal esophagus to create a barrier to the

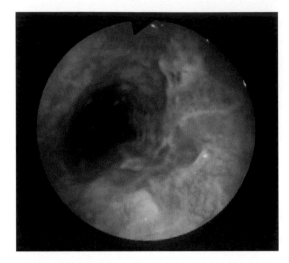

Figure 2.37 *Stage III esophagitis caused by hyperemesis.*

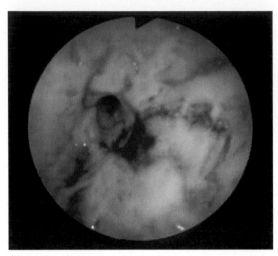

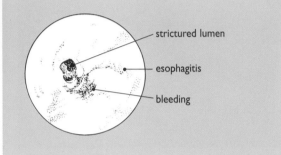

Figure 2.38 *Stage IVa reflux esophagitis. Here, a stricture and evidence of esophagitis are apparent. Bleeding is also present just proximal to the stricture over an area of ulceration.*

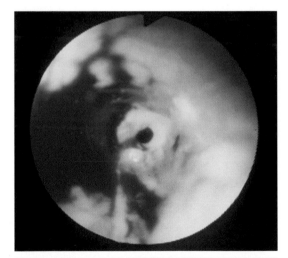

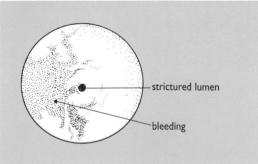

Figure 2.39 *This patient with Zollinger-Ellison syndrome presents with severe stricture and stage IVa reflux esophagitis. The residual esophageal lumen is very stenotic. Blood covers the area of ulceration or erosion.*

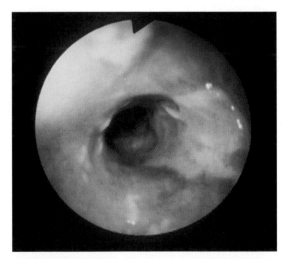

Figure 2.40 *Stage IVa reflux esophagitis. An ulcer as sociated with this severe form appears in the distal esophagus. The ulcer has a white base and covers approximately one-third of the circumference. At the time of this endoscopy, this ulcer had been treated and was beginning to heal, thus accounting for the relative inactivity of the surrounding mucosa.*

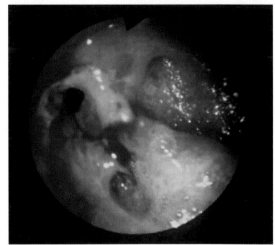

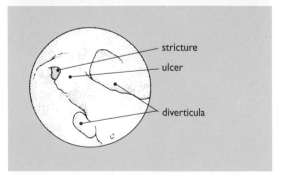

Figure 2.41 *Stage IVa reflux esophagitis. The tight esophageal stricture has associated ulceration and pseudodiverticula formation.*

reflux of acid from the stomach into the esophagus. The competence of the fundoplication can be assessed endoscopically by determining whether the esophagitis is healing and by passing the instrument through the esophagogastric junction and retroflexing it to examine the cardia. One can then determine whether the tissue of the cardia is snug around the endoscope as a result of the surgery (Figs. 2.44–2.46). An ulcer may occur within the fundoplication wrap (Fig. 2.47).

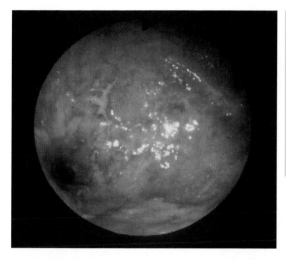
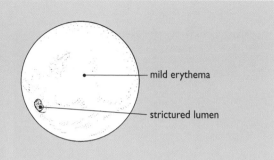

Figure 2.42 Stage IVb reflux esophagitis. Note the reflux-associated benign esophageal stricture. The mucosa is slightly red and demonstrates inflammation caused by stasis. No ulcers are present.

Grading of reflux esophagitis

Grade 0
No evidence of reflux-induced damage: crisp, sharply delineated squamocolumnar mucosal junction (SCMJ).
No friability: distal esophageal mucosa squamous smooth and shiny.

Grade 1
Mild, patchy or more diffuse erythema at the level of the SCMJ; slight blurring of the SCMJ; minor friability; loss of shininess of the distal squamous mucosa. Such abnormalities are equivocal and cannot be interpreted as genuinely characteristic of reflux-induced damage. There is no apparent break in the mucosa.

Grade 2
One or more discrete superficial erosions, seen as red dots or streaks, with or without adherent whitish exudate. Such linear erosions are usually small and often on top of the esophageal folds. They involve less than 10% of the mucosal surface of the distal 5 cm of the squamous segment of the esophagus above the gastroesophageal junction.

Grade 3
Confluent but noncircumferential erosions seen as defects that merge either longitudinally or laterally. There may be additional exudate covering the erosive defects or slough formation. Less than 50% of the overall mucosal surface of the distal 5 cm is involved.

Grade 4
Circumferential erosions or exudative lesions at the level of the SCMJ, regardless of the extent along the distal esophagus.

Grade 5
Deep ulceration anywhere along the esophagus.

Grade 6
Various degrees of stricturing, prohibiting passage of a standard (>9 mm) or small-caliber (<9 mm) endoscope.

Grades 1–6 can be present with or without a segment of columnar metaplasia.

All reflux-grading systems, including the two shown, have major shortcomings. The Los Angeles grading system for reflux esophagitis aims to describe the extent of mucosal damage as simply and unambiguously as possible. This system avoids words open to interpretation and terminology that implies assumptions about the process. The recording of complications or minimal changes is kept separate from the scoring of the extent of the esophagitis.

Los Angeles system for classification of reflux esophagitis

Grade A	One or more mucosal breaks each no longer than 5 mm.
Grade B	At least one mucosal break more than 5 mm long, but not continuous between the tops of two mucosal folds.
Grade C	At least one mucosal break that is continuous between the tops of two or more mucosal folds, but which is not circumferential.
Grade D	Circumferential mucosal break.

Figure 2.43 Table showing two systems for grading of reflux esophagitis.

Another now rarely performed surgical approach to reducing reflux is to insert a silicone (Angelchik) prosthesis around the distal esophagus. The effect of this prosthesis is to make the gastroesophageal junction competent. This can be assessed endoscopically by retroflexing the tip of the endoscope to perform the U-turn maneuver to visualize the cardial tissue. The tissue with the prosthesis should be snug around the endoscope (Fig. 2.48). Complications have been reported with the use of this prosthesis, including perforation of the prosthesis into the esophagus and perforation with migration of the prosthesis into the stomach (Fig. 2.49 and 2.50).

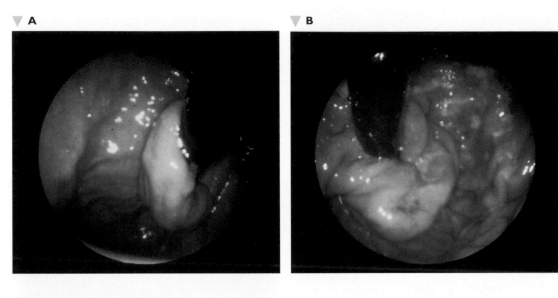

Figure 2.44 (A and **B)** Two examples of Nissen fundoplication for reflux. The endoscope is retroflexed in the stomach to examine the cardia. Abundant cardial tissue is snug around the endoscope, indicating that the Nissen wrap is competent in each of these patients.

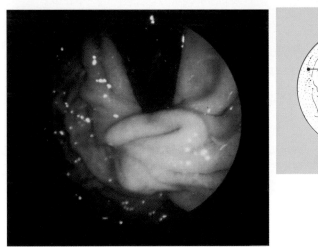
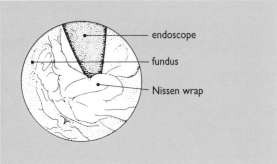

endoscope

fundus

Nissen wrap

Figure 2.45 Nissen fundoplication for reflux. Here, cardial tissue again appears snug around the endoscope. In fact, this Nissen wrap was supercompetent, causing the patient some difficulty with belching and some dysphagia. It is not possible to determine whether the Nissen wrap is too tight using this endoscopic inspection; symptoms are a better correlative factor.

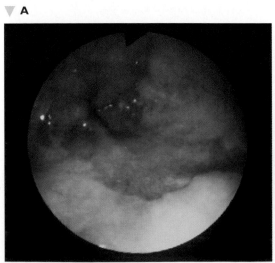
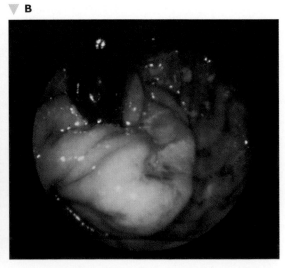

Figure 2.46 (A) This patient with prior severe reflux esophagitis had a Nissen fundoplication performed. The ora serrata appears in the distal esophagus, and there is little evidence of esophagitis as healing continues. **(B)** This same case viewed from below with the endoscope retroflexed reveals that the cardial tissue is snug around the endoscope.

Reflux-Associated Complications

Several complications of reflux can occur, including strictures, ulcers, and Barrett's metaplasia.

STRICTURES

Strictures develop in approximately 15% of patients with reflux esophagitis. Characteristically, there is a long duration of reflux symptoms, an incompetent LES, and impaired esophageal clearing. The usual presenting symptom is dysphagia, initially to solid foods but gradually progressing to liquids as the lumen narrows. If dysphagia is present and there are no other symptoms of reflux, one must consider both a peptic stricture and esophageal cancer in the differential diagnosis because some patients may develop a reflux-related stricture with few or no reflux symptoms.

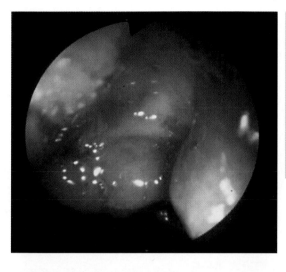
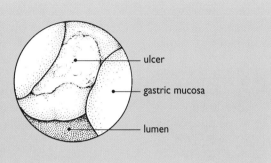

Figure 2.47 Ulcer in the area of a fundoplication.

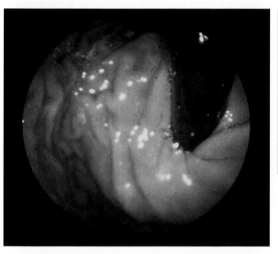
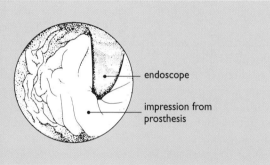

Figure 2.48 Angelchik prosthesis around the distal esophagus, viewed from below with the endoscope retroflexed.

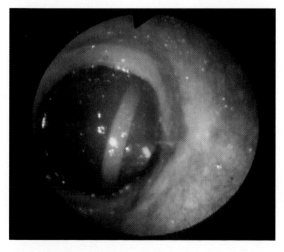
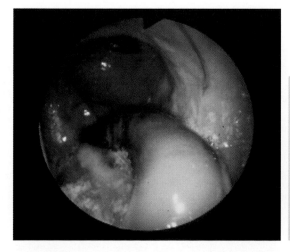
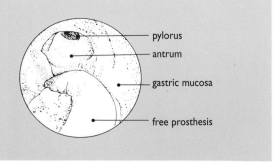

Figure 2.49 Angelchik prosthesis perforating into the esophagus, causing esophageal obstruction.

Figure 2.50 This is a complication of the Angelchik prosthesis. The entire prosthesis has migrated into the stomach and is free in the gastric lumen.

Strictures occur when circumferential inflammation of the esophageal wall extends to the submucosa and a fibrous reaction takes place, resulting in the formation of scar tissue that can narrow the esophageal lumen and shorten the esophagus. In the absence of Barrett's metaplasia, strictures usually occur in the distal esophagus, often proximal to a hiatal hernia. If Barrett's metaplasia is present, the squamocolumnar junction migrates proximally in the esophagus, and a stricture may be noted proximal to the displaced junction. Proximal strictures may also be found in esophaged injury resulting from trauma to the esophagus, suchas with caustic ingestion or medication-related esophageal injury associated with ulceration.

Strictures tend to be short, although they may occasionally be 5 or 10 cm long, especially in nasogastric-tube-related strictures. A barium esophagram will usually detect the stricture, but careful observation is required to define its length. As with webs and rings, a bolus swallow may be required during the x-ray study to demonstrate the obstruction.

A small-caliber endoscope may be helpful in evaluating strictures because it can be passed through the stricture to permit biopsies and cytologies along the entire length of the stricture. Also, when retroflexed, the endoscope will allow visualization of the esophagogastric junction below the stricture. Endoscopy combined with biopsy and brush cytology allow one to differentiate a benign reflux stricture from a cancer. Occasionally it may be necessary to dilate a stricture so that biopsies and cytologies can be obtained along its length. By knowing the diameter of the instrument, one can calibrate the diameter and determine the length of the stricture and the distance from the incisors. Observed endoscopically, strictures vary from predominant involvement of a portion of the wall, seen as a white crescent-like area covered with an exudate, to circumferential involvement. There may also be varying amounts of reflux-associated change and superficial ulceration. The caliber of the lumen varies from fairly wide with minimal dysphagia (1.2–1.3 cm in diameter) to very tight with nearly complete esophageal obstruction.

The initial therapy for reflux strictures is to treat the underlying reflux esophagitis. Some investigators feel that all strictures should be dilated initially over a guidewire or with a balloon. Others try to dilate a stricture initially with rubber mercury-filled bougies. If the stricture is exceptionally tight or tortuous, a springtip guidewire can be passed through the stricture under endoscopic guidance (Fig. 2.51). Fluoroscopy confirms that the tip of the wire is in the stomach. Then, dilators of gradually increasing size are passed over the wire. The guidewire reduces the chances of an esophageal perforation. Endoscopy immediately after dilation will often reveal a small amount of bleeding when the stricture has been stretched. Endoscopy is rarely helpful immediately after dilation except to permit biopsy and cytology in the strictured area if these examinations could not be adequately performed before dilation. Commonly used dilators, guided over a guidewire, are of the Savary-Gilliard type; olive-shaped metal dilators of gradually increasing size are used less frequently.

Balloons can either be inserted over a guidewire (OTW) or can be advanced via the instrumentation channel of the endoscope (TTS; through the scope). The catheter is passed into the stricture and then the balloon is expanded under direct vision to dilate the stricture (Fig. 2.52).

Ulcers

Ulcers in the esophagus are rare. They usually occur as a result of injection sclerotherapy for esophageal varices, but may also appear in association with reflux esophagitis, Barrett's metaplasia, and esophageal infections such as candida, herpes, and HIV. Quite often ulcers are deep and extend into the muscle layers of the esophagus (Fig. 2.53). Manifestations include severe pain or moderate-to-severe upper gastrointestinal bleeding.

Ulcers may also develop in patients on medication (e.g. antibiotics, especially tetracycline) if the pills are ingested without liquid and remain in the esophagus for a prolonged period. This cause of ulceration is dealt with in detail in Chapter 4.

Esophageal ulcers can usually be detected by barium esophagraphy (Fig. 2.53). Endoscopic examination reveals deep, white-based lesions, usually in the distal esophagus. There may be an associated stricture or reflux mucosal injury. Bleeding may be noted; occasionally, it may be massive.

Barrett's Metaplasia or Columnar Metaplasia

In patients with chronic reflux esophagitis, the normal squamous esophageal mucosa may become replaced with metaplastic columnar epithelium. This occurrence has been associated with a number of conditions, including esophagitis, proximal esophageal strictures, esophageal ulcers, mucosal dysplasia, and adenocarcinoma.

Some investigators feel that a rare type of Barrett's metaplasia is caused by a congenitally short esophagus in the presence of a hiatal hernia. Many now feel that nearly all cases of Barrett's metaplasia are acquired. The current theory is that chronic reflux esophagitis produces a chronically inflamed esophageal mucosa, which desquamates and is gradually replaced by columnar epithelium. As this replacement occurs, the squamocolumnar junction (ora serrata) migrates in a cephalad direction and may be found in the upper third of the esophagus in patients with this condition. The junction may

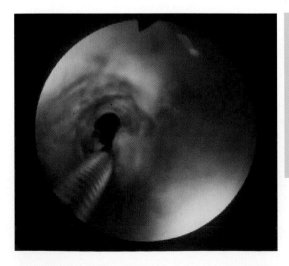

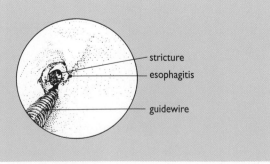

stricture
esophagitis
guidewire

Figure 2.51 *Tight esophageal stricture caused by reflux. A guidewire has been passed under endoscopic guidance to direct dilators and reduce the likelihood of a perforation during dilation.*

▼ **A** ▼ **B**

▼ **C** ▼ **D**

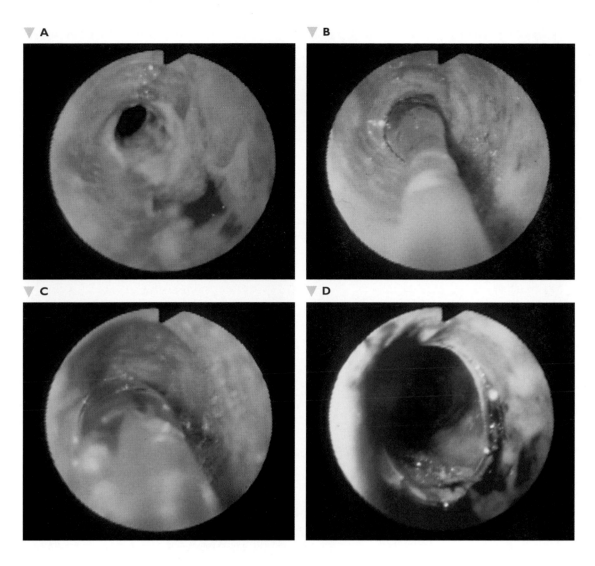

Figure 2.52 Tight esophageal stricture caused by stage IVa reflux esophagitis **(A)** Dilation by passage of mercury-filled bougies would be difficult, so a balloon-tipped catheter has been passed into the stricture under endoscopic guidance **(B)**. Then the balloon is inflated to stretch the stricture **(C)**. Finally, inspection of the stricture after dilation shows that the lumen is open **(D)**. The minimal bleeding was caused by the dilation. (Courtesy of Dr Eric Harder)

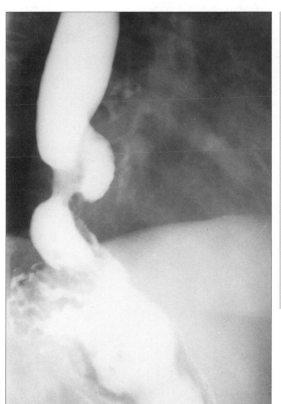

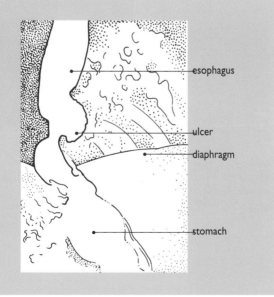

Figure 2.53 Barium esophagram shows a large esophageal ulcer in the distal third of the esophagus. The ulcer extends into the tissue adjacent to the esophagus. (Courtesy of Dr Charles Rohrmann)

appear normal or it may be indistinct, or it may exhibit the characteristic changes of reflux esophagitis. In other cases, the junction may be very irregular, with mixed islands of squamous and columnar mucosa (Figs. 2.54–2.56). The segment of Barrett's metaplasia may be short, only extending 2–3 cm up the esophagus (Fig. 2.57).

There are three types of columnar epithelium: (1) fundal mucosa, identical to that found in the gastric fundus, with parietal and chief cells; (2) cardial-type mucosa, with pylorocardial glands and a foveolar epithelial sur-

face; and (3) metaplastic mucosa of the specialized Barrett's type or intestinal type. There may also be a mosaic presentation with various cell and tissue types. It is this latter metaplastic mucosa that is felt to be the tissue in which dysplasia and adenocarcinoma may develop. The characteristic distribution of these types of mucosa seems to be specialized-type mucosa cephalad, just distal to the proximally migrated squamocolumnar junction; then, moving distally, a variable segment of cardial mucosa; finally, most distally, fundal-type mucosa. The cardial and fundal mucosa usually occur in the

▼ **A**

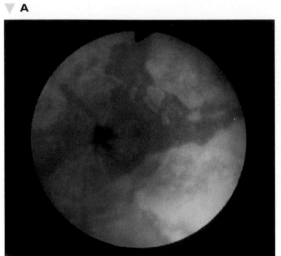

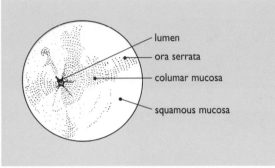

▼ **B**

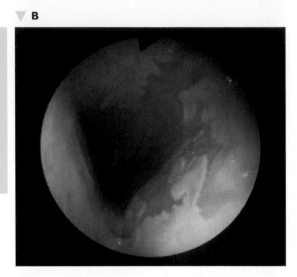

Figure 2.54 (A and **B)** Barrett's metaplasia. The squamocolumnar junction has moved proximally in the esophagus. It is distinct but irregular, with islands of columnar mucosa.

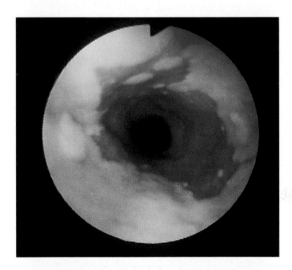

Figure 2.55 Barrett's metaplasia. The proximal junction is slightly irregular, with islands of squamous and columnar tissue.

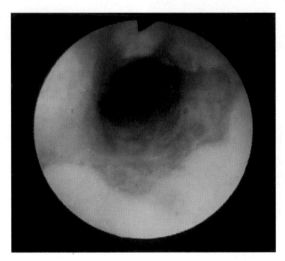

Figure 2.56 Barrett's metaplasia. The squamocolumnar junction is located at 20 cm from the incisor teeth. The ora serrata is regular and would appear normal except for its proximal position.

Figure 2.57 Distinct ora serrata in the distal esophagus. The mucosa with a gastric appearance was found to be Barrett's metaplastic mucosa, which was seen in a 'short segment', extending 2–3 cm up the esophagus.

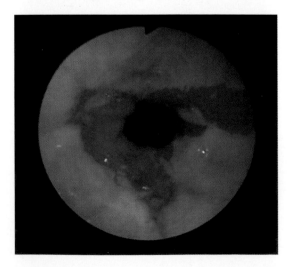

distal 2–3 cm of the esophagus. The pathophysiologic sequence is thought to start with reflux, which causes inflammation, followed by desquamation, replacement with metaplastic mucosa, and finally dysplasia and carcinoma. Biopsies along the length of the esophagus are essential to identify the types of mucosa present and to establish the presence of Barrett's metaplasia, as well as dysplasia and early adenocarcinoma.

The typical endoscopic appearance of a Barrett's esophagus is normal, pink esophageal mucosa proximally, an ora serrata in the upper or middle third of the esophagus, and a salmon-pink segment of Barrett's metaplasia below the ora serrata. This latter mucosa runs down and joins the similar-looking mucosa of the stomach (Figs 2.58–2.60). The esophagus in the Barrett's segment is devoid of folds, and submucosal blood vessels can occasionally be seen.

In the distal esophagus one may see the zone in which the ora serrata used to be located before its cephalad migration (Figs. 2.61 and 2.62). This is recognized by a semicircular ridge of tissue and by gastric folds that run

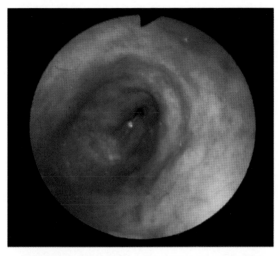
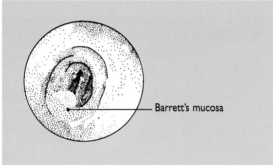

Figure 2.58 Barrett's metaplasia in the midesophagus, just below the ora serrata. The mucosa appears slightly irregular, but there are no endoscopically visible areas suggesting carcinoma or adenoma. Vessels are not well seen. Biopsy is indicated to verify mucosal type and detect possible dysplasia.

Barrett's mucosa

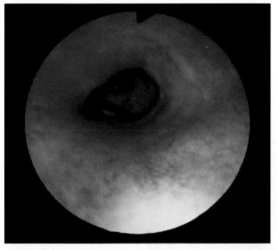
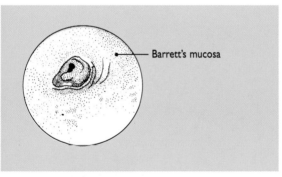
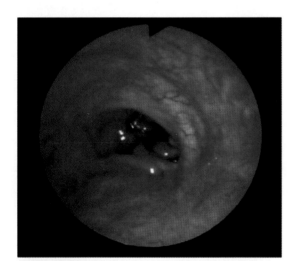

Barrett's mucosa

Figure 2.59 This Barrett's segment can be seen as a fine, erythematous mucosal pattern.

Figure 2.60 The color of this Barrett's mucosa is typical; atypically, blood vessels can be seen.

Figure 2.61 In this case of Barrett's metaplasia, the area of the former LES can be seen. This physiologic narrowing is not a stricture but represents the area where the ora serrata used to be located. The ora serrata is now located cephalad.

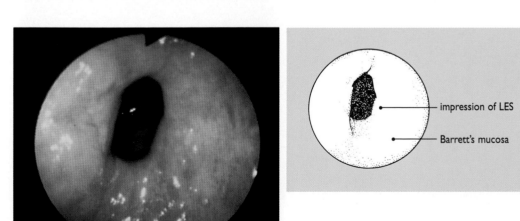

impression of LES

Barrett's mucosa

vertically and end just below the ridge. The transition from the stomach to the tubular esophagus is determined by the location of the proximal extent of the gastric folds, which is an important landmark (Fig. 2.62).

A hiatal hernia may be seen – directly (Fig. 2.63) and with the endoscope retroflexed (Fig. 2.64) – just below the ridge. Therefore, if the ridge and the gastric folds are seen and identified but the squamocolumnar junction is more than 1 cm proximal to that area, the endoscopist should suspect Barrett's metaplasia. Because neoplasia only occur in specialized or intestinal type columnar metaplastic mucosa, efforts are made to diagnose Barrett's columnar metaplasia by biopsying this abnormal appearing mucosa in the distal esophagus. It is important to make this diagnosis regardless of the extent of the metaplasia.

On occasion, one will see islands of whitish-pink squamous epithelium in the otherwise uniform salmon-pink Barrett's segment.

As mentioned earlier, a number of conditions have been associated with Barrett's epithelial change. Esophagitis may be noted in the squamous mucosa proximal to the squamocolumnar junction (Fig. 2.65). This esophagitis is similar in appearance to typical, distal reflux esophagitis. The mucosa may be red and friable, with erosions, exudation, and bleeding. There may also be some degree of friability and erythema in the Barrett's segment.

Strictures typically occur in the esophagus at or just proximal to the ora serrata. Therefore, the mucosa distal to a stricture is always columnar. As the ora serrata migrates cephalad, so does the location of strictures (Figs. 2.66 and 2.67). An exception is when a stricture occurs in the distal esophagus in association with a deep esophageal ulcer, with resulting fibrous tissue formation. In this case, the strictured area may remain in the distal esophagus, even as the squamocolumnar junction migrates cephalad (Fig. 2.68). If a stricture is found distally, the differential diagnosis should include a fibrous

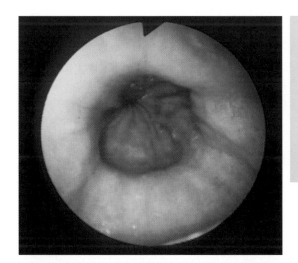

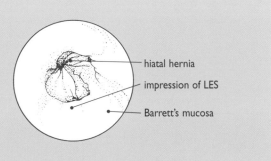

Figure 2.62 *In this case, the LES can be seen. Although the typical squamocolumnar junction is not present, the narrow area can be appreciated. There is also a hiatal hernia just below the LES. The folds inside the hernia terminate just below the narrowed area.*

▼ A ▼ B ▼ C

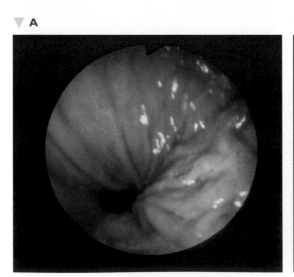

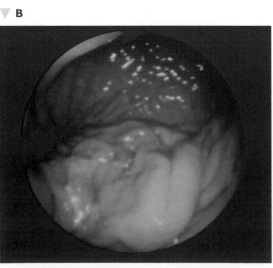

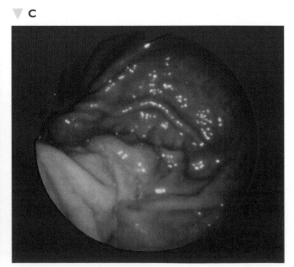

Figure 2.63 *(A–C) Examples of hiatal hernias in cases of Barrett's metaplasia, seen under direct endoscopic view as the tip is advanced past the area of the LES.*

stricture that has remained in the distal esophagus because of associated ulceration with fibrosis or an infiltrating adenocarcinoma occurring with a stricture.

Of patients with reflux, approximately 15% develop stricture. If the stricture is located in the distal esophagus, it is usually associated with a hiatal hernia or Barrett's metaplasia. If the stricture is in the middle or the upper third of the esophagus, it is almost always associated with Barrett's metaplasia.

Ulcers occur in Barrett's metaplasia and may be found anywhere along the Barrett's segment (Fig. 2.69). These ulcers typically appear in the lower esophagus; they may be deep and may bleed. The ulcers are never totally surrounded by squamous mucosa; there is always at least a portion of the ulcer margin that is lined by columnar epithelium.

An ulcer may occur at the squamocolumnar junction (Fig. 2.70). Then, as the junction migrates in a cephalad direction, the ulcer remains in its original position and is gradually and increasingly surrounded by columnar epithelium. In an area of Barrett's metaplasia, it may be difficult to differentiate an island of squamous mucosa from an ulcer (Figs. 2.71 and 2.72), although one can usually make this distinction because the ulcer has depth whereas the squamous mucosa is flat.

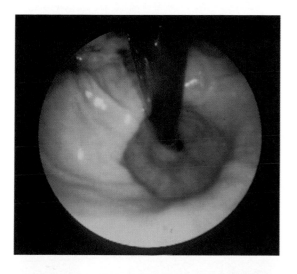

Figure 2.64 *This hiatal hernia in this case of Barrett's metaplasia is seen from below with the endoscope retroflexed.*

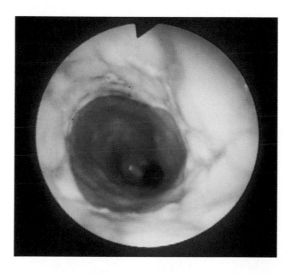

Figure 2.65 *Barrett's metaplasia, with a mucosal junction located abnormally high in the esophagus. There is evidence of inflammation and ulceration at the mucosal junction.*

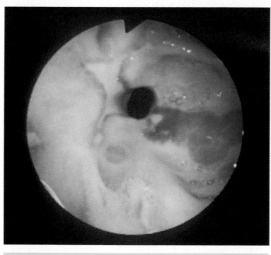

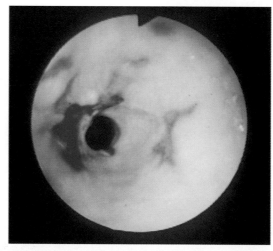

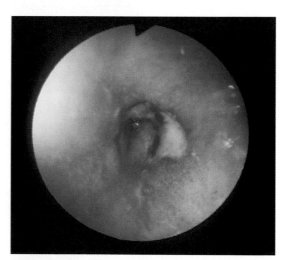

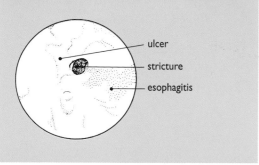

Figure 2.66 *Barrett's metaplasia. A stricture is present at the proximal squamocolumnar junction, with associated evidence of esophagitis and ulceration. The stricture moved proximally with the mucosal junction.*

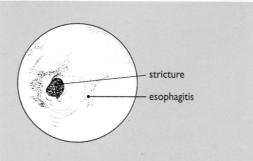

Figure 2.67 *Barrett's metaplasia. This stricture is located at 20 cm from the incisor teeth, having migrated proximally with the mucosal junction. There is associated esophagitis, ulceration, and bleeding.*

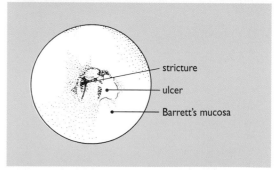

Figure 2.68 *Barrett's metaplasia. The ora serrata has moved proximally, but this ulceration and associated stricture remain in the distal esophagus at the location of the LES.*

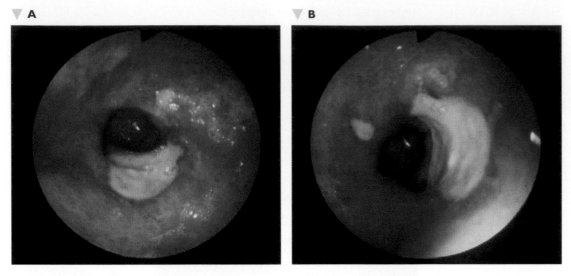

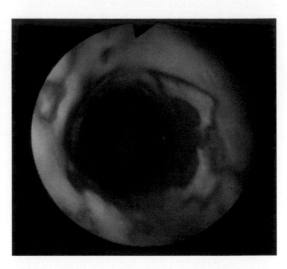

Figure 2.69 **(A)** *Barrett's metaplasia, with kissing ulcers in the Barrett's segment. The ulcers appear benign, with white bases and smooth margins. Biopsy and cytology were performed to rule out a malignancy.* **(B)** *A close-up view.*

Figure 2.70 *Multiple ulcers at the squamocolumnar junction in a patient with Barrett's metaplasia.*

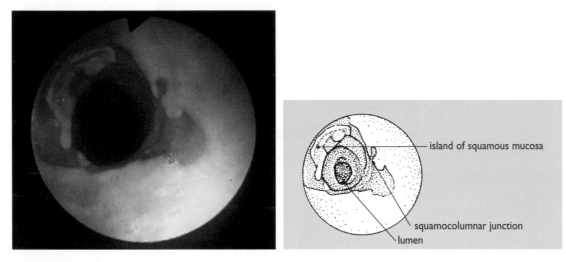

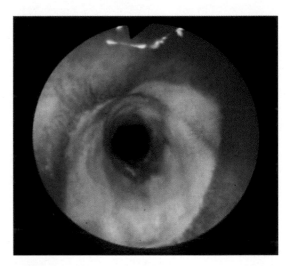

Figure 2.71 *Barrett's metaplasia and proximal squamocolumnar junction. An island of squamous mucosa is seen surrounded by metaplastic Barrett's epithelium.*

Figure 2.72 *Patch of squamous mucosa in the middle of a long segment of Barrett's metaplasia. The squamous mucosa is flat and does not resemble an ulcer.*

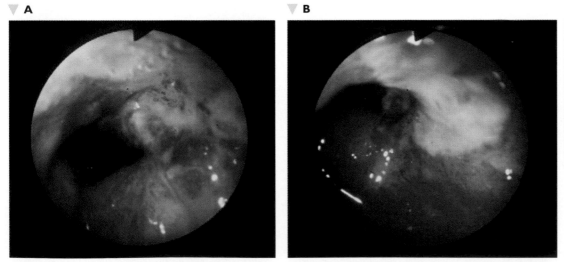

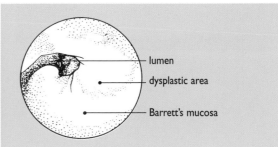

Figure 2.73 *This patient has Barrett's metaplasia, with carcinoma and severe dysplasia proximal to the cancer. Here we see two views (**A** and **B**) of the dysplastic area demonstrating an irregular, discolored surface. A small amount of exudate appears to be present.*

Barrett's metaplasia is a premalignant condition. In approximately 8% of patients who first present with Barrett's metaplasia, an adenocarcinoma is found to be present. Dysplasia of the mucosa is also an associated condition. This raises the question as to whether all patients with Barrett's metaplasia need to be periodically screened for the development of dysplasia or adenocarcinoma.

The dysplastic area may be irregular, with a villous surface (Fig. 2.73), or the mucosal surface may appear similar to the adjacent columnar mucosa. A mosaic of abnormalities may occur. When the dysplastic type of mucosa occurs in elevated bumps, some consider these areas to be adenomas – a rarity in Barrett's metaplasia.

Dysplasia is diagnosed histologically. In surveying patients with Barrett's metaplasia, some recommend a series of biopsies, starting in the area of the gastric cardia and extending throughout the length of the esophagus, to detect dysplasia and foci of adenocarcinoma.

There is increasing interest in diagnosing early adenocarcinoma in Barrett's metaplasia because these lesions may be treatable with surgical resection. Adenocarcinoma may occur in areas of columnar metaplasia mucosa that are minimally abnormal endoscopically or that appear indistinguishable from other areas of metaplastic mucosa (Figs. 2.74–2.76). Carcinoma may be discovered by performing multiple biopsies during periodic surveillance (Fig. 2.77).

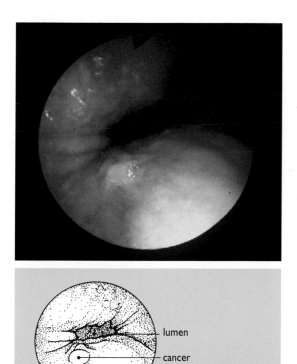

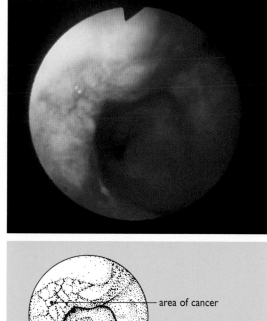

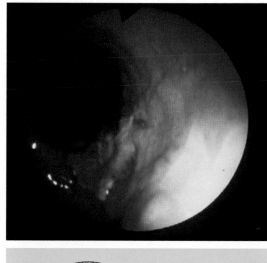

Figure 2.74 *Very early adenocarcinoma in a patient with Barrett's metaplasia.*

Figure 2.75 *Nearly invisible adenocarcinoma in patient with Barrett's metaplasia.*

Figure 2.76 *Barrett's metaplasia with mucosal irregularity that proved on biopsy to be an adeno carcinoma.*

Figure 2.77 *Barrett's metaplasia with proximal squamocolumnar mucosa. A minute ulcer was found on surveillance endoscopy and proved to be an adenocarcinoma.*

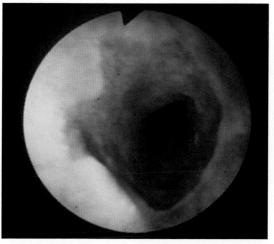

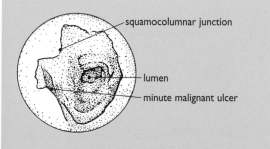

Adenocarcinomas in Barrett's metaplasia are usually found in the middle or distal third of the esophagus (Figs. 2.78 and 2.79). Proximal esophageal cancer is less common but does occur (Fig. 2.80). Most esophageal adenocarcinomas are felt to be associated with Barrett's metaplasia. Other etiologies of adenocarcinoma are thought to be cancer in esophageal sub-mucosal glands or congenital ectopic gastric mucosa in the esophagus (Figs. 2.81–2.83).

Adenocarcinomas vary in configuration from flat (infiltrating) to polypoid. They frequently ulcerate and may bleed. Occasionally, the tumor may obstruct the lumen (Figs. 2.84–2.86). Metastases may occur in the esophageal wall

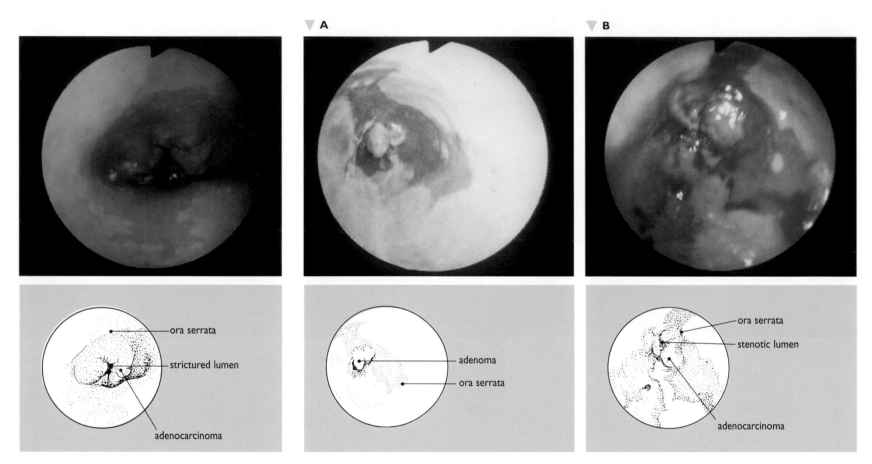

A

B

Figure 2.78 *Barrett's metaplasia, with an irregular ora serrata and an adenocarcinoma just below the mucosal junction. The cancer is infiltrating and has caused a stricture.*

Figure 2.79 *(A) Esophageal adenoma in a patient with Barrett's metaplasia. Because of underlying medical problems, this was removed endoscopically using a polypectomy technique. (B) 2 years later, an adenocarcinoma was found in the same area. The tumor was superficial but had metastasized.*

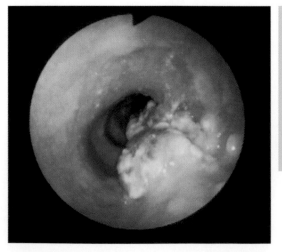

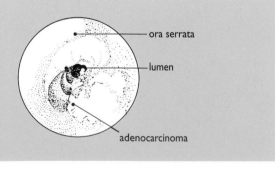

Figure 2.80 *Barrett's metaplasia. An adenocarcinoma is seen in the proximal esophagus at the squamocolumnar junction. The area of the cancer is elevated and covered with an exudate.*

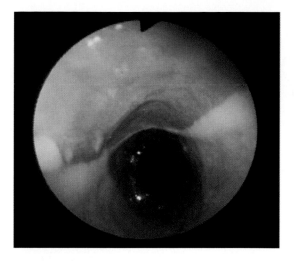

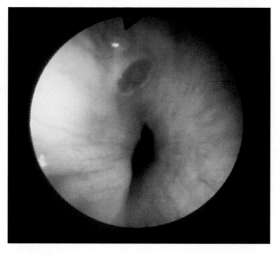

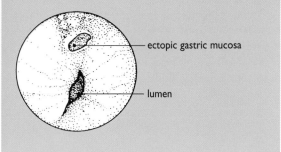

Figure 2.81 *Ectopic gastric mucosa in the proximal esophagus. The color is similar to gastric mucosa.*

Figure 2.82 *Small area of ectopic gastric epithelium in area of upper esophageal sphincter.*

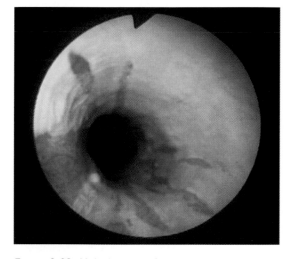

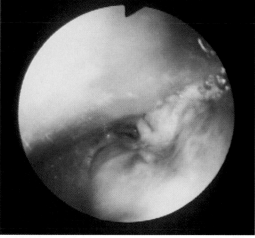

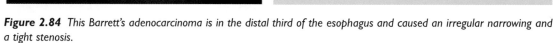

Figure 2.83 *Multiple areas of ectopic gastric mucosa in the esophagus, surrounded by pearly white esophageal squamous mucosa. The color of the ectopic mucosa is typical of gastric mucosa.*

Figure 2.84 *This Barrett's adenocarcinoma is in the distal third of the esophagus and caused an irregular narrowing and a tight stenosis.*

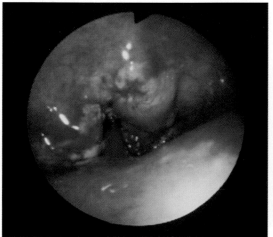

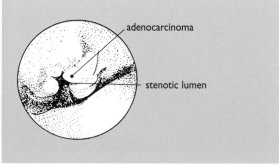

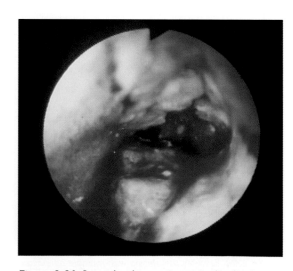

Figure 2.85 *Obstruction of the distal esophagus by a Barrett's adenocarcinoma. Here, the tumor is friable and irregular.*

Figure 2.86 *Barrett's adenocarcinoma in the distal esophagus, with tight stenosis and friability.*

adjacent to the carcinoma (Fig. 2.87). In some cases, multiple adenocarcinomas may be found (Fig. 2.88). In cases of stenosing carcinoma, an endoscopic prosthesis may be passed as palliative treatment (Figs. 2.88 and 2.89). The endoscopic appearance of esophageal and cardial adenocarcinomas is considered in greater detail in Chapter 3.

Barrett's metaplasia is a premalignant condition and periodic surveillance for dysplasia and carcinoma is appropriate. Screening may reveal one of the following three categories of biopsy: Barrett's metaplasia with no dysplasia, high grade dysplasia without carcinoma, or indefinite or low grade dysplasia. Biopsies should be taken every 2 cm throughout the Barrett's segment and from all four quadrants per station as well as from any

endoscopically visible abnormality. If metaplasia only is seen (Fig. 2.90), surveillance with endoscopy and biopsy must be repeated in 1–2 years. In high grade dysplasia (Fig. 2.91) it is recommended that the patient be reendoscoped within 1 month for extensive rebiopsy. If dysplasia is noted again without cancer, the choice is surgery or repeat endoscopic surveillance, with biopsies every 3 and then every 6 months thereafter. If a carcinoma is found, usually adjacent to an area of high grade dysplasia, surgery is the best option if it is clinically feasible.

Biopsies should always be reviewed by a gastrointestinal pathologist experienced in interpreting Barrett's mucosal biopsies before the initiation of definitive therapy. For patients in the intermediate risk category it is often

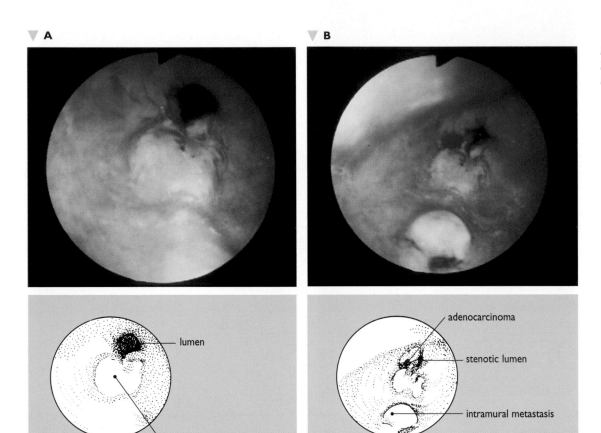

Figure 2.87 **(A)** Distal adenocarcinoma associated with Barrett's metaplasia. The tumor is diffusely infiltrating. **(B)** Intramural metastasis from the carcinoma on the left.

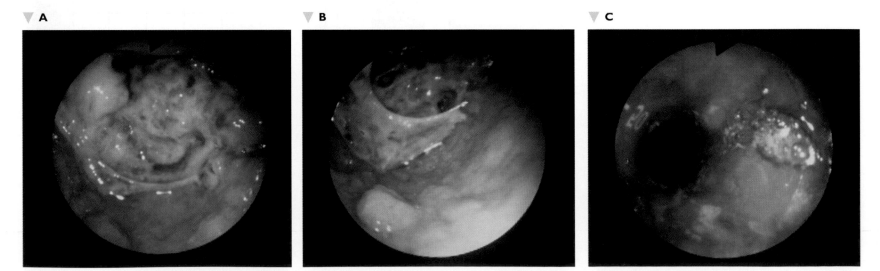

Figure 2.88 Barrett's metaplasia with multiple adenocarcinomas. **(A)** A large distal cancer is seen. This tumor is infiltrating and obstructing the lumen. **(B)** Proximal to the distal cancer, this smaller adenocarcinoma is seen. **(C)** The smaller, proximal adenocarcinoma is seen through the wall of a transparent Tygon prosthesis, placed for palliation.

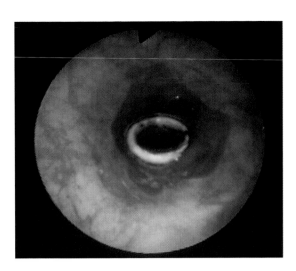

Figure 2.89 *In this case of Barrett's carcinoma with stenosis, an esophageal prosthesis has been passed. The proximal, wide flange of the tube can be seen just distal to the ora serrata. The tumor is located just beyond the flange.*

recommended that surveillance endoscopy and biopsy be repeated every 6–12 months. If the endoscopist sees what appears to be cancer, even if the biopsies are actually negative, the procedure should be repeated and the area rebiopsied.

Other factors to be considered with regard to possible neoplasm are the presence and extent of any endoscopic abnormality and the results of histological examination of biopsies of the area. Flow cytometry may be useful in identifying patients at risk of future progression. It can be used to identify a normal diploid DNA population (Fig. 2.92) or abnormalities such as tetraploid or aneuploid populations (Fig. 2.93).

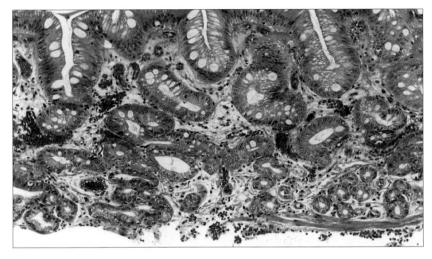

Figure 2.90 *Barrett's specialized metaplastic epithelium. This tissue is characterized by goblet cells and mucus-containing cells in the surface epithelium. The deep portion of the biopsy shows pylorocardiac gastric-type glands. (Courtesy of Brian Reid MD, PhD, and Rodger Haggitt MD)*

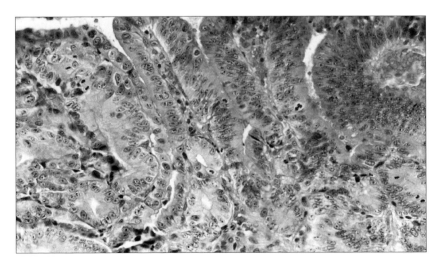

Figure 2.91 *High grade dysplasia in Barrett's epithelium. The dysplasia is characterized by cells with nuclei that appear polymorphic and stratified. Compared with Barrett's metaplastic epithelium there is less mucus seen in the epithelial cells and areas of architectural abnormalities with back to back glands. (Courtesy of Brian Reid MD, PhD, and Rodger Haggitt MD)*

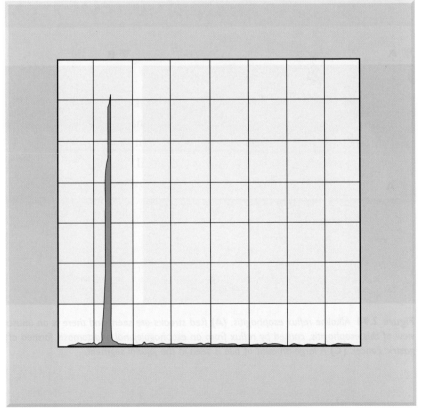

Figure 2.92 *Normal DNA content flow histogram from a patient with Barrett's metaplasia without dysplasia. The majority of the cells contain a diploid DNA content (G1). The S-phase and G2 fractions are normal. (Courtesy of Brian Reid MD, PhD and Peter Rabinovitch MD, PhD)*

appearance is subtle. If any lesion or suspicious area is seen, biopsy and cytology are essential. In a patient presenting with dysphagia, it is necessary to inspect the cardia from above and below, and a cardial cancer should always be included in the differential diagnosis of a distal esophageal narrowing. Tumors at the cardia may simulate achalasia. Therefore, in patients with suspected achalasia, an endoscopic inspection of the cardia usually precedes

balloon dilation because the latter is not performed for carcinomatous obstruction of the esophagogastric junction. Also, with adenocarcinoma at the esophagogastric junction one may find above normal gastric acid production (as noted with a history of duodenal ulcer and an endoscopic appearance of prominent areae gastricae in the fundus of the stomach) and Barrett's metaplasia.

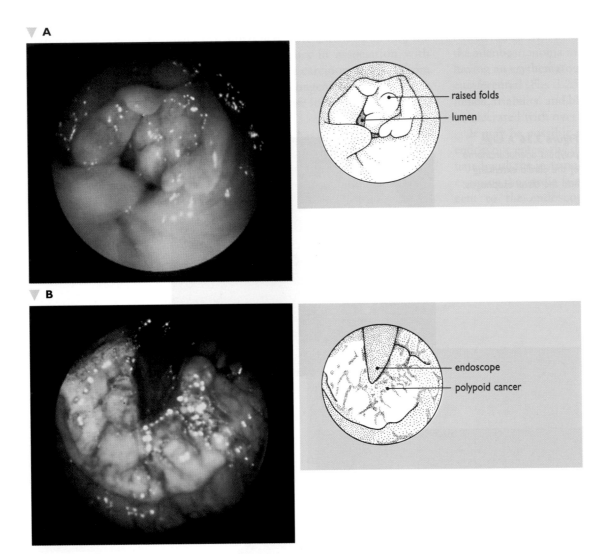

Figure 3.29 (A) On direct view, this adenocarcinoma in the distal esophagus demonstrates heavy folds, with a raised and somewhat irregular mucosa. (B) On retroflexed view, the cancer is better seen. The tumor appears polypoid and friable. Now the cause of the obstruction and symptomatic dysphagia is clearly evident.

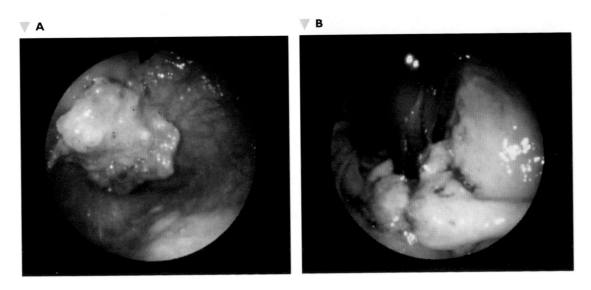

Figure 3.30 (A) Cardial adenocarcinoma seen from above in an elderly patient who presented with dysphagia. (B) With the endoscope retroflexed in the stomach, the infiltrating mass can be observed adjacent to the instrument.

Adenocarcinoma arising in Barrett's metaplasia may present as a polypoid, exophytic mass with exudation, friability, and bleeding (Figs. 3.31 and 3.32). A more common appearance is that of an infiltrated lesion causing a stricture. It is often located a few centimeters distal to the new proximal squamocolumnar junction; therefore, the cancer is often in the middle third of the esophagus. As with infiltrative squamous-cell carcinoma, the mucosa may appear intact down to the level of the stricture, making the endoscopic diagnosis of a malignant stricture difficult. Tumor nodules and abnormal mucosa with erythema and exudation may be visible at the cephalad margin of the stricture. The margin may be abrupt, suggesting tumor. In all cases of Barrett's-associated adenocarcinoma, biopsies of the mucosa adjacent to the tumor will determine whether Barrett's metaplasia is present. In some cases this diagnosis of Barrett's metaplasia is obvious, but when the squamocolumnar junction is indistinct, biopsy of adjacent mucosa is essential to diagnose Barrett's metaplasia. Biopsy and cytology of the mass is also essential to diagnose a carcinoma.

Early Esophageal Cancer

At present the diagnosis of esophageal cancer is usually made when the cancer is at an advanced stage and surgical resection for cure is not possible.

Clearly, the early diagnosis of esophageal cancer is essential. In certain geographic areas with a high incidence of esophageal cancer, screening programs for symptomless patients have led to early detection and, consequently, to an excellent chance of surgical cure and a reasonable 5-year survival rate.

The appearance of early esophageal cancer is not as obvious as with larger, further advanced squamous-cell and adenocarcinomas. In fact, there are early cancers that are invisible to the naked eye and cannot be detected endoscopically. These occult cancers may be encountered when a wash cytology is positive yet no lesion is seen endoscopically (squamous-cell), or in Barrett's metaplasia when high grade dysplasia or a small focus of adenocarcinoma is detected on biopsy but the endoscopy does not reveal an area that suggests cancer.

Early Squamous-Cell Cancer

Early squamous-cell carcinoma may have four characteristic appearances. The first is that of localized mucosal erosions, seen in approximately 50% of cases (Fig. 3.33). The mucosa is red, eroded, and friable, often in a geographic pattern, surrounding areas of more normal mucosa. The second type consists of circumscribed mucosal protuberances, seen in 25% of cases. These lesions show an irregular, thickened mucosa with a polypoid, nodular, or papillary

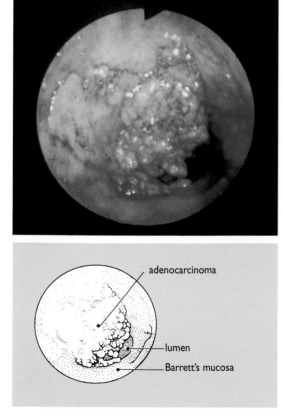

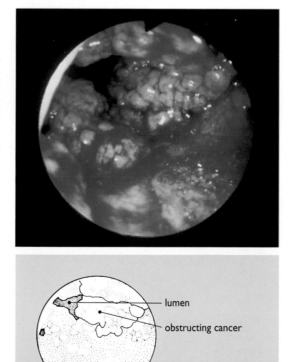

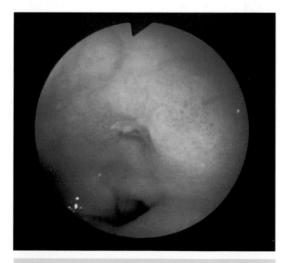

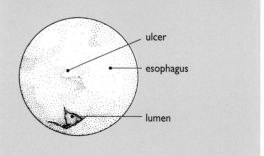

Figure 3.31 *Adenocarcinoma of the esophagus, arising in an area of Barrett's metaplasia. The tumor is an exophytic, polypoid mass that is friable and bleeding.*

Figure 3.32 *Extensive adenocarcinoma in Barrett's metaplasia with obstruction of the lumen and bleeding.*

Figure 3.33 *Early squamous-cell carcinoma. Note the tiny ulcer, which proved on biopsy to be malignant (1 of 20 positive).*

configuration (Fig. 3.34). The mucosa over the surface is often eroded or ulcerated, and friable. The third type is a focal area of erythema (occasionally with red spots), congestion and coarseness of the mucosa, which bleeds easily; this type is seen in approximately 13% of cases (Fig. 3.35). Finally, the fourth type, seen in approximately 9% of cases, appears as white mucosal plaques that are not friable, are single or multiple, and may be confluent (Fig. 3.36). If no lesion is visible, toluidine blue staining in vivo may help reveal areas of early squamous-cell cancer as these areas stain dark blue.

Endosonography of Early Esophageal Cancer

The poor outcome associated with esophageal cancer could be greatly improved by early diagnosis – detecting the cancer before it has spread beyond the esophageal wall to involve lymph nodes, adjacent structures or distal organs. By identifying high risk individuals and screening them with ultrasound, early resectable cancers may be detected. On ultrasound an early tumor may appear as a focal area of mucosal thickening with an intact muscularis propria beneath it, and no evidence of abnormal lymph nodes. Endosonographic staging is reported to be more accurate than CT (Fig. 3.37).

Early Adenocarcinoma

Early adenocarcinoma is occasionally noted in patients with Barrett's metaplasia of the esophagus (Fig. 3.38). Routine biopsies as part of a screening program may reveal high grade dysplasia or a focus of invasive adenocarcinoma in an area that did not appear abnormal endoscopically. A small nodule, erosion, friable area, or ulcer may be noted, or the area may appear the same as the surrounding Barrett's metaplastic mucosa. The only method to detect these early and potentially resectable cancers is to biopsy patients with Barrett's metaplasia as part of a screening program. The ideal frequency for this program is not known. Certainly, these patients should be examined periodically and endoscoped if symptoms change or if new symptoms develop. High grade dysplasia in a patient with Barrett's metaplasia is an indication for surgery or depending on the situation, for frequent endoscopy and biopsy (every 3–6 months).

Early cardia adenocarcinoma may occur as a small polypoid mass at the squamocolumnar junction that may at first appear as a thickened fold (Fig. 3.39).

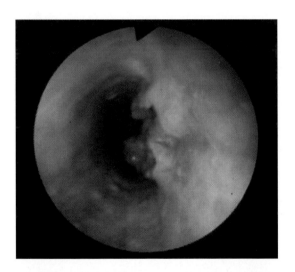

Figure 3.34 *Early squamous-cell carcinoma with the nodular or papillary surface configuration.*

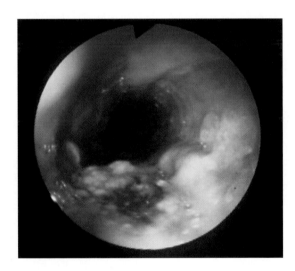

Figure 3.35 *Early squamous-cell carcinoma of the esophagus appearing as an area of erythema and coarsening of the mucosa. Small nodules are noted.*

▼ **A** ▼ **B**

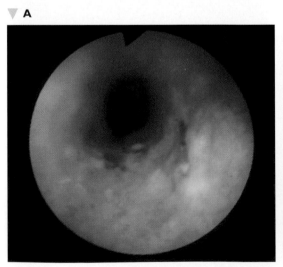

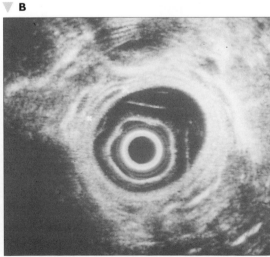

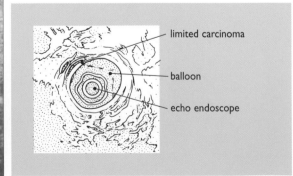

Figure 3.36 *(A) Early squamous-cell esophageal cancer appearing as mutliple white mucosal plaques. (B) Endoscopic ultrasound of this early cancer shows a tumor of the wall that is limited and does not extend beyond the wall.*

▼ A   ▼ B

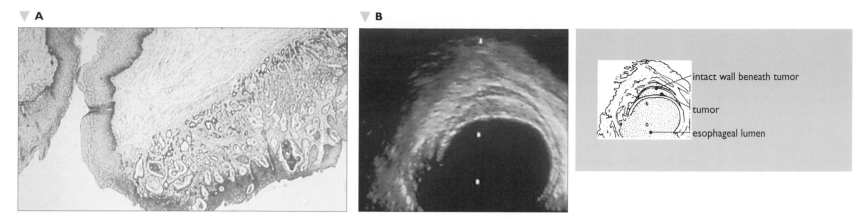

Figure 3.37 *(A) Histology of early squamous-cell carcinoma. (B) Ultrasound shows the lesion as a mucosal thickening but with intact layers of esophageal wall beneath the lesion.*

▼ A   ▼ B

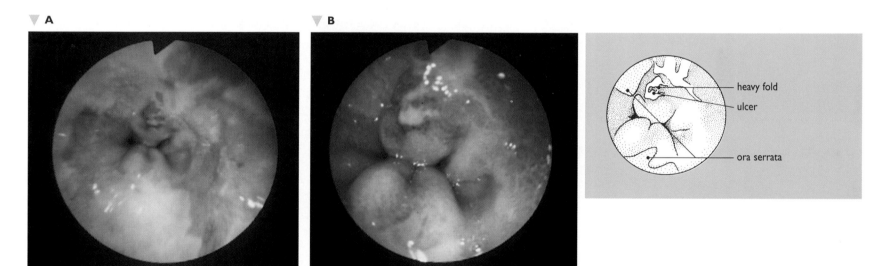

Figure 3.38 *Early adenocarcinoma. (A) A slightly enlarged fold can be observed at the squamocolumnar junction of a patient with Barrett's metaplasia. Biopsy revealed malignancy. (B) A close-up view. The small ulcer resulted from a previous biopsy.*

▼ A   ▼ B

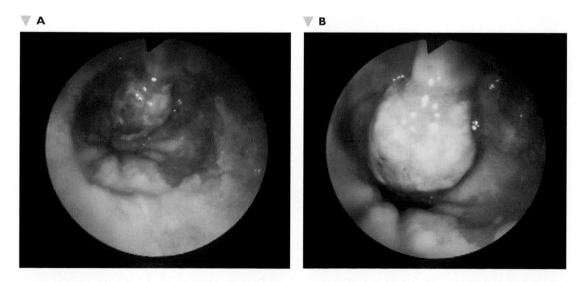

Figure 3.39 *(A) Early adenocarcinoma of the cardia just distal to the ora serrata. What appeared to be a thickened fold is seen to be a mass as the endoscope is advanced into the distal esophagus. (B) A close-up view.*

Biopsy and Cytology in Esophageal Cancer

The mucosa surrounding an esophageal cancer may have a marked inflammatory reaction. Therefore, biopsy of that mucosa may not reveal cancer cells but rather reactive tissue. If multiple biopsies are taken (up to 8–10) and if the biopsies are carefully planned to include areas that may contain tumor tissue, the true-positive biopsy rate may be as high as 80–90%. Rates of positive biopsies as low as 60% were reported in the past, but this has improved considerably with current techniques.

Another essential aspect to diagnosis is the use of endoscopic sheathed brush cytology. The brush is passed down the channel, opened, and then passed over the surface of the lesion, thus sampling a wide area of tumor. When multiple biopsies are used in conjunction with this type of brush cytology, a true-positive diagnosis rate of 95% can be attained. Exfoliative wash cytology can also aid in precise diagnosis if an expert cytologist is available.

When a stricture is present, it may be difficult to biopsy the area inside the narrowed segment. In such cases it may be possible to pass a cytology brush gently through the stricture to sample the mucosa. Occasionally, a biopsy forceps can be guided through the narrowed lumen to sample the narrowed segment. If these techniques are not possible or are negative although the endoscopic appearance is that of a cancer, another technique is to dilate the stricture gently over a wire placed via the endoscope and confirmed fluoroscopically, and then repeat the biopsy and brushings along the length of the suspicious area (Fig. 3.40). It is also possible to use a sclerotherapy needle to obtain an aspiration cytology. This may be important when one encounters what appears to be an infiltrating malignancy covered by normal mucosa.

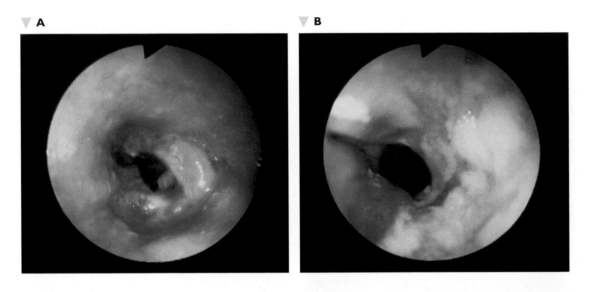

▼ A ▼ B

Figure 3.40 **(A)** *This stricture was suspected of being caused by a squamous-cell carcinoma. The mucosa just proximal to the narrowed area is slightly nodular and red, but biopsies in this area have failed to reveal tumor.* **(B)** *When the tip of the endoscope is advanced into the narrowing after gentle dilation, the obvious squamous-cell carcinoma with ulceration is seen.*

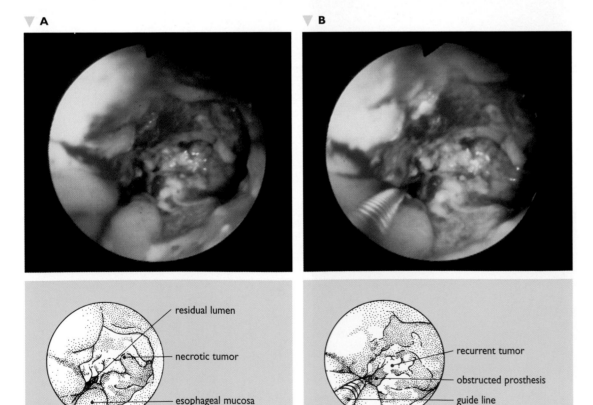

▼ A ▼ B

Figure 3.41 **(A)** *A large necrotic tumor can be observed. The stenotic residual lumen is eccentric and not easily seen.* **(B)** *Under endoscopic guidance, a guidewire is introduced into the tumor. This wire can safely route dilators through the stenotic lumen and reduce the likelihood of a perforation.*

Endoscopic Management of Malignant Strictures

Patients with esophageal carcinomas may present with very tight, irregular strictures. Dilation of the stricture may be essential to allow adequate biopsy and cytology, and also to initiate treatment for relief of symptoms. Under endoscopic guidance, a guidewire with an atraumatic tip can be passed through the lumen of the stricture into the stomach (Fig. 3.41), the position of the wire confirmed radiographically. Metal, olive-shaped dilators or catheter dilators with single or multiple tapers can then be passed over the wire to dilate the stricture. The guidewire reduces the risk of perforation. By using dilators of gradually increasing size, it is possible to dilate the stricture progressively. The endoscope can also be used to guide balloon-tipped catheters into a tight stricture for balloon dilation under direct endoscopic guidance.

For patients with recurrent or unresectable carcinomas, palliative therapy is often appropriate. This can be accomplished in one of several ways: a stent, laser treatment, bipolar electrocoagulation, or endoluminal radiation therapy. Nonexpandable stents are placed by dilating the esophagus and inserting a plastic, tubular esophageal prosthesis. The upper and lower margins of the tumor can be located and the distance from the teeth measured to determine the length and correct position of the prosthesis. The endoscope can then be used as a guide for insertion of the prosthesis (Fig 3.42). After insertion, the endoscope can evaluate the position of the prosthesis relative to the carcinoma (Fig. 3.43). This prosthesis may be useful in occluding a tracheoesophageal fistula, but should be avoided in very proximal esophageal lesions. Complications may include overgrowth of the tumor, obstruction of

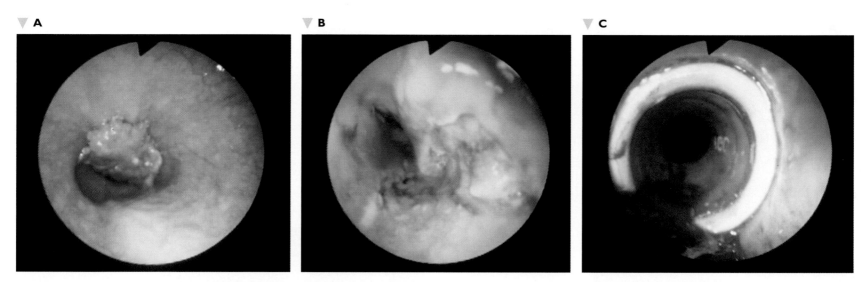

Figure 3.42 (A) Squamous-cell carcinoma of the esophagus, with an ulcerated area seen in the distance. **(B)** On close-up view, the ulcer is found to be deep and infiltrating. **(C)** Under endoscopic guidance, a prosthetic stent was placed through the narrowed area, with the top of the stent just above the tumor.

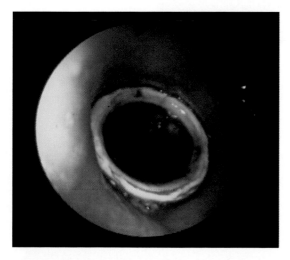

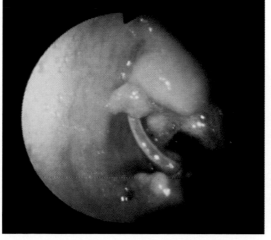

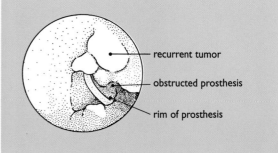

Figure 3.43 A prosthesis in position in the esophagus of a patient with adenocarcinoma associated with Barrett's metaplasia. The wide proximal flange of the prosthesis is located just cephalad to the stenosing carcinoma.

Figure 3.44 A carcinoma has grown extensively and is now obstructing a prosthesis proximally. Only a small rim of the prosthesis is still visible.

the proximal lumen (Figs. 3.44 and 3.45), reflux with bleeding (Fig. 3.46), migration of the prosthesis (Fig. 3.47), and the pressure necrosis of the esophageal wall (Fig. 3.48). Another type of esophageal stent is a metal self-expanding stent. This type of stent is configured to a small diameter and can often be inserted without prior dilation of the malignant growth. The stent is accurately placed over a guidewire. When the constraining membrane is removed, the stent expands and gradually opens up the lumen. Often, no dilation is needed before insertion, so this may be less traumatic than other types of stenting procedures.

▼ A

▼ B

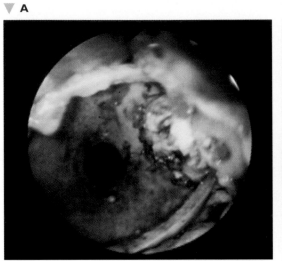

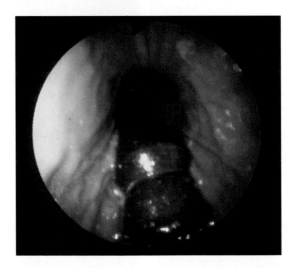

Figure 3.45 (A) *Prosthesis passed to palliate unresectable squamous-cell carcinoma of the esophagus is partially occluded by tissue overgrowth.* **(B)** *The overgrowth was removed by treatment with a Nd:YAG laser.*

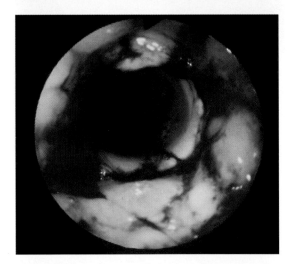

Figure 3.46 *Reflux esophagitis above a prosthesis with evidence of friability and bleeding.*

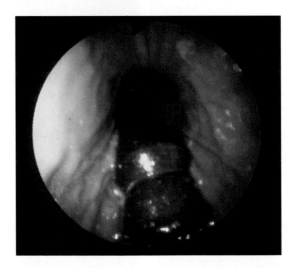

Figure 3.47 *A prosthesis placed to palliate an esophageal cancer has migrated into the stomach.*

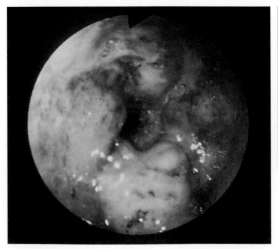

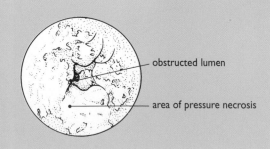

obstructed lumen

area of pressure necrosis

Figure 3.48 *This squamous-cell carcinoma had been treated with a prosthesis. However, the prosthesis has produced pressure necrosis of the esophageal wall. The mucosa is inflamed, and an ulcer can be faintly observed.*

Another approach to the palliation of recurrent or unresectable esophageal cancers is to use the endoscope to direct a Nd:YAG laser at the tumor. This laser can destroy tumor tissue and re-establish the lumen (Figs. 3.49 and 3.50). Alternative methods of destroying cancerous tisue include argon plasma electcoagulation and intratumoral injection of recrotizing agents,

such as absolute ethsnol. Radiation therapy can also be delivered locally with the application of endoluminal radiation. This therapy can open an obstructed lumen (Fig. 3.51) but may be associated with ulceration, bleeding (Fig. 3.52), necrosis (Fig. 3.53) and stenosis (Fig. 3.54).

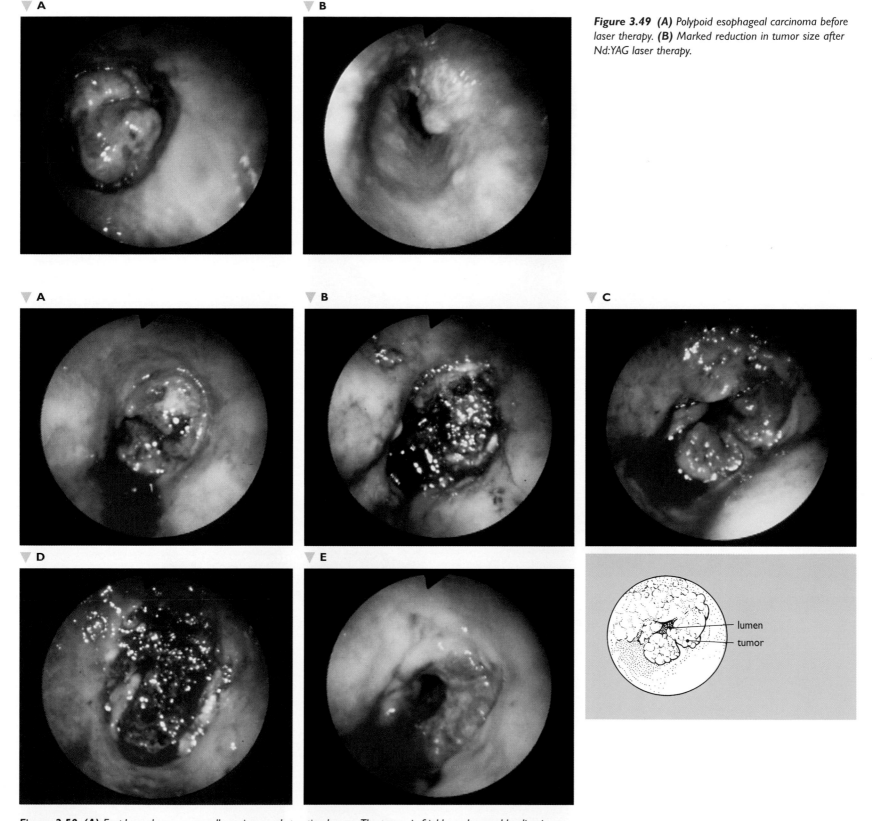

Figure 3.49 **(A)** Polypoid esophageal carcinoma before laser therapy. **(B)** Marked reduction in tumor size after Nd:YAG laser therapy.

Figure 3.50 **(A)** Esophageal squamous-cell carcinoma obstructing lumen. The tumor is friable and some bleeding is present. **(B)** Immediately after the first Nd:YAG laser treatment, tumor surface is coagulated and necrotic, with minimal bleeding. **(C)** Before the second laser treatment the tumor is smaller and a lumen has been re-established. **(D)** Immediately after the second therapy, coagulated necrotic tumor is seen. **(E)** Several days after the second treatment the tumor is smaller and the lumen is wider. The tumor is still minimally friable.

Other Esophageal Malignancies

Other esophageal malignant tumors include lesions that can be recognized because of characteristic endoscopic features, for example, pigment visible in a primary melanosarcoma (Fig. 3.55). Melanosarcoma may also present in a polypoid form with pigment less evident (Fig. 3.56). In other instances tumors may be difficult or impossible to distinguish endoscopically, but the biopsy may permit diagnosis of tumors other than squamous-cell or adenocarcinomas, for example, esophageal myoblastoma granulare (Fig. 3.57). Kaposi's sarcoma may be noted in the esophagus (Fig. 3.58) and in the mouth (Fig. 3.59). An adenoid cystic carcinoma is an esophageal tumor originating from the salivary glands (Fig. 3.60).

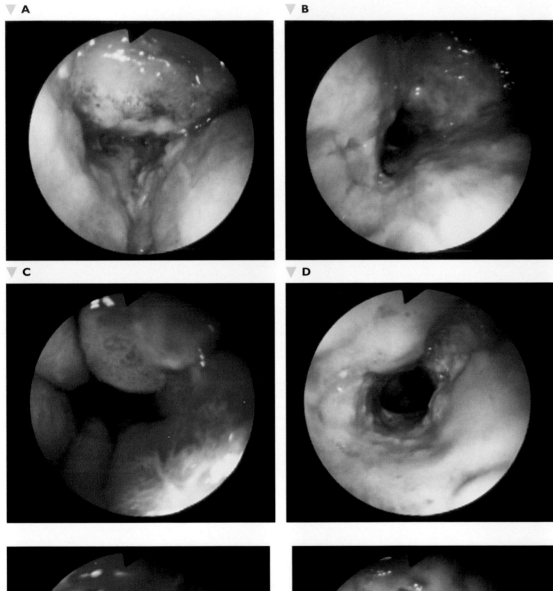

Figure 3.51 **(A)** This obstructing esophageal carcinoma was treated with endoluminal radiation therapy. **(B)** Two weeks after therapy the tumor is reduced in size and the lumen is beginning to open. **(C)** Two months after endoluminal radiation the lumen is narrow but open and the tumor is less apparent. **(D)** One year later the tumor remains reduced in size and the lumen is open.

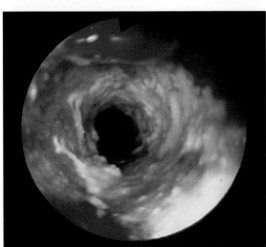

Figure 3.52 Ulceration and bleeding 3 weeks after a course of endoluminal radiotherapy for esophageal cancer.

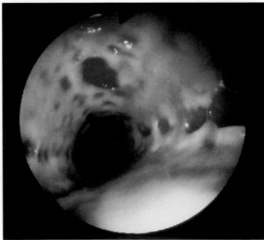

Figure 3.53 Extensive mucosal necrosis and ulceration after two sessions of endoluminal radiation therapy.

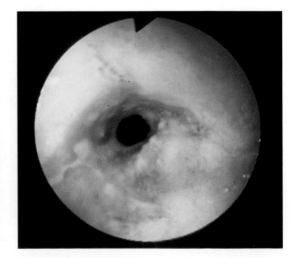

Figure 3.54 Esophageal stricture after endoluminal radiotherapy for esophageal cancer. The lumen is markedly narrowed and ulceration is present.

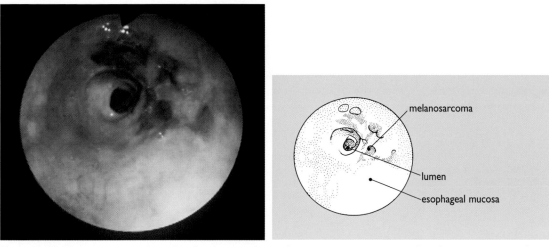

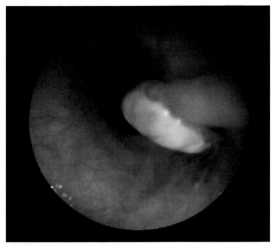

Figure 3.55 *This primary esophageal melanosarcoma has a charactersitic appearance, with melanin-pigment noted. The lumen is narrowed in the area of the tumor.*

Figure 3.56 *Metastatic melanosarcoma in the esophagus in a polypoid form. Pigment is less evident.*

▼ **A**

▼ **B**

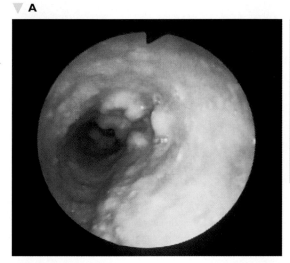

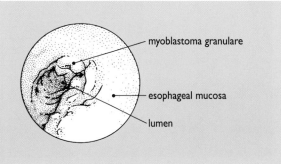

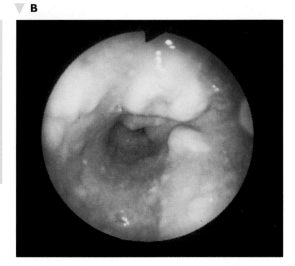

Figure 3.57 *(A) This lesion in the distal esophagus occurs with several masses, one of which has a depressed center suggesting that the tumor in the center might have outgrown its blood supply. The mucosa overlying the masses appears slightly pale. On biopsy, the tumor proved to be an esophageal myoblastoma granulare. (B) A close-up. The multiple masses can be seen, and the depressed center of the largest mass can be appreciated.*

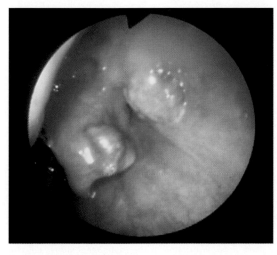

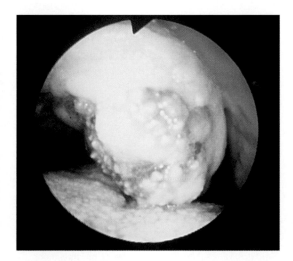

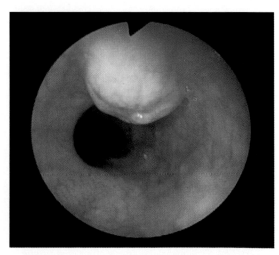

Figure 3.58 *Kaposi's sarcoma in an AIDS patient involving the esophagus.*

Figure 3.59 *Kaposi's sarcoma involving the mouth in a patient with AIDS.*

Figure 3.60 *Adenoid cystic carcinoma of the esophagus. The tumor appears polypoid with a central indentation.*

Extrinsic Compression on the Esophagus by Adjacent Neoplasms

Carcinomas of the thyroid, lymph nodes or lung, and metastases to the mediastinum may occur with extrinsic compression of the esophagus, causing dysphagia (Figs. 3.61 and 3.62). Endoscopically, the esophagus may appear to have a smooth indentation in one wall, whereas the overlying esophageal mucosa is usually normal. Metastases may also involve the esophageal wall directly. These result from tumors of other organs such as breast cancer (Fig. 3.63) or other tumors (Fig. 3.64 and 3.65). Metastases to the tissue around the esophagus may cause extrinsic esophageal narrowing, though the mucosa through the area appears normal (Fig. 3.66). Lesions may occur at a distance from primary tumors (Fig. 3.67) or adjacent to the primary tumor, with satellite nodules and, in some cases, submucosal spread (Figs. 3.68 and 3.69).

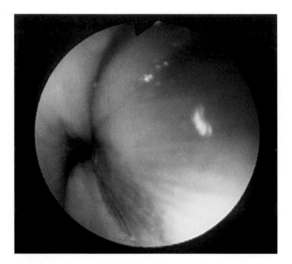

Figure 3.61 *Distal esophageal narrowing caused by a bronchogenic carcinoma adjacent to the esophagus.*

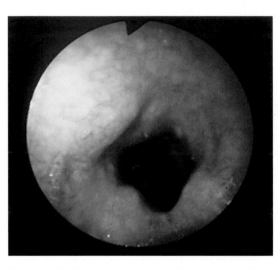

Figure 3.62 *Extrinsic compression of the esophageal wall caused by an enlarged lymph node in the mediastinum. The covering mucosa is normal.*

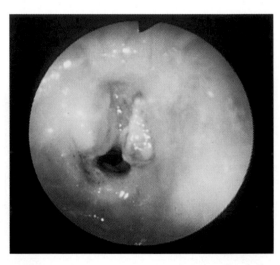

Figure 3.63 *Breast carcinoma that metastasized to the esophageal wall. The area of the metastasis is slightly erythematous, with a small nodule. The lumen is narrowed. A prosthesis that had been inserted previously is invisible because of this overgrowing tumor.*

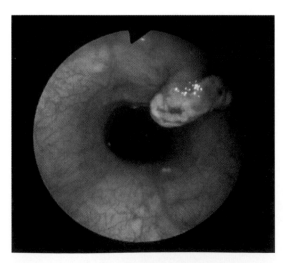

Figure 3.64 *Esophageal metastasis of melanosarcoma, as evidenced by a small amount of pigment.*

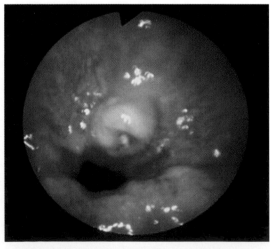

Figure 3.65 *Esophageal metastases of an amelanotic melanosarcoma. No pigment is noted, the surface is umbilicated.*

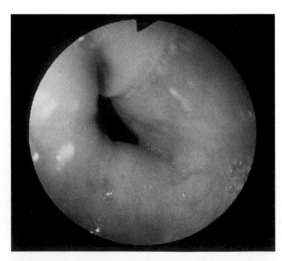

Figure 3.66 *Narrowing of the esophageal lumen, caused by breast carcinoma metastasizing to the mediastinum adjacent to the esophagus. The overlying mucosa appears normal.*

▼ A

▼ B

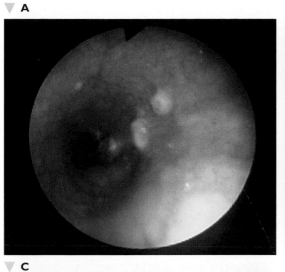

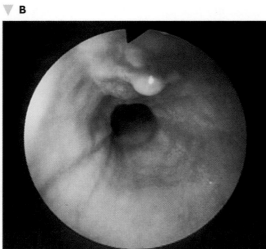

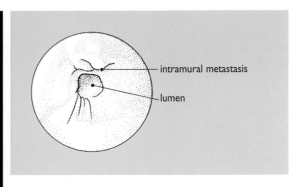

▼ C

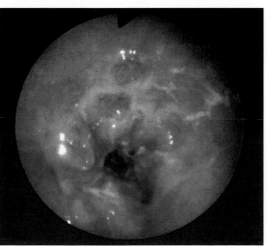

Figure 3.67 **(A)** *Intramural metastasis from esophageal squamous-cell carcinoma, and* **(B)** *cardial adenocarcinoma. (see drawing).* **(C)** *Cardial carcinoma associated with proximal intramural metastases seen in this photograph.*

Figure 3.68 *These tiny satellite lesions are intramural metastases from an adenocarcinoma in the distal esophagus. The primary tumor is located just distal to these lesions.*

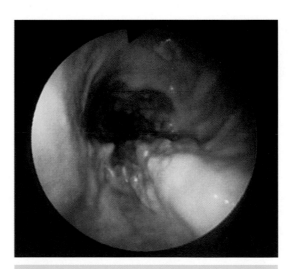

Figure 3.69 *Proximal intraluminal extension of esophageal squamous-cell carcinoma.*

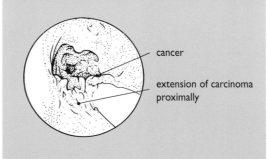

One of the most feared complications of esophageal cancer is a tracheoesophageal fistula, which may cause very troublesome and disabling symptoms for the patient. These fistulas may occur after radiation-therapy-associated injury to the esophagus (Fig. 3.70). Endoscopy may allow the physician to visualize the cancer and the fistula directly (Figs. 3.71–3.74). In some cases it may be possible to see the pleural cavity and visualize lung tissue at the base of the fistula (Fig. 3.75) or look into the necrotic tumor cavity (Fig. 3.76). A tracheoesophageal fistula may be an indication for an esophageal prosthesis. Squamous-cell carcinoma may be noted in a patient with portal hypertension and esophageal varices (Fig. 3.77).

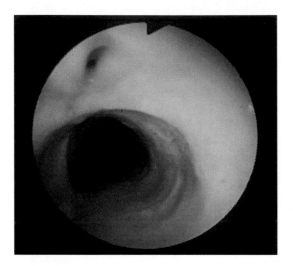

Figure 3.70 Tracheoesophageal fistula after radiation therapy. The surrounding mucosa appears normal.

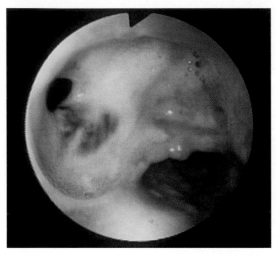
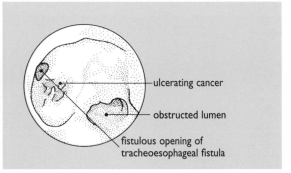

Figure 3.71 Tracheoesophageal fistula, caused by an ulcerating esophageal squamous-cell carcinoma. The fistulous tract orifice is clearly seen.

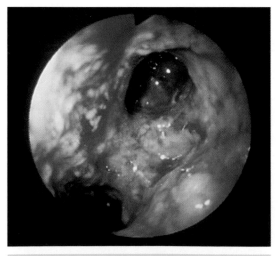

Figure 3.72 This squamous-cell carcinoma is seen as a large, necrotic tumor, with a narrowed lumen and a large fistula to the lung.

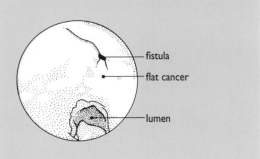

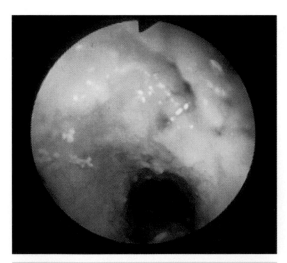

Figure 3.73 This flat squamous-cell carcinoma displays less exudation and friability than the cancer shown in Fig. 3.72. The mucosa appears diffusely abnormal, and the orifice of a small fistula to the lung is seen.

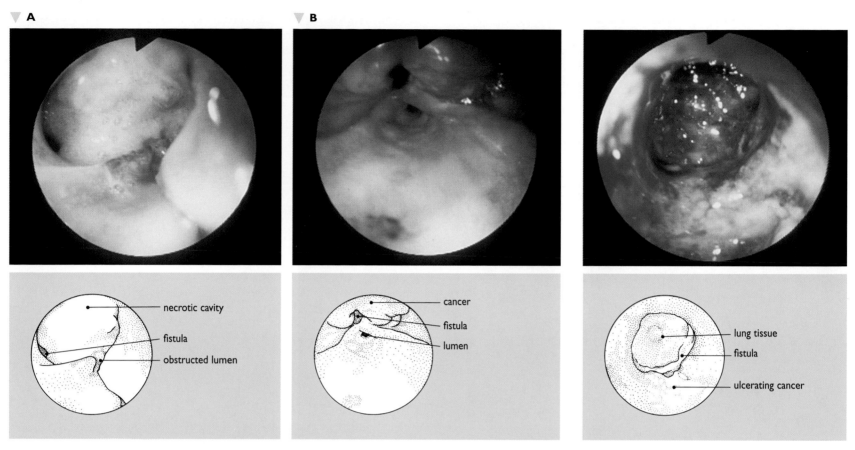

Figure 3.74 (A) *This cancer appears with a large necrotic cavity in the lung and a tracheoesophageal fistula.* **(B)** *With the endoscope at a slightly different position, the fistula orifice is better seen.*

Figure 3.75 *At the base of this large, ulcerating squamous-cell carcinoma is a tracheoesophageal fistula, with lung tissue visible at the base.*

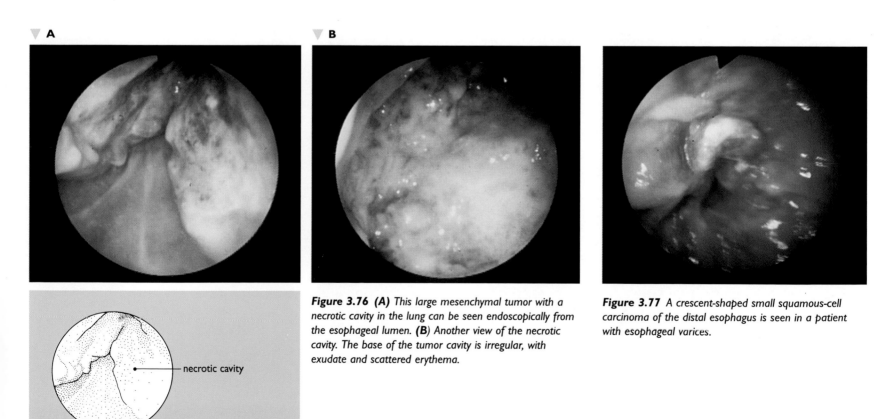

Figure 3.76 (A) *This large mesenchymal tumor with a necrotic cavity in the lung can be seen endoscopically from the esophageal lumen.* **(B)** *Another view of the necrotic cavity. The base of the tumor cavity is irregular, with exudate and scattered erythema.*

Figure 3.77 *A crescent-shaped small squamous-cell carcinoma of the distal esophagus is seen in a patient with esophageal varices.*

Endosonography in Esophageal Cancer

Endoscopic ultrasound can be used to determine the extent of esophageal wall involvement with a tumor. The depth of invasion can be an indicator of whether the tumor is early and limited to the mucosa, or extends into the wall through the submucosa or muscularis propria. Involvement of adjacent structures such as the aorta can often be detected. Lymph nodes can be seen, although it is difficult to determine whether a lymph node is normal or involved with the tumor. Factors such as size, smoothness of the margin, and structural heterogeneity are taken into consideration. More studies are necessary (Figs. 3.78–3.81).

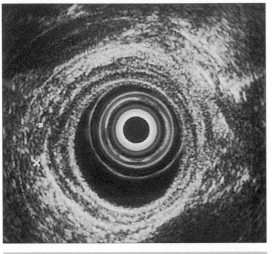

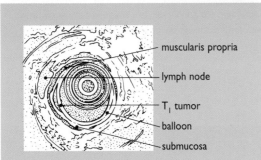

Figure 3.78 Localized esophageal carcinoma. A tumor limited to the mucosa and submucosa is seen. The muscularis propria is intact. The lymph node seen is not suspicious for cancer. This is a T_1 tumor. (Courtesy of Dr TL Tio)

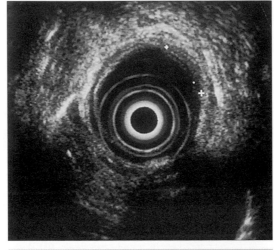

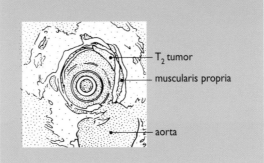

Figure 3.79 This esophageal cancer penetrates into the muscularis propria of the esophageal wall. This is a T_2 tumor. (Courtesy of Dr TL Tio)

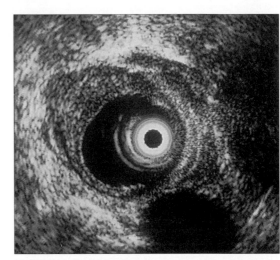

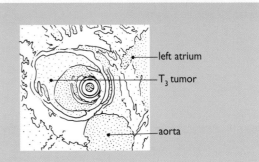

Figure 3.80 This esophageal cancer is more extensive and extends through the wall into adjacent tissue. This is a T_3 tumor. (Courtesy of Dr TL Tio)

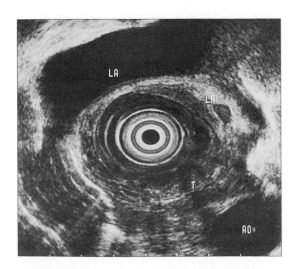

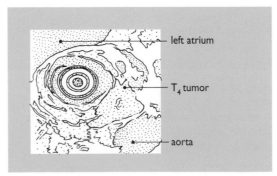

Figure 3.81 Extensively infiltrating esophageal cancer. The tumor involves the structures adjacent to the esophageal wall, including the aorta. This is a T_4 tumor. (Courtesy of Dr TL Tio)

INFECTIOUS DISEASES OF THE ESOPHAGUS

Several types of infectious agents can involve the esophagus and produce symptoms that vary from mild discomfort to severe life-threatening clinical problems. These diseases often occur in patients who are immunosuppressed from underlying medical illnesses. For some of these infections, there are now specific therapeutic measures available, making precise diagnosis essential. For other infections, treatment of the underlying disorder may result in an improvement of the symptoms.

The three most commonly encountered infections of the esophagus are herpetic esophagitis, candida esophagitis, and cytomegaloviral esophagitis. These diseases must be distinguished from esophagitis caused by gastroesophageal reflux and, in bone marrow transplant patients, from the esophageal changes of chronic graft-versus-host disease. There are characteristic endoscopic features to each type of esophageal infection, but it is still often difficult to differentiate one from the other and several diseases may coexist. Therefore, biopsies, brushings, and cultures may be necessary.

Many patients suspected of having esophageal infections are immunosuppressed. The approach to endoscopy and biopsy must take into account the patient's coagulation status and platelet count. Many investigators feel that biopsy should only be performed if the platelet count is above 50 000 per millilitre and can be supported at that level for several days after the procedure. Even longer periods of platelet support may be needed in patients on chemotherapy, which interferes with the epithelial healing process.

HERPETIC ESOPHAGITIS

One of the most commonly encountered infections involving the esophagus is caused by herpes simplex virus. This infection may be confused with or coexist with candidiasis of the esophagus or cytomegalovirus infection. The incidence of herpetic esophagitis is increasing, especially in the immunocompromised host with leukemia, lymphoma, a bone marrow transplant, etc. However, the infection may also occur in patients without severe underlying illness. The clinical presentation often includes odynophagia, dysphagia, and heartburn. There may be a history of a herpetic lesion on the lip preceding the onset of odynophagia by several days. Examination of the oropharynx may be normal or may show vesicles in the mouth and pharynx. Radiologic examination of the esophagus may or may not be normal depending on the severity of mucosal involvement.

Herpetic esophagitis evolves in several phases. In the first phase, the lesion is vesicular (Fig. 3.82). The following phase is marked by sharply demarcated small ulcers with raised margins (Fig. 3.83). These ulcers are typically in the middle or upper third of the esophagus, and may show a gray or yellowish necrotic material in the base. The mucosa surrounding the ulcer is often erythematous, with normal mucosa surrounding the erythema. These ulcers will enlarge and may begin to coalesce. Finally, there is a necrotic phase during which the infected epithelium is diffusely involved, resulting in a diffuse esophagitis with confluent ulcers (Fig. 3.84). Smear of the surface of the esophagus fails to reveal mycelia of *Candida*.

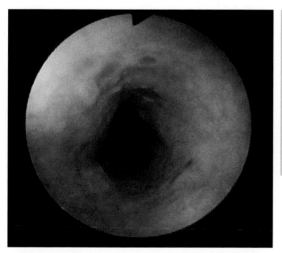

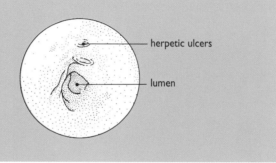

Figure 3.82 Early herpetic esophagitis. Ulcers are small and slightly depressed, with a minimally raised margin.

▼ A

▼ B

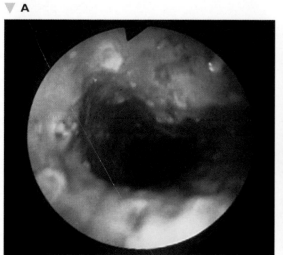

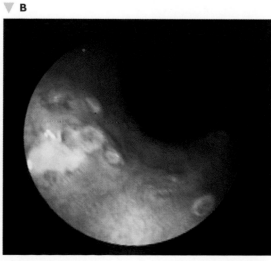

Figure 3.83 (*A* and *B*) Two examples of herpetic esophagitis with strongly demarcated ulcers. The ulcer bases have an exudative appearance.

Diagnosis is made by examining tissue from esophageal mucosa. Biopsy specimens reveal typical cytopathic changes of replicating viruses. As these changes are most marked at the margin of the herpetic ulcer, biopsies should be taken there. The base of the ulcer usually does not contain virus and biopsies are not productive from that site.

Biopsy specimens will reveal multinucleated giant cells and ballooning degeneration of cells; these cells are marked by basophilic nuclei with a 'ground glass' inclusion and chromatin margination (Fig. 3.85). One may also observe cells with eosinophilic intranuclear inclusions surrounded by a halo. No cytoplasmic inclusions are seen.

These cytopathic changes may also be found on brushings obtained from the area at the margin of the ulcer, in cells obtained by exfoliative cytology, and in tissue culture after 1 week. Recently, the use of monoclonal antibodies in herpetic esophagitis has simplified the diagnosis, as these specific antibodies will identify the presence of herpes virus in the involved tissue. It is important to remember that cytopathic changes may not be obvious unless one is looking for them. Therefore, the pathologist should be alerted to the possibility of herpetic esophagitis so that these characteristic changes may be sought.

Clinically, the usual consideration is whether the patient has reflux esophagitis (which should be treated with appropriate antireflex measures), or candida esophagitis (which should be treated with antifungal drugs). Herpetic esophagitis, cytomegaloviral esophagitis and varicella zoster virus (VZV) esophagitis are all treatable with antiviral agents. In patients who have undergone a bone marrow transplant, chronic graft-versus-host disease (which can be treated with increased dosages of immunosuppressive agents) must also be included in the differential diagnosis.

CANDIDA ESOPHAGITIS

Candida is a fungus that can proliferate anywhere along the gastrointestinal tract, and candida esophagitis is being increasingly diagnosed. This increase may be due to improved detection through endoscopy and the increasing number of immunosuppressed patients, including patients with organ transplants, those undergoing cancer chemotherapy, and those with other causes for immunosuppression such as AIDS. Other predisposing illnesses to candida infection include diabetes mellitus and malignancy. Significant symptomatic esophageal candidiasis has also been reported in patients with no underlying illness. In the years before the application of endoscopy, diagnosis was made by barium swallow radiograph that demonstrated irregular outlines of exudates, ulcers, strictures, aperistalsis, etc. However, in candida esophagitis, the x-ray may appear normal (lack of sensitivity). If an abnormality is seen on x-ray it may not be fungal in origin (lack of specificity). Endoscopy is a far better diagnostic method for candida esophagitis.

The presenting symptoms of candida esophagitis are usually dysphagia and odynophagia. In addition, esophageal obstruction from debris may occur. Diagnosis is made from the endoscopic appearance of the esophageal mucosa and from examination of brushings taken with endoscopic guidance. The likelihood of finding esophageal candidiasis is increased if oral thrush is present.

▼ A   ▼ B

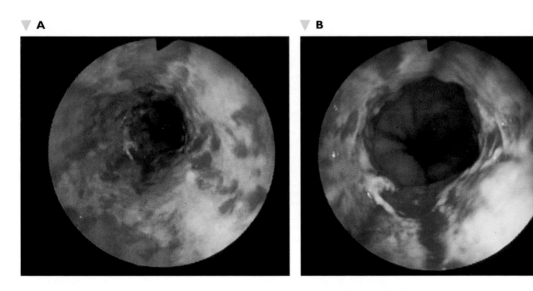

Figure 3.84 (A) Severe, herpetic esophagitis. There is evidence of diffuse involvement of the mucosa with confluent ulcers, friability, and exudation. **(B)** A close-up view. One can see that the mucosa of the stomach, just distal to the ora serrata, is normal, but the esophageal mucosa is severely involved.

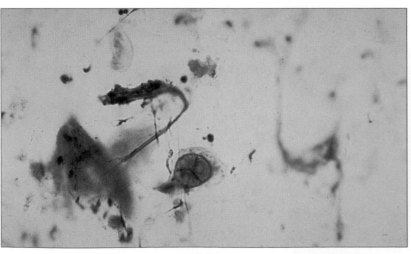

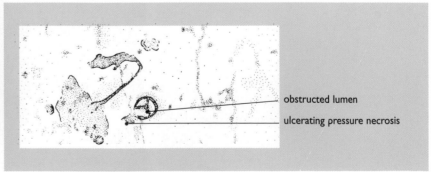

obstructed lumen

ulcerating pressure necrosis

Figure 3.85 Photomicrograph shows cells with the typical cytopathic changes of herpes virus: intranuclear inclusions but no cytoplasmic inclusions. (Courtesy of Dr George McDonald)

A grading scale for esophageal candidiasis has been proposed by Kodsi (Fig. 3.86). Endoscopic examination of early, mild candida esophagitis demonstrates small amounts of a white, cream-like exudate; the surrounding mucosa may be erythematous or fairly normal in appearance (Fig. 3.87). As the disease increases in severity, larger amounts of exudate become evident, with more obvious mucosal erythema and early ulceration. With further progression, the entire circumference of the esophagus becomes involved (Fig. 3.88). These changes are characteristic but not pathognomonic. The under-lying esophageal mucosa becomes increasingly erythematous and friable, and exudation becomes severe (Fig. 3.89). The gastric mucosa just beyond the squamocolumnar junction usually is normal in appearance (Fig. 3.90).

Ultimately, the increased inflammation and debris may narrow or obstruct the esophagus (Fig. 3.91). At this point marked friability, bleeding, and ulceration may be noted. The endoscopic differential diagnosis includes herpetic esophagitis and reflux esophagitis; each may present with similar endoscopic appearances. Other rare esophageal infections include *Torulopsis glabrata*,

---

Grades of Esophageal Candidiasis

Grade I
A few small (up to 2 mm) white and raised plaques with hyperemia but no evidence of ulceration or edema.

Grade II
Multiple raised plaques over 2 mm with edema and hyperemia. No ulcers are noted.

Grade III
Linear and nodular elevated confluent plaques with hyperemia and ulceration.

Grade IV
Grade III plus mucosal friability which may be associated with luminal narrowing.

Adapted with permission from Kodsi et al. Gastroenterology, 1976; 71:715-719.

Figure 3.86 *Grades of Esophageal Candidiasis.*

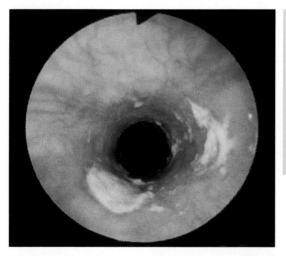

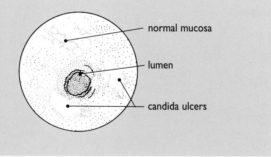

normal mucosa

lumen

candida ulcers

Figure 3.87 *Candida esophagitis. Ulcers are noted, with fairly normal surrounding mucosa. A white exudate covers the ulcers.*

▼ **A**

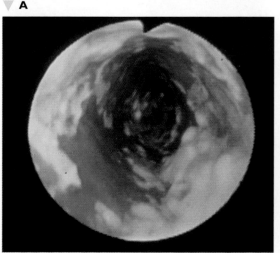

▼ **B**

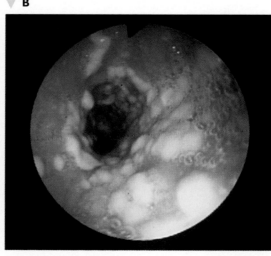

Figure 3.88 *(**A** and **B**) Two cases of moderate to severe candida esophagitis. Here the entire circumference of the esophagus is involved, with erythema of the mucosa and white exudate clearly evident.*

Pneumocystis carinii and *Lactobacillus acidophilus*. There are now reported cases of aphthous ulcers of the esophagus in AIDS patients that only contain HIV and no other viral pathogens. This may now be in the differential diagnosis. After *Candida* treatment, evidence of residual mucosal abnormalities may be noted (Fig. 3.92).

▼ **A**

▼ **B**

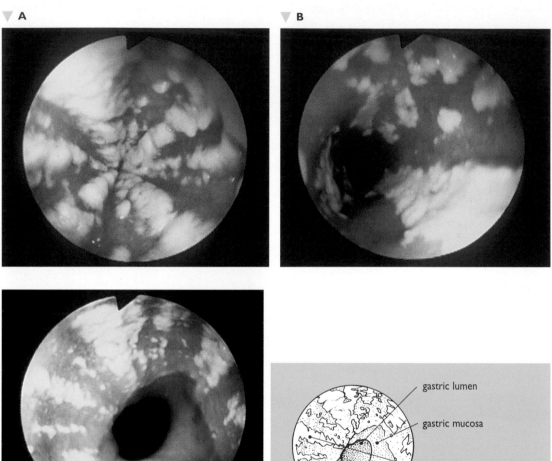

Figure 3.89 (A and **B)** *Two cases of severe candida esophagitis in patients with AIDS. The underlying mucosa is erythematous, and the linear exudate is typical of this infection.*

gastric lumen

gastric mucosa

severe candida esophagitis

squamocolumar junction

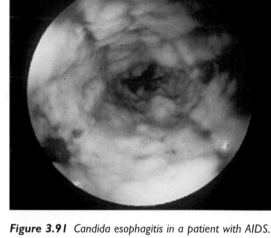

Figure 3.90 *Severe candida esophagitis in a patient with AIDS. The gastric mucosa just beyond the squamocolumnar junction is normal.*

Figure 3.91 *Candida esophagitis in a patient with AIDS. The combination of exudate and severe edema of the mucosa may compromise the esophageal lumen.*

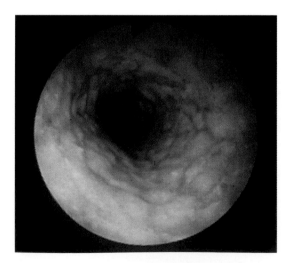

Figure 3.92 *Residual mucosal irregularity after treatment of severe candida esophagitis.*

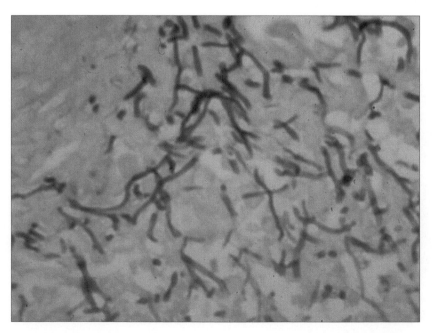

Figure 3.93 *This strained brushing from the exudate of a patient with candida esophagitis shows large numbers of candida mycelia. (Courtesy of Dr Eric Harder)*

Diagnosis is usually made by examining the mucosal brushings obtained during endoscopy. A sheathed cytology brush is passed, and plaque or exudate is brushed. After staining the slides with Gram's stain, mycelia and/or yeast forms can be seen (Fig. 3.93). Biopsies can be obtained and examined for invasive *Candida*, especially in patients presenting with ulcerative mucosa, but this method is not as commonly used or as productive as the smear technique.

Cultures are not relied upon since *Candida* is normally found in 35–50% of oral pharyngeal washings and in 65–90% of stool samples. Thus, a positive culture is not indicative of disease. If a culture is desired, a sterile cytology brush can be passed and exudate sampled. The brush is then rubbed directly onto Sabouraud's agar or washed in normal saline followed by culture of the saline. Serology can also be used to determine invasive *Candida*, but the sensitivity and specificity of the serologic approach is still not satisfactory because of the occurrence of false-positive results.

CYTOMEGALOVIRUS ESOPHAGITIS

Cytomegalovirus (CMV) is another viral agent that causes esophagitis. These infections may occur secondary to damaged epithelium, as is seen in chronic graft-versus-host disease. However, in primary CMV infections the esophageal mucosa has a relatively characteristic appearance: superficial erosions with a geographic, serpiginous, nonraised border (Fig. 3.94). This distinguishes CMV lesions from the raised lesions seen in herpes simplex virus. In CMV, the erosions may be large (1–3 cm in diameter) but very superficial. The centers of these erosions are diffusely involved and have a reticulated appearance (Fig. 3.95). When these changes are noted at the gastroesophageal junction, the appearance of the mucosa may be similar to that of reflux esophagitis. However, the mucosal changes are distinctive when surrounded by normal mucosa. Deep ulcers with raised margins, caused by CMV, may also be noted (Fig. 3.96). Ulceration may be severe (Figs. 3.97 and 3.98). Large CMV esophageal ulcers are often observed in AIDS patients and in bone marrow transplant patients.

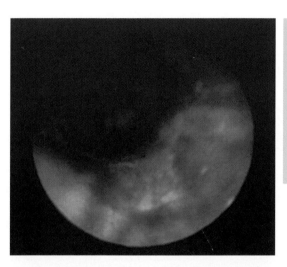

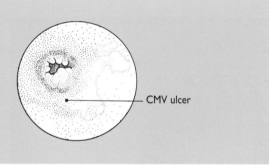

Figure 3.94 *This is the characteristic appearance of esophageal mucosa infected with cytomegalovirus (CMV): large, superficial erosions with a geographic pattern; the margins of the erosions are not raised. (Courtesy of Dr George McDonald)*

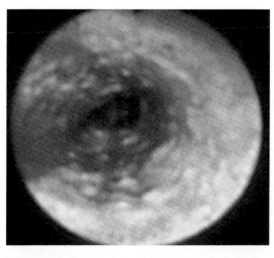

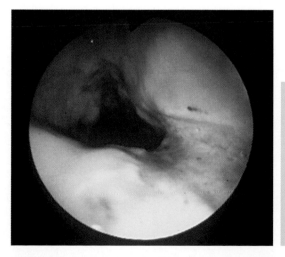

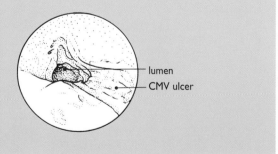

Figure 3.95 *In this severe case of cytomegaloviral esophagitis, there is evidence of diffuse involvement of the esophageal mucosa, with a characteristic flat, reticulated surface. (Courtesy of Dr George McDonald)*

Figure 3.96 *AIDS patient with large cytomegalovirus (CMV) ulcer of the esophagus.*

Diagnosis of CMV is made by obtaining tissue from biopsies or cytologic brushings, and evaluating the tissue for typical cytopathic changes. The changes include a characteristic cellular appearance with a basophilic intranuclear inclusion, a clear halo surrounding the nucleus, and the presence of multiple, smaller intracytoplasmic inclusions (Fig. 3.99). Cultures for the virus can also be obtained; cytopathic effects are seen in tissue culture after 3 weeks. CMV may occur simultaneously with graft-versus-host disease and herpetic esophagitis.

HIV ESOPHAGITIS

HIV can be associated with ulcers in the esophagus. Recent studies have shown HIV viruses in the base of esophageal ulcers with no other pathogens found. These ulcers only respond to immunosuppressive agents, primarily steroids. Other studies have shown that the immunomodulating drug thalidomide may also be useful in HIV ulcers. These ulcers may be large and may cause bleeding (Fig. 3.100)

NEW TECHNIQUES FOR EVALUATION OF SUSPECTED INFECTIOUS ESOPHAGITIS

A variety of viruses can cause esophagitis and ulceration including CMV, herpes, Epstein-Barr (EBV), varicella zoster virus (VZV) and HIV. One of the most important technical considerations for accurate diagnosis of infectious esophagitis is the site of biopsy (Fig. 3.101). In cases of herpes, it is important to biopsy the squamous mucosa around an ulcer rather than the base of the ulcer itself. In CMV, the biopsy must be taken at the base of an esophageal ulcer, as the virus is only detectable in the submucosal tissue, it is not present in the stratified squamous epithelium of the esophagus. In CMV of the stomach and duodenum, the virus is often present in both the columnar epithelium surrounding the ulcer and the deeper tissue at its base. Finally, in cases of *Candida,* biopsies are rarely necessary and diagnosis is made based on a smear of the exudate showing branching hyphae or budding yeast.

Obtaining cultures is also an important consideration in suspected infectious esophagitis. Herpes simplex and varicella zoster viruses are cultured rapidly from tissue, however, it can take 2–3 weeks for a cytomegaloviral viral culture to become positive. A major advance in the culture of the herpes group viruses (herpes simplex, CMV and varicella zoster) is the Shell vial culture technique. In this technique, the tissue is cultured in a monolayer of cells and stained after 1 day with monoclonal antibodies. This is a very rapid means of diagnosing CMV and marks a real advance in the management of this disease. Cultures of exudate for *Candida* are not helpful as this is often a commensal organism and a positive culture does not necessarily indicate tissue infection.

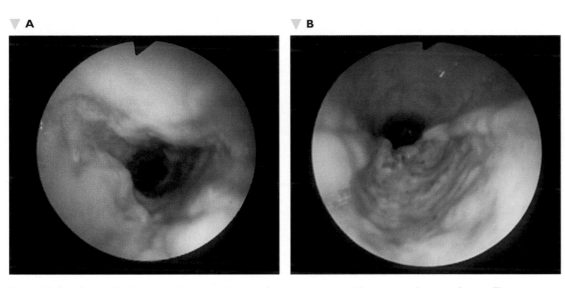

Figure 3.97 (A and B) *Two cases of large, severe esophageal ulcers causal by cytomegalovirus infection. The case on the right **(B)** is in a patient with AIDS.*

Figure 3.98 *Severe cytomegalovirus infection and ulceration of the esophagus.*

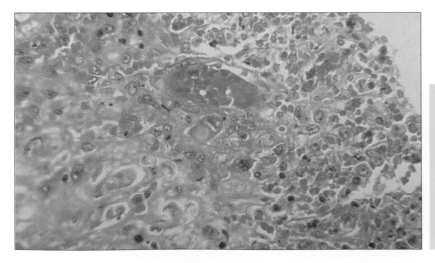

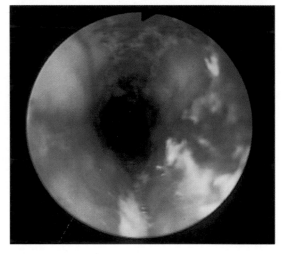

intranuclear inclusion with halo

intracytoplasmic inclusion

Figure 3.99 *Photomicrograph shows the typical cellular changes associated with cytomegaloviral infection. The cell has an intranuclear inclusion, a halo surrounding the nucleus, and mutliple intracytoplasmic inclusions. (Courtesy of Dr George McDonald)*

Tissue is routinely examined by culture and histology, but now new tests capable of detecting the presence of virus in tissue are attracting increasing interest. The type of fixative used for biopsy tissue when testing for viral antigens, DNA or RNA varies for different tests and must be carefully considered before proceding. Tissue can be examined with monoclonal or polyclonal antibodies to detect viral antigens of CMV, herpes simplex virus, Epstein-Barr virus and varicella zoster virus. This test can be performed either on a smear of exudate or on a tissue biopsy. In-situ DNA or RNA hybridization or the polymerase chain reaction can also be used to detect the presence of viral DNA or RNA in the tissue.

The time is approaching when tissue or exudate will be able to be tested rapidly and infectious agents identified with minimal delay. Advances such as those described above will significantly assist in the management of these often critically ill patients.

Deep ulcers may occur in HIV-positive patients who are negative for CMV, herpes, *Candida,* etc. Ulceration may be severe and may only respond to steroids (Fig. 3.100).

GRAFT-VERSUS-HOST DISEASE

Bone marrow transplant is a therapeutic technique being used with increasing frequency for several hematologic disorders, including aplastic anemia and leukemia. After transplantation, patients often experience esophageal problems, including viral infections (herpes and CMV), fungal infections with *Candida,* and reflux esophagitis. Later in the course of recovery, these patients may develop severe retrosternal pain, dysphagia, and odynophagia caused by an epithelial reaction of the esophageal mucosa as part of chronic graft-versus-host disease.

Viral esophagitis occurs approximately 10 weeks after bone marrow transplantation. Chronic graft-versus-host disease involving the esophagus has a median onset of approximately 250 days after transplantation, with a range of approximately 70 days to more than 2 years. As a further complication, these patients may present with a combination of chronic graft-versus-host disease of the esophagus and viral or fungal infection.

In a recent study, 8 out of 63 patients with chronic graft-versus-host disease developed severe esophageal symptoms. At endoscopy, 7 out of the 8 patients showed mucosal changes characteristic of graft-versus-host disease. The first and most commonly seen change is desquamation marked by superficial peeling of the erythematous mucosa (Figs. 3.102 and 3.103). Severe involvement is marked by erythema and exudation, and may demonstrate

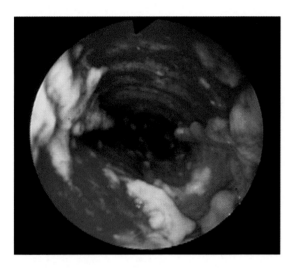

Figure 3.100 *Patient with AIDS and severe esophageal ulceration, which responded to steroid therapy.*

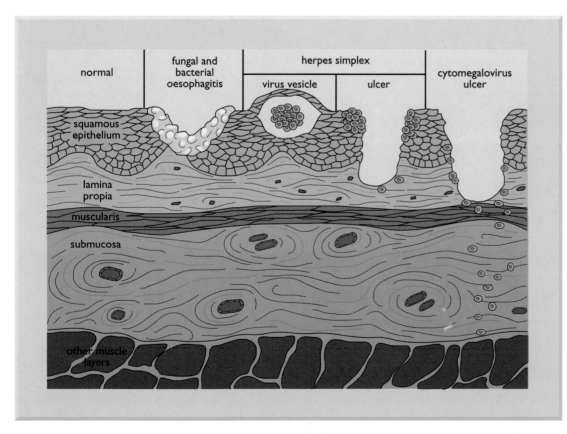

Figure 3.101 *Biopsy site for identification of possible esophageal infection. (Adapted with permission from McDonald Gastrointestinal Diseases: Pathophysiology, Diagnosis, Management 4th edn. W.B. Saunders, 1989, pp 640–656.)*

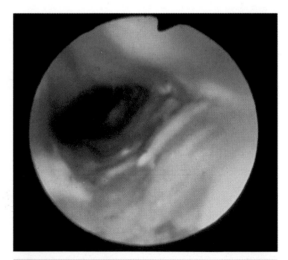

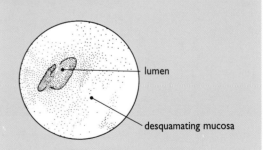

Figure 3.102 *In the early stages of graft-versus-host disease (GVHD), desquamation of the mucosa can be noted. (Courtesy of Dr George McDonald)*

mucosa hanging in shreds (Figs. 3.104–3.106). This latter change is often found in the upper esophagus and is occasionally confluent with chronic graft-versus-host disease involving the oral mucosa. Even in the presence of these severe changes, the distal esophagus may appear normal.

Other characteristic findings are webs, strictures, and rings (Fig. 3.107).

These abnormalities can cause severe dysphagia. In one case, severe webs obstructed the upper esophagus, and retrograde endoscopy via a gastrostomy was necessary to evaluate the area (Fig. 3.108). Abnormal peristalsis may also be noted in association with poor acid clearing from the esophagus, leading to changes of reflux esophagitis.

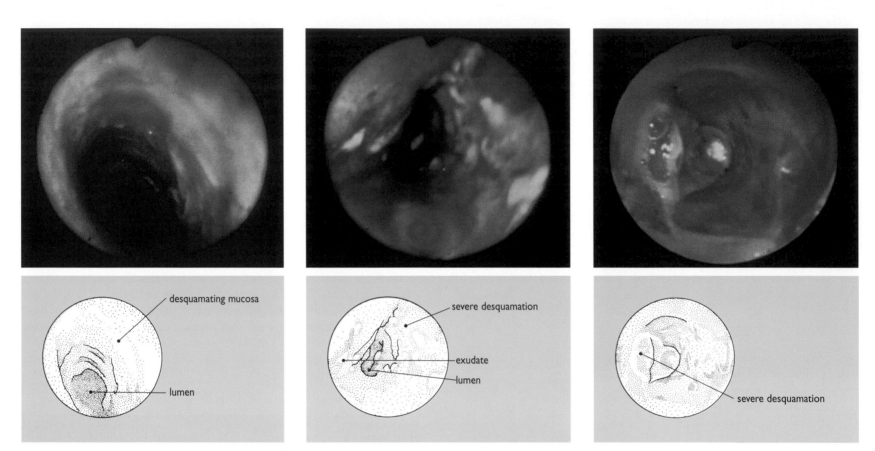

Figure 3.103 GVHD. In this early stage, mucosal desquamation and erythema are evident. (Courtesy of Dr George McDonald)

Figure 3.104 GVHD. As the disease progresses, one may note severe desquamation, with erythema, shredding mucosa, bleeding, and marked exudation. (Courtesy of Dr George McDonald)

Figure 3.105 GVHD. In severe disease, one may note marked, diffuse mucosal erythema in association with severe desquamation. (Courtesy of Dr George McDonald)

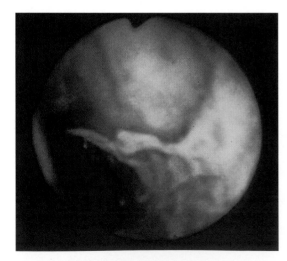

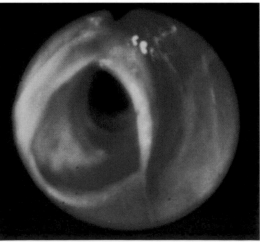

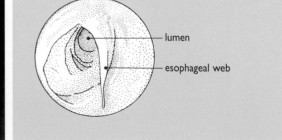

Figure 3.106 This patient presented with substernal esophageal pain and dysphagia approximately 250 days after bone marrow transplantation. Endoscopic examination reveals shredded desquamated mucosa, indicative of graft-versus-host disease. (Courtesy of Dr George McDonald)

Figure 3.107 An esophageal web with mucosal erythema, a characteristic finding in graft-versus-host disease. (Courtesy of Dr George McDonald)

Diagnosis is based on clinical presentation and endoscopic appearance. Biopsies show cellular infiltration and fibrosis, which can be distinguished by its submucosal location from the fibrosis seen in progressive systemic sclerosis that usually involves the muscularis propria.

Treatment is usually to increase immunosuppressives (e.g. steroids and azathioprine). Esophageal changes often regress with this therapy. Webs, strictures, and rings may require dilation but one must be very cautious because there is an increased risk of esophageal perforation from dilation in these patients. As bone marrow transplants increase, clinicians will see increasing numbers of patients with the aforementioned esophageal abnormalities. As the symptoms are severe and the treatments very different, the characteristic presentation, specific diagnostic methods, and differential diagnosis will become increasingly important.

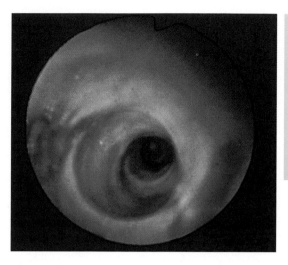

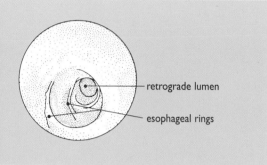

retrograde lumen

esophageal rings

Figure 3.108 *Retrograde study via a gastrostomy reveals multiple esophageal rings and mucosal erythema that caused total obstruction of the upper third of the esophagus. (Courtesy of Dr George McDonald)*

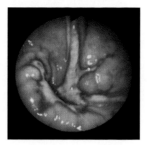

Esophagus III: Motor Dysfunction, Vascular Abnormalities, and Trauma

In this chapter we consider disorders of the esophagus for which endoscopy has a role in diagnosis and therapy. The esophagus has a simple function: to pass food and liquids into the stomach and to keep them there. When the esophagus malfunctions, the disability to the patient may be striking. Among the causes of dysfunction are motor disorders, vascular abnormalities, and injury by a variety of mechanisms.

NORMAL ESOPHAGEAL ANATOMY AND FUNCTION

The wall of the esophagus contains striated muscle in the upper one-third and smooth muscle in the lower two-thirds. In its normal resting state the cricopharyngeus sphincter seals the entrance to the esophagus to prevent the negative intrathoracic pressure from drawing air into the esophagus. The lower esophageal sphincter (LES) remains closed at rest to prevent reflux of gastric acid, pepsin, bile, and swallowed food into the esophagus.

At the start of a swallow the hypopharynx generates a high spike of pressure and the cricopharyngeus sphincter temporarily relaxes to allow the bolus of food or liquid to pass. Simultaneously, the LES relaxes until the bolus passes into the stomach. The muscle of the esophageal wall propels the bolus down the esophagus in a process called peristalsis. Primary peristalsis is the normal peristalsis initiated by a swallow. Secondary peristalsis is an orderly peristalsis that occurs in response to distension of the esophagus. For example, when food refluxes from the stomach into the esophagus, a peristaltic wave is initiated to clear this potentially noxious material from the distal esophagus. Tertiary peristalsis is abnormal peristalsis. These random nonorderly contractions of the esophageal musculature occur sporadically in localized segments of the esophagus and may be associated with pain.

DISEASES AFFECTING ESOPHAGEAL MOTILITY

Many disease states can affect the esophagus and its motility. Prominent among these are diffuse esophageal spasm, achalasia, and scleroderma. Endoscopy may be useful for diagnosis of these diseases and associated complications.

DIFFUSE ESOPHAGEAL SPASM

Diffuse esophageal spasm describes a clinical condition caused by tertiary esophageal contractions. The patient may experience sudden regurgitation of swallowed liquids and may have difficulty swallowing solids. This contrasts with dysphagia caused by organic narrowing, in which symptoms initially are associated with solids and gradually progress to liquids as the lumen narrows. Symptoms of esophageal spasm may be intermittent, may be brought on by hot or cold liquids, and may be relieved by a Valsalva type maneuver. The spasm may produce severe chest pain radiating to the back, resembling the pain of coronary artery disease. Therefore, coronary angiography and investigations of the esophagus may be necessary to make the diagnosis.

Endoscopic Examination

Esophageal motility is difficult to evaluate endoscopically; one may observe peristaltic contractions and have the general impression that it is moving distally, but the movement is difficult to confirm. Teriary esophageal contractions appear as contractions of the esophageal wall with transient narrowing of the lumen. The mucosa is normal (Fig. 4.1). Spasms of the LES is an associated finding (Fig. 4.2), and diverticula may be present (Fig. 4.3). The esophageal lumen may appear eccentric, especially distally, and retained food debris may be noted (Fig. 4.4).

Better methods of evaluating esophageal motor function include fluoroscopic studies and manometry. Using fluoroscopy, a radiologist can watch a column of barium pass through the hypopharynx, cricopharyngeus sphincter, and into the esophagus. This process can be videotaped for later study. The radiologist can then determine whether hypopharyngeal coordination is normal, whether pulmonary aspiration occurs, and whether normal peristalsis is present. Tertiary contractions can be diagnosed, and the function of the LES can be evaluated. A tertiary contraction observed by fluoroscopy and associated with chest pain supports the diagnosis of esophageal spasm.

Manometry is the other commonly used diagnostic method for motility problems. An esophageal catheter with single or multiple pressure transducers is used. Peristalsis can be recorded, the height and the duration of the wave determined, the relationship of the peristaltic wave to a swallow studied, and the progression of the contraction down the esophagus evaluated. The LES can be studied with regard to baseline pressure, whether it relaxes normally with swallowing, etc. These probes can be combined with pH-sensitive transducers to determine simultaneously whether reflux is present and whether it triggers the esophageal contractions and symptoms. Technology is available to permit 24-hour pH and pressure monitoring.

ACHALASIA

Achalasia is a disease in which a hypertensive LES fails to relax adequately with swallowing. The smooth muscle portion of the esophagus is aperistaltic. Contractions may occur but do not do so in an orderly manner. The esophagus eventually dilates because of the combination or poor propulsion and the hypertensive LES.

The cause of achalasia is not known. However, in most cases the number of Auerbach's ganglia in the body of the esophagus is reduced, with inflammatory cells surrounding the remaining cells. In the LES area there may be normal or reduced numbers of ganglia.

A column of fluid may be present in the dilated esophagus, which is seen on routine chest x-ray as an air–fluid level in the esophagus. A barium esophagram is performed next and suggests the diagnosis of achalasia.

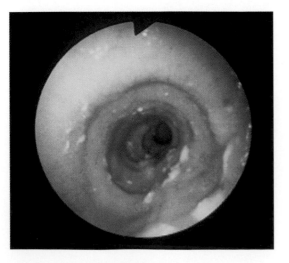

Figure 4.1 Ring-like esophageal contractions caused by diffuse spasm. The overlying mucosa is normal.

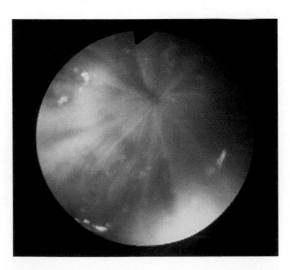

Figure 4.2 Diffuse esophageal spasm. Here, the LES is tightly closed.

Barium empties slowly only after a tall column of barium forms. The barium column has a 'beak-like' appearance at the LES. The diagnosis of achalasia is supported by esophageal manometry. Aperistalsis of the smooth muscle portion of the esophagus is seen; the LES has an elevated resting pressure and does not relax with swallowing. In most cases the diagnosis is confirmed by endoscopy, which rules out a neoplasm as a cause of the patient's symptoms.

A variety of medications should be tried including calcium channel blockers, anticholinergics, and nitrates. If these fail, symptomatic relief is obtained by reducing LES pressure. This is accomplished using balloon-dilation catheters. If this technique fails, surgical myotomy may be necessary. Early treatment halts the progression of the symptoms. Preliminary research notes that endoscopic injection of botulina toxin into the esophageal wall muscle may relieve symptoms. Further studies are necessary to establish safety and efficacy.

Endoscopic Examination

Endoscopy is of value in achalasia, both for diagnosis and for evaluation of the complications of the disease. Carcinoma infiltrating the area of the LES may produce symptoms, radiographic findings, and manometry similar to achalasia. Endoscopy is essential to exclude this possibility. Some endoscopists perform endoscopy on any patient who presents with achalasia, but all would endoscope a patient over the age of 40 years with atypical symptoms, rapid onset or progression, or with known achalasia who has a worsening or change in symptoms, because such a patient has an increased chance of cancer.

In achalasia, retained food and liquids in the dilated esophagus may increase the risk of aspiration of esophageal contents during endoscopy. Therefore, in patients with known or suspected achalasia, the esophagus should be routinely emptied with a large-caliber lavage tube before the examination. This also improves the quality of the endoscopic examination.

Endoscopically, the esophagus is dilated and aperistaltic, and the mucosa may have a white appearance (Fig. 4.5). Stasis of food is often noted (Fig. 4.6). The LES appears closed (Fig. 4.7), but with gentle pressure on the tip of the endoscope and after momentary resistance, the endoscope can be passed into the stomach. The mucosa of the LES segment appears normal. The squamocolumnar junction is usually within the level of the LES. The endosope is then routinely retroflexed to evaluate the cardia of the stomach from below. The cardia appears snug with otherwise normal-appearing gastric mucosa (Fig. 4.8). This maneuver is essential to exclude the possibility of a carcinoma at the gastroesophageal junction. Another mucosal change noted in achalasia is hypertrophy of the esophageal mucosa in response to the chronic stasis (Fig. 4.9).

▼ **A**

▼ **B**

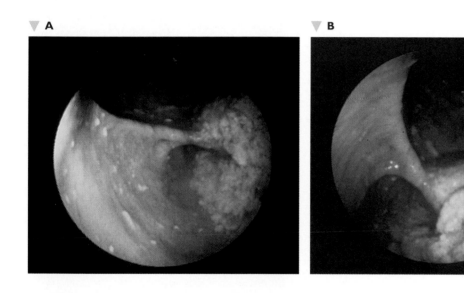

Figure 4.3 (A and **B)** Large epiphrenic diverticulum associated with diffuse esophageal spasm. Note the retained food in the distal esophagus.

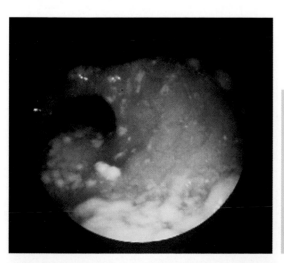

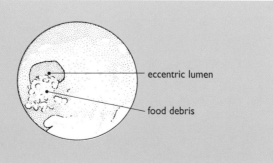

eccentric lumen

food debris

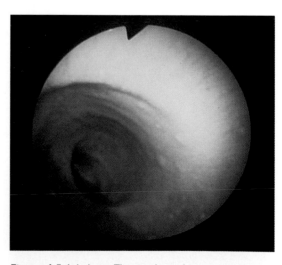

Figure 4.4 In this case of severe diffuse spasm, the lumen appears eccentric with evidence of stagnation and food debris.

Figure 4.5 Achalasia. The esophageal mucosa appears white.

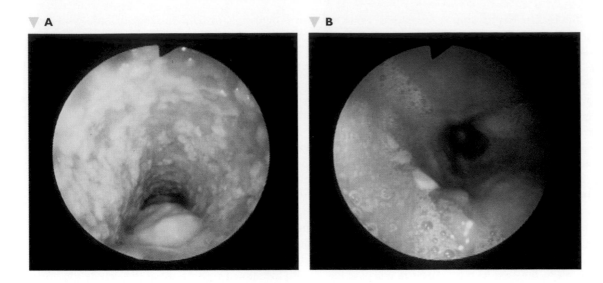

Figure 4.6 *Achalasia.* **(A)** *The esophageal lumen is wide, and food residue from the long-standing obstruction can be noted.* **(B)** *An aperistaltic esophagus with food stagnation.*

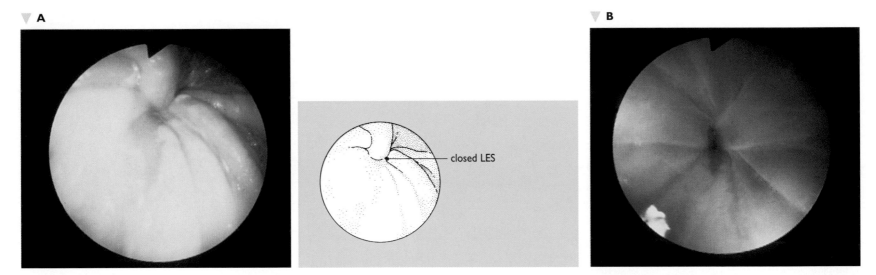

Figure 4.7 *Achalasia.* **(A)** *The LES is closed and remains closed until the tip of the endoscope is advanced against it and into the stomach.* **(B)** *Another example of a tight LES.*

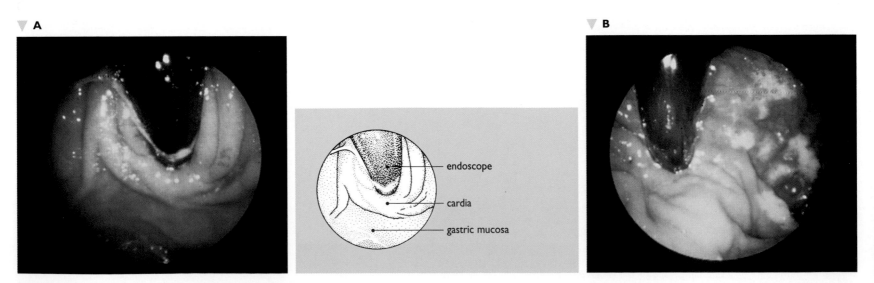

Figure 4.8 *Two views of the cardia in patients with achalasia* **(A)** *and vigorous achalasia* **(B)***, seen with the endoscope retroflexed. In both cases the cardia appears snug around the endoscope.*

Tumors that can produce an achalasia-like picture include primary gastric carcinoma of the cardia and metastases from another primary site such as lung or breast. If the endoscope will not pass into the stomach, the likelihood of a cancer is increased. This may be a difficult diagnosis because initially the overlying mucosa appears relatively normal as the endoscope is passed into the stomach. Examination of the gastric cardia from below is the best method for diagnosing this problem (Fig. 4.10). In some cases initial studies may only detect relatively normal-appearing mucosa overlying the tumor, but cytology and biopsy can usually establish the diagnosis.

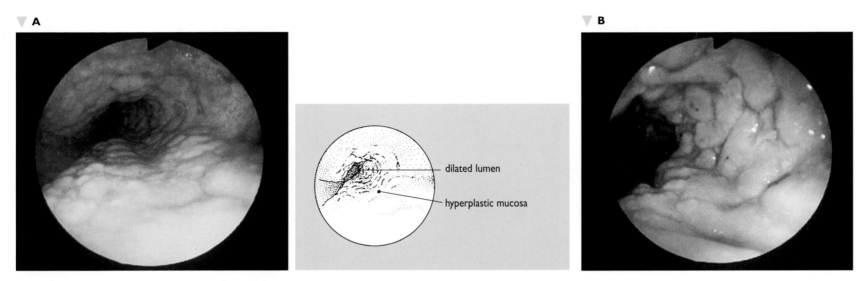

Figure 4.9 (A and B) *A wide lumen and hyperplastic mucosa are evident in these two cases of achalasia.*

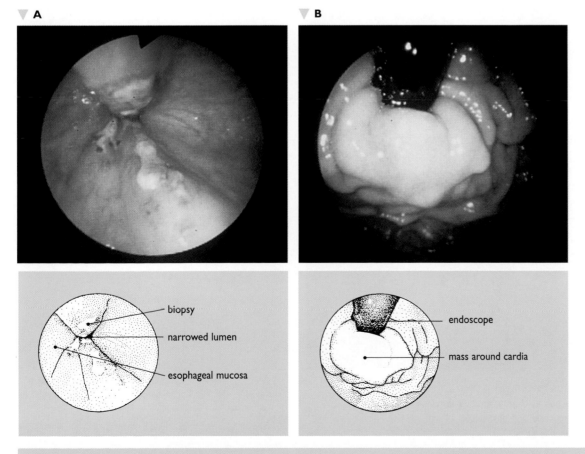

Figure 4.10 (A) *This achalasia-like appearance was caused by pulmonary cancer surrounding the distal esophagus. The small, white ulcer-like lesions are the result of a previous biopsy several days earlier. There is the suspicion of a mass or heavy folds in the LES area.* **(B)** *With the tip of the endoscope retroflexed, a snug mass is seen surrounding the endoscope. The mucosa over the mass is pale and slightly discolored.*

Some patients with achalasia have high pressure waves in the esophagus that appear as contractions. This is called vigorous achalasia. Small pseudodiverticular outpouchings sometimes occur just above the LES in patients with achalasia (Fig. 4.11). They may complicate treatment of the achalasia with balloon dilation because it may be difficult to position the balloon catheter in the high pressure area.

There is reportedly a slightly increased incidence of squamous-cell carcinoma of the esophagus in achalasia, especially after 10 years of disease (Fig. 4.12). These cancers occur in the distal two-thirds of the esophagus. Cancer may still occur in patients treated adequately with dilation or with surgery to disrupt the hypertensive LES. Therefore, patients with achalasia may benefit from periodic endoscopic screening every few years. Recurrent symptoms of dysphagia, chest pain, or weight loss warrant immediate investigations to exclude another cause such as a stricture or a cancer.

The usual initial therapy for achalasia after a trial of drug therapy fails to relieve symptoms is to disrupt the hypertensive LES using balloon dilation under fluoroscopic guidance. If balloon dilation fails, a surgical myotomy is often the next treatment. Both of these treatments can result in compli-

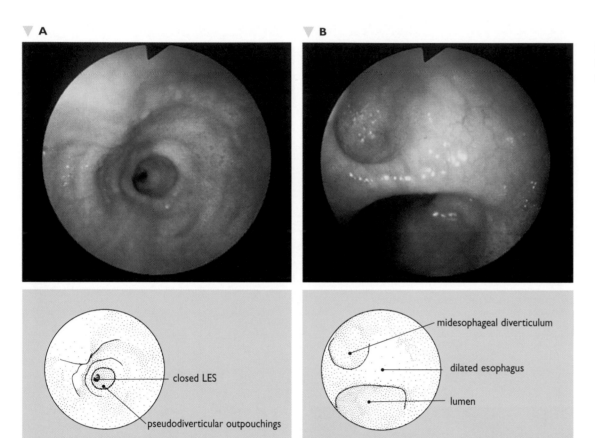

Figure 4.11 (A) Pseudodiverticular outpouchings above the closed LES in a patient with achalasia. *(B)* A midesophageal diverticulum in a patient with achalasia.

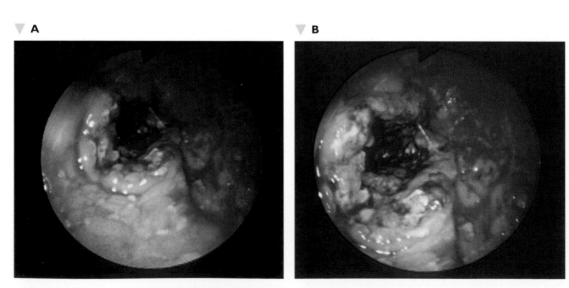
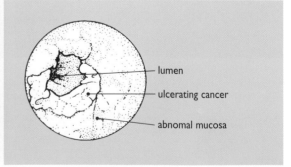

Figure 4.12 (A) This patient with long-standing achalasia developed recurrent dysphagia. A distal esophageal mass surrounding a deep ulcer is seen. *(B)* This mass, on closer inspection, is a squamous-cell carcinoma. The mucosa surrounding the mass is abnormal as a result of long-standing achalasia and obstruction.

cations. Chronic gastroesophageal reflux may result from balloon dilation, producing esophagitis with erythema, erosions, linear ulcerations, and strictures (Fig. 4.13). Myotomy can result in incompetence of the LES, producing severe reflux esophagitis and stricture (Fig. 4.14). Other surgical procedures include esophagectomy with an interposed colonic segment (Fig. 4.15).

SCLERODERMA

Diseases of connective tissue may affect esophageal function; the most severe problems are seen in scleroderma, in which peristalsis is absent or marked-

ly decreased in the lower two-thirds of the esophagus. In addition, the LES has low or absent pressure and fails to function as a sphincter. The combination of aperistalsis and severe reflux of gastric contents into the esophagus gravely injures the esophageal mucosa. Fibrosis may occur in the esophageal wall in conjunction with many forms of motor abnormalities. Esophageal dysfunction often progresses even when the cutaneous manifestations of the disease are quiet or regress.

▼ **A**

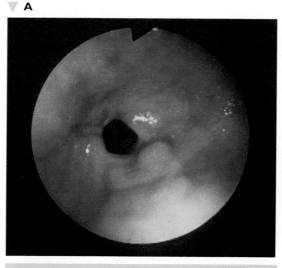

erythema

lumen through LES

erosion

▼ **B**

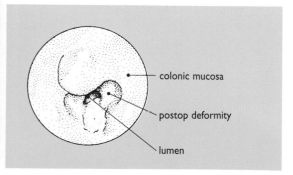

Figure 4.13 (A) Achalasia treated with pneumatic balloon dilation. Reflux resulted, with erosions and an esophageal stricture; *(B)* a close-up view.

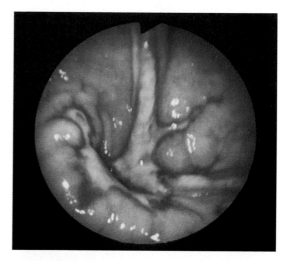

Figure 4.14 Achalasia treated with a Heller myotomy. Severe reflux resulted, with nonhealing, linear, white-based ulcer.

▼ **A**

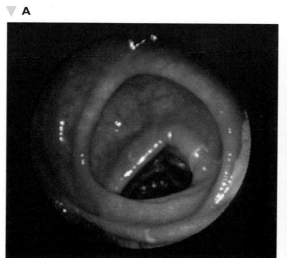

▼ **B**

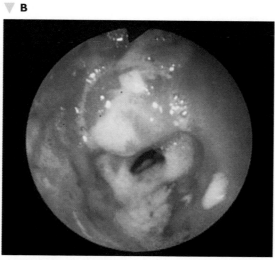

colonic mucosa

postop deformity

lumen

Figure 4.15 Achalasia and a colonic interposition. *(A)* The colonic segment appears normal with haustral folds and normal mucosa. *(B)* The anastomosis of the colon and stomach is narrowed, with evidence of postoperative changes in the form of mucosal deformity and exudates.

Endoscopic Examination

The endoscopic appearance is that of severe reflux with ulceration, erythema, and often tight strictures (Fig. 4.16). The esophagitis may extend into the proximal esophagus. The esophagus may appear aperistaltic (Fig. 4.17), and the LES may appear open without evidence of physiologic narrowing. The main role of endoscopy is the management of complications. Endoscopy is also indicated to exclude other causes of dysphagia such as concomitant esophageal candidiasis or a carcinoma.

VASCULAR ABNORMALITIES

Several types of esophageal vascular problems are evaluated endoscopically. The most important is esophageal varices. Others include angiodysplastic lesions, phlebectasias, and dysphagia lusoria.

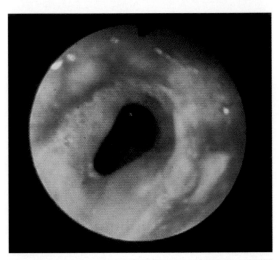

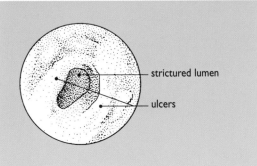

strictured lumen

ulcers

Figure 4.16 Scleroderma with evidence of esophageal reflux in the form of erythema and ulceration. A stricture is also present. (Courtesy of Dr Eric Harder)

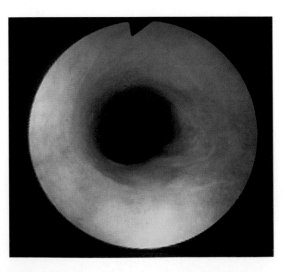

Figure 4.17 Scleroderma with an aperistaltic esophagus. The mucosa appears normal.

ESOPHAGEAL VARICES

As a result of cirrhosis or other diseases affecting the portal circulation, such as thrombosis of the portal vein, increased portal vein pressure causes the portal venous blood to seek collateral pathways to bypass the liver and enter the systemic circulation. Venous collaterals of the anterior abdominal wall, rectal vasculature, and retroperitoneal pathways account for the majority of decompressive flow. However, dilated veins – or varices – in the submucosa of the esophagus also serve as collateral pathways. To reach the systemic circulation, blood flows from the short gastric and coronary veins into the esophageal varices and then to the azygous system (Fig. 4.18). Consequently, varices usually occur in the distal half of the esophagus but, in cases of severe portal hypertension, can extend up into the proximal esophagus (Fig. 4.19). There may be associated varices of the cardia and fundus of the stomach.

Esophageal varices cause grave problems clinically. Approximately 10% of patients with upper gastrointestinal bleeding have bleeding esophageal varices. When these veins bleed there is a substantial risk of death from the bleeding (30–40%). There is also a significant risk of rebleeding (approximately 75% over the next 2 years).

Varices may have a characteristic appearance on a barium esophagram, but endoscopy is more accurate. Endoscopy is more precise because it can distinguish between folds and vascular structures. In addition, endoscopy allows assessment of gastric varices. Endoscopy can also estimate the risk of rebleeding and enables treatment by injection sclerotherapy or esophageal banding.

Endoscopic Examination

In most cases the diagnosis of varices can be made endoscopically without difficulty as they have a characteristic endoscopic appearance. The veins appear as irregular, serpiginous, often bluish structures running longitudinally in the submucosa of the esophageal wall (Fig. 4.20). They are usually most prominent distally. Occasionally it may be difficult to determine whether a structure is a fold or a small varix. Clues include the color, tortuosity, and variations with respiration.

Color

Varices are usually blue, although the color in some instances may be white or normal esophageal color, especially if the varices are small, not bleeding, or have been previously treated.

In some instances, a portion of the surface of the varix appears red. Termed the red color signs, these findings correlate with risk of hemorrhage. There are four subcategories of red signs.

- The red wale sign: dilated venules appearing like red streaks on the surface of the varix (Fig. 4.21); this has previously been referred to as varices on varices
- Small cherry red dots, less than 2 mm in diameter (Fig. 4.22)
- A hematocystic spot: a larger, solitary red spot on the varix (Fig. 4.23)
- A diffuse redness on the area of a varix.

Overall, any red color sign increases the risk of bleeding from 12–52% Of the four signs, diffuse redness and hematocystic spots correlated most highly with the risk of bleeding.

Types of Varices

Varices can be straight (Fig. 4.24), bead-like and markedly large, or nodular and tortuous (Fig. 4.25). Straight varices have only a 7% risk of bleeding whereas the risk with large tortuous varices is as high as 60%. Varices are also graded by extent of protrusion into the lumen. Grade 1 is less than 1 mm, grade 2 is up to 2 mm, grade 3 is up to 3 mm, and grade 4 is over 3 mm. The largest varices may occupy more than one-third of the lumen and may seem to occlude the lumen; small early varices may simply bulge into the lumen (Fig. 4.26).

Location

The location of the varices is predictive of bleeding risk. Varices are categorized as those above the tracheal bifurcation, those in the middle section, and those in the lower third of the esophagus. Varices that extend proximally have the highest risk of bleeding; the risk with varices limited to the distal third of the esophagus is lowest. Examining the location of varices is thought to be important because, after injection sclerotherapy, varices first disappear proximally, and this may be a useful marker for successful therapy. Downhill

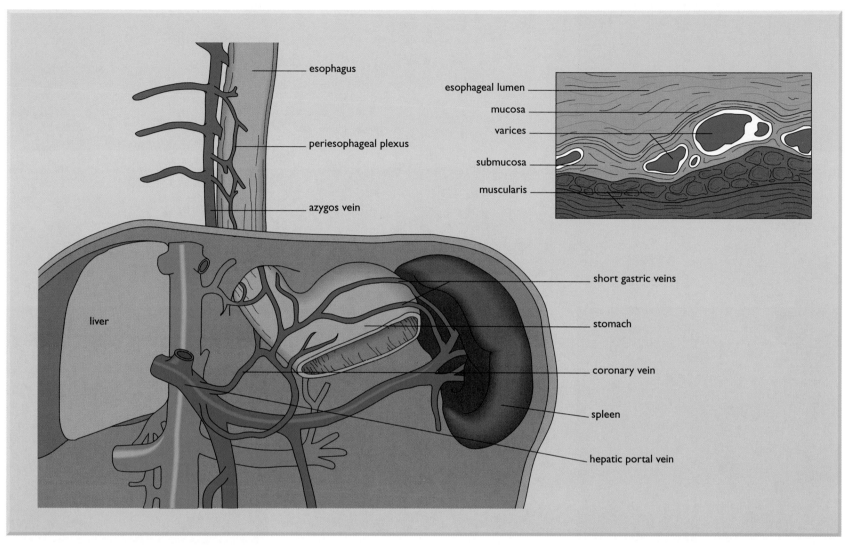

Figure 4.18 Diagram of esophageal varices.

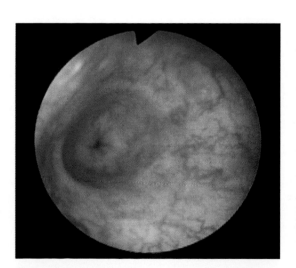

Figure 4.19 This patient has portal hypertension and esophageal varices. The proximal esophageal vascularity is pronounced.

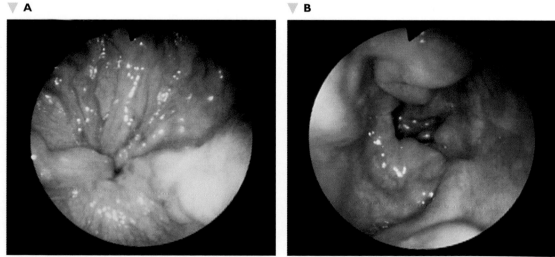

Figure 4.20 (A and B) Two views of esophageal varices. Color variations range from pale covering mucosa to blue. The varices bulge into the lumen and are serpiginous.

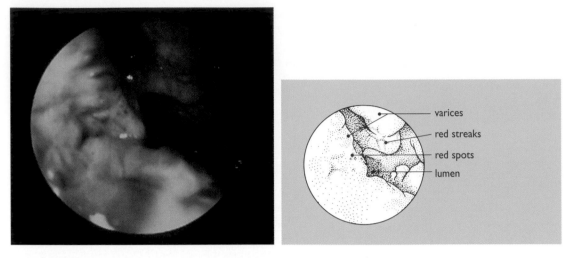

Figure 4.21 The red wale sign. Red spots are seen on areas of erythema, and streaks cover the tops of the varices in the background.

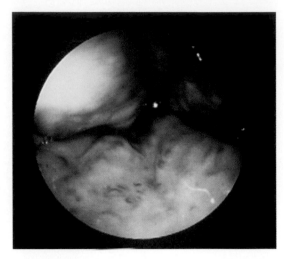

Figure 4.22 Large esophageal varices that appeared with an upper gastrointestinal bleed. The varices are bluish and show evidence of cherry red spots over the surface, suggesting recent active variceal hemorrhage.

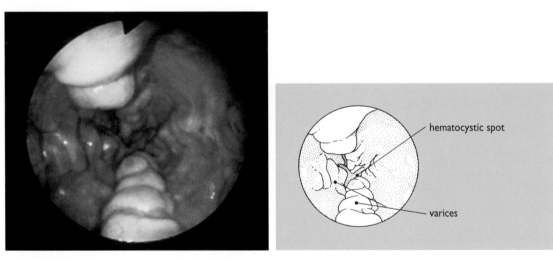

Figure 4.23 Varices with positive red signs and, possibly, a hematocystic spot, indicating recent bleeding.

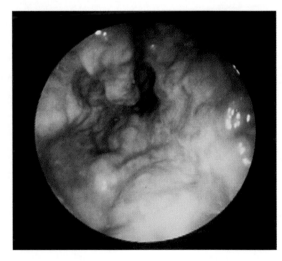

Figure 4.24 Large varices that are relatively straight.

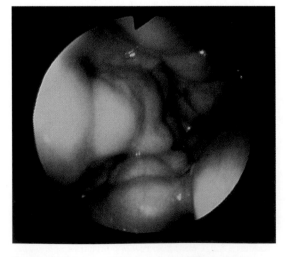

Figure 4.25 Large, nodular, tortuous varices of the esophagus that seem to occlude the lumen.

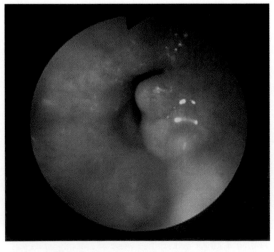

Figure 4.26 A small varix bulging into the lumen.

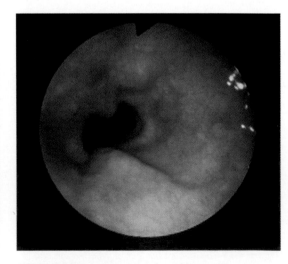

Figure 4.27 Downhill varices in a patient with non-Hodgkin's lymphoma.

varices may occur in patients with mediastinal disease when esophageal varices bypass a superior vena caval obstruction (Fig. 4.27).

To summarize, the following endoscopic observations of varices connote an increased likelihood of bleeding.

- Diffuse redness
- Hematocystic spot
- Large, tortuous varices
- Proximal extension
- Esophagitis.

Often, active variceal bleeding can be observed, varying from an ooze to a massive torrential hemorrhage. Active spurting may be seen (Fig. 4.28). Actively bleeding varices are usually seen in the distal esophagus but may be noted in the proximal esophagus, especially in the presence of large varices from high portal pressures. Even if no active bleeding is seen, the presence of the above factors or an adherent clot may indicate that the varices are the likely source of bleeding.

Occasionally it may be difficult to determine whether a structure is a varix covered with normal mucosa or an esophageal fold. In this circumstance an endoscopic Doppler probe or endosonography may be helpful to detect flow acoustically or image the varices in and adjacent to the esophageal wall.

The application of these devices may be the best method of deciding at endoscopy whether a structure is a varix or a fold. These same methods may help determine whether flow is still present after injection sclerotherapy. Another technique is to distend the esophagus gradually with air while watching endoscopically. A fold tends to flatten and disappear, whereas varices remain visible. Occasionally, as the pressure varies, one may see the varices empty and then refill and distend in a cephalad direction.

Associated gastric varices resemble gastric folds and are more difficult to diagnose (Figs. 4.29 and 4.30). Using an endoscopic Doppler probe or ultrasound endoscopy to generate an image of the wall and adjacent structures may be helpful for diagnosis.

The entire upper gastrointestinal tract should be inspected in a patient with upper gastrointestinal bleeding varices because 30–70% of patients with known varices have bleeding from other lesions such as gastritis or ulcers. Diagnosis of the bleeding site is further complicated if blood refluxes from the proximal stomach into the esophagus, leading to a false diagnosis of esophageal bleeding. On occasion this differential diagnosis remains a problem. In a patient with upper gastrointestinal bleeding, if the source of bleeding is in doubt but no lesion other than varices is seen, many feel that the varices may be assumed to be the source of bleeding. In these circumstances, the presence of endoscopic factors predictive of high bleeding risk such as the red signs are important and increase the likelihood that the source of hemorrhage is the varices.

Endoscopic Sclerotherapy

All treatments of bleeding esophageal varices have some risk. Currently, injection sclerotherapy is the most frequently used therapy for control of the acute hemorrhage.

Injection sclerotherapy controls bleeding immediately in about 85–90% of patients. Treated patients require fewer blood transfusions and have a reduced incidence of rebleeding. The technique for sclerosing varices is far from standardized. Rigid and flexible endoscopes are used. Some endoscopists use a balloon at the tip of the endoscope to compress the varix after injection. Some inject into the varix whereas others inject next to it. There are many variations in the sites injected, the volume of sclerosant injected, types of sclerosing agent used, and the schedule for reinjection. Some endoscopists use an overtube with a notch to enable a single varix to be isolated and injected.

Once the target varix is selected, an injection needle catheter is passed down the biopsy channel of the endoscope. A large-caliber endoscope is generally used because the large channel facilitates removal of blood and fluid.

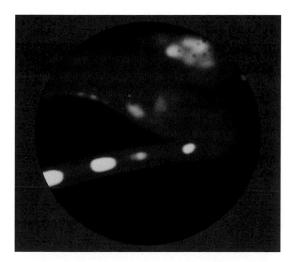

Figure 4.28 An esophageal varix with active, spurting bleeding.

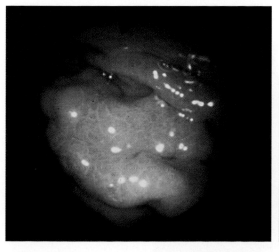

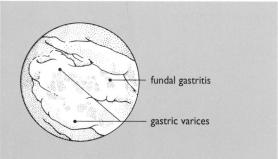

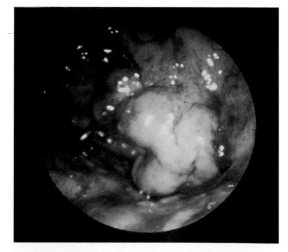

Figure 4.29 Gastric varices in a patient with severe portal hypertension. The covering mucosa is erythematous. Differentiating these varices from gastric folds may be difficult. This is an example of fundal congestive gastropathy.

Figure 4.30 Large fundal varices showing evidence of recent bleeding.

The catheter is passed into view and the needle advanced from the tip. The needle is then passed into the wall of esophagus, into or next to the varix (Fig. 4.31). Varices are usually injected initially 1–2 cm above the esopha-gogastric junction. Three injections are made in a ring at this level around the esophagus. In some instances, a second set of injections is made 3–5 cm more proximally in the esophagus.

After injection of sclerosing agent, the needle is withdrawn. The varix often turns pale or white. There may be some back-bleeding after the needle is removed (Fig. 4.32), which usually stops after several minutes or after rein-jection. A volume limit is usually placed on the amount of sclerosant to be injected. Agents injected to plug varices include cyanoacrylates, such as Histoacryl (Fig. 4.33). In some instances the cyanoacrylate is seen as a white plug over the varix and injected site (Figs. 4.34 and 4.35). The cyanoacry-late is injected immediately adjacent to the bleeding point in an esophageal or gastric varix and bleeding often stops at once.

If bleeding persists, a Sengstaken-Blakemore tube may be required. This tube has a gastric balloon, which anchors it in place, and an esophageal bal-loon that, when inflated, compresses the varices and stops the bleeding. Additional lumens are available for suction of the stomach and suction of the esophagus above the esophageal balloon to remove swallowed saliva and reduce the chance of aspiration. The Sengstaken-Blakemore tube is not always effective and may be associated with complications such as aspira-tion and laceration of the esophageal wall (Fig. 4.36).

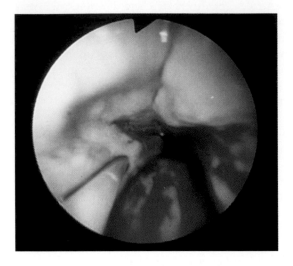

Figure 4.31
Sclerotherapy needle is inserted into varix in a patient who is actively bleeding.

▼ **A**

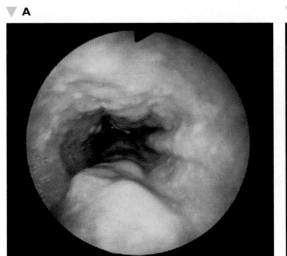

▼ **B**

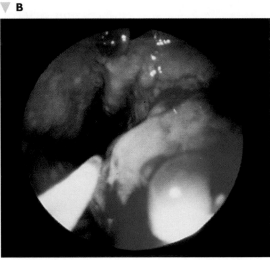

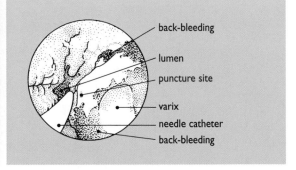

Figure 4.32 (A) *Large grade 4 esophageal varices.* **(B)** *After the injection needle is withdrawn from the varix, some back-bleeding occurs. The injected varix is slightly larger than before injection. The puncture site is seen just adjacent to the tip of the needle.*

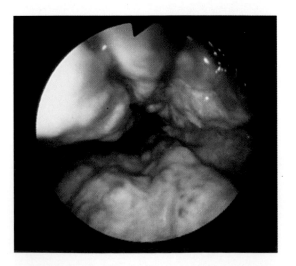

Figure 4.33 *Giant esophageal varices with mucosal red dots after cyanoacrylate injection.*

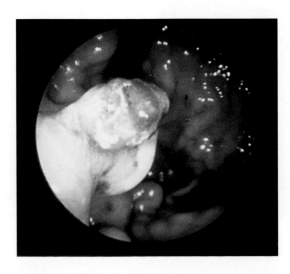

Figure 4.34 *Varices obliterated with cyanoacrylate injection. The varix is slightly white and some cyanoacrylate is seen on the surface.*

The goal of sclerotherapy is the complete obliteration of the varices. This is accomplished by a series of injections every few days initially and then monthly until the varices have disappeared. After several days, thrombosed varices may appear pale (Fig. 4.37) and gradually decrease in diameter as the injections progress. An area of variceal necrosis may be seen. An endoscopic Doppler probe may help in determining whether the varix is thrombosed.

An esophageal ulcer forms at the injection site in more than 30% of patients (Figs. 4.38–4.41). The ulcers may be single or multiple, deep or superficial. They are often sharply demarcated and show evidence of recent hemorrhage with a clot at the base. The base may be white with an exudate, or gray with necrotic material (Fig. 4.42). Esophageal ulcers are difficult to treat and are associated with a considerable risk of mortality when they bleed. Esophageal strictures also form after sclerotherapy in approximately 5–10% of patients and may require dilation. Esophageal perforation occurs in approximately 1% of patients (Figs. 4.43 and 4.44). Sclerotherapy is usually not effective for controlling bleeding gastric varices.

▼ **A**

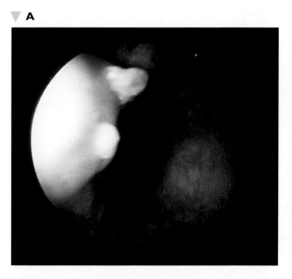

▼ **B**

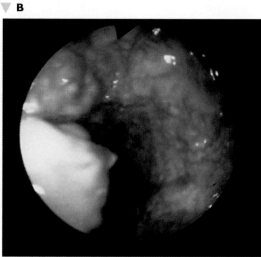

Figure 4.35 (A and **B)** *Histoacryl injection stopped massive esophageal variceal bleeding. Plugs of the Histoacryl are seen at the injection sites. Residual varices are noted.*

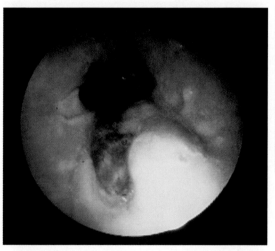

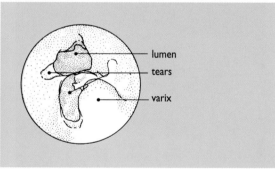

Figure 4.36 *Laceration of the esophageal mucosa caused by a Sengstaken-Blakemore tube used to stop bleeding from esophageal varices.*

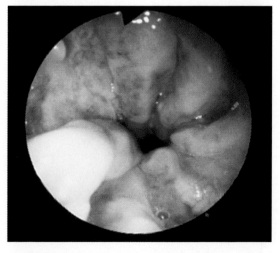

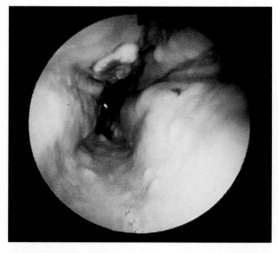

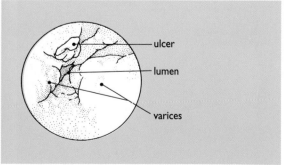

Figure 4.37 *After several sclerotherapy injection sessions varices appear pale and fibrosed.*

Figure 4.38 *An ulcer is seen with overlying necrotic tissue in the distal esophagus 7 days after injection sclerotherapy. In this case varices are still visible.*

A new type of therapy for esophageal varices is called banding. In this technique a cylindrical hood is placed on the tip of an end-viewing endoscope. An overtube is used to allow the endoscope to be passed into the esophagus repeatedly with reduced patient discomfort and gagging. A rubber band is placed on the hood over the endoscope tip. When a varix is visualized, suction is applied via the endoscope biopsy channel, drawing the varix into the hood. The rubber band is then advanced over the varix and is tightly applied to the base of the varix (Figs. 4.45 and 4.46). This technique has been

▼ **A**

▼ **B**

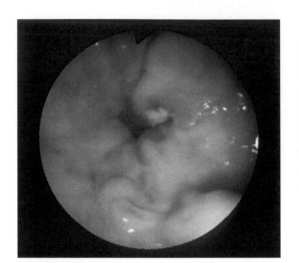

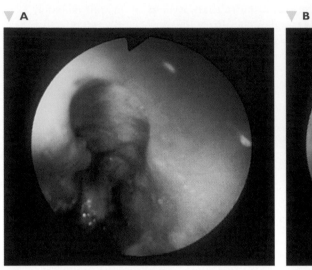

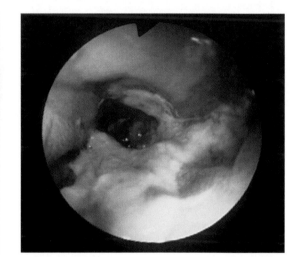

Figure 4.39 *Small ulcer in distal esophagus after injection sclerotherapy for varices.*

Figure 4.40 (A) *An acute, deep esophageal ulcer after sclerotherapy.* **(B)** *Two months later, the ulcer is small but still present. No clear varices are seen.*

▼ **A**

▼ **B**

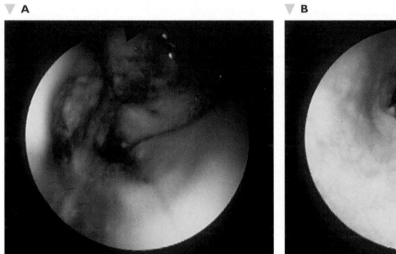

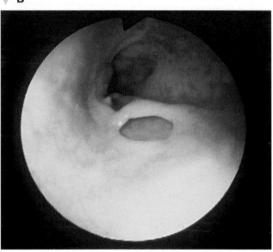

Figure 4.41 (A) *After sclerotherapy there was a severe inflammatory reaction with mucosal necrosis that led to the ulcerations seen here.* **(B)** *After healing, an area of mucosal bridging is noted. (Different patients in **A** and **B**.)*

Figure 4.42 *Large esophageal ulcer seen after injection sclerotherapy. An exudative coating is noted on the ulcer surface.*

Figure 4.43 *Mediastinal fistula after variceal sclerotherapy.*

varices
fistula
lumen

shown to control variceal bleeding same extent as sclerotherapy. More ulcers are noted with banding but fewer rebleeding episodoe occur and the number of sessions required to obliterate varices is fewer with banding than with sclerotherapy. Some clinicians use both techniques rather than exclusively one or the other.

Other Therapeutic Procedures

Surgical treatment of varices includes shunt surgery, esophageal transection, or esophageal resection with a colonic interposition. Shunt surgery should be followed by endoscopic confirmation that the varices are decompressed. Esophageal transection with the placement of a Boerema or Murphy button is a method that disrupts the varices and prevents further bleeding. However, this button may create a visible defect in the esophagus (Fig. 4.47). An inter-

position of the colon can also be used to interrupt the varices, but because the surgery does not correct the underlying portal hypertension, the varices may recur (Fig. 4.48). New treatments include decompressing the portal system by using a stent placed percutaneously via the jugular vein. The stent is advanced under fluoroscopic guidance and shunts between a hepatic vein and the portal system. This procedure is referred to as TIPS (transjugular intrahepatic portosystemic shunt).

OTHER VASCULAR DISORDERS

Angiodysplastic lesions may be noted in the esophagus as part of the spectrum of vascular malformations of the intestine. Phlebectasias are small vascular lesions covered with normal-appearing mucosa that protrude into the esophageal lumen. They appear similar to other submucosal lesions but

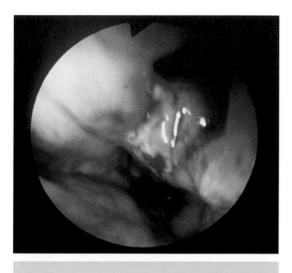

Figure 4.44 Esophageal wall necrosis and perforation after sclerotherapy.

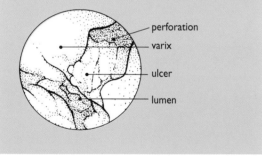

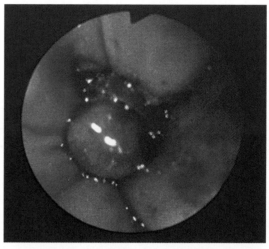

Figure 4.45 A band has just been placed on a varix. The varix appears as a ball of tissue as seen in this photograph.

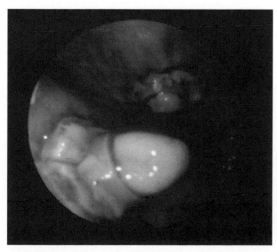

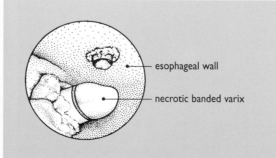

Figure 4.46 Appearance of necrotic varix several days after banding.

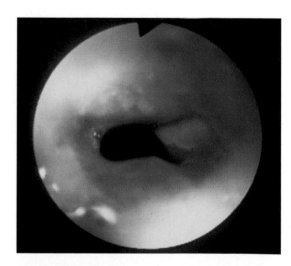

Figure 4.47 A fibrotic ring is seen in the distal esophagus after esophageal transection and insertion of a Boerema button to treat varices.

are small and may have a bluish color suggesting a vascular lesion (Figs. 4.49 and 4.50). Dysphagia lusoria is a condition in which an aberrant origin of the right subclavian artery crosses behind the esophagus and compresses the esophagus against the trachea, producing dysphagia. Endoscopically, a smooth indentation of the esophageal lumen is seen covered with normal mucosa.

ESOPHAGEAL INJURY

INJURY BY RADIATION

Radiation delivered to neoplasms of the lung or mediastinum may injure the esophageal mucosa at doses as low as 30 Gy. Chemotherapeutic drugs such as Adriamycin, which are often used in conjunction with radiation therapy, potentiate the effect of radiation, causing more severe injury. After intraluminal radiation therapy necrosis may be extensive.

Endoscopic Examination

Acute radiation injury manifests itself as acute esophagitis. Erythema and exudation are seen in the area maximally exposed to the radiation (Figs. 4.51 and 4.52). Ulceration and necrosis of the tumor may be seen (Figs. 4.53 and 4.54). Later, telangiectasias may be noted in the damaged area (Figs.

4.55–4.57). Tight strictures with a peculiar whitish and opalescent color may form and may require dilation to relieve dysphagia (Fig. 4.58). Often the esophagus is dilated proximal to the stricture.

Tracheoesophageal fistula is a serious complication of radiation injury (Figs. 4.59 and 4.60). Lung tissue may be visible at the base of the fistula. When fistulas occur in conjunction with ulceration and stricture, treatment becomes difficult. A guidewire passed endoscopically under fluoroscopic control reduces the chance of esophageal perforation during dilation and during attempts to position an endoprosthesis to treat the fistula (Fig. 4.61). Strictures and tracheoesophageal fistulas may be caused by recurrent tumor as well as radiation damage. Thoracic computed tomography or endoscopic ultrasonography may be useful to determine whether tumor mass is present in the area of the fistula or stricture.

INJURY BY NOXIOUS AGENTS

Ingestion of substances such as lye or acid may injure the esophagus, causing severe retrosternal pain. The extent of injury may be difficult to judge from examination of the oropharynx or by general examination of the patient. An endoscopist is occasionally called upon to evaluate the extent of injury. In the past, endoscopists were reluctant to endoscope these patients because of the risk of perforating a severely injured gut wall. Now, early

▼ **A**

▼ **B**

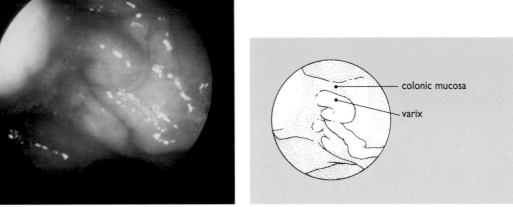

Figure 4.48 (A) Colonic interposition was performed to treat esophageal varices after splenic vein thrombosis. **(B)** Submucosal varices have recurred in the interposed colon.

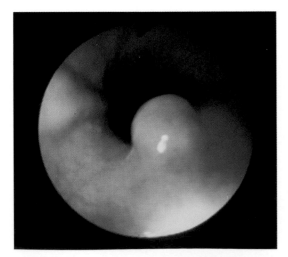

Figure 4.49 This small submucosal bump is vascular in appearance and is presumed to be a small dilated vessel or phlebectasia.

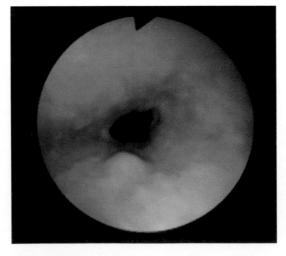

Figure 4.50 This small submucosal lesion in an otherwise normal-appearing distal esophagus was thought to be venous in nature.

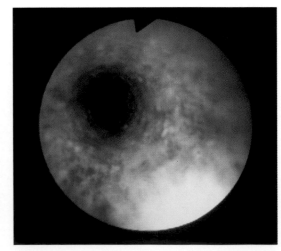

Figure 4.51 Acute radiation esophagitis 4 weeks after cessation of radiation therapy. Erythema, punctate hemorrhage, and exudation are evident.

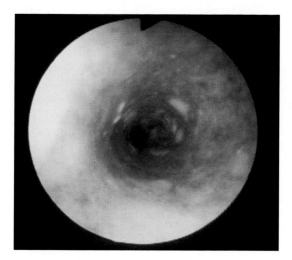

Figure 4.52 *Exudative esophagitis 3 weeks after completion of radiation therapy for lung cancer.*

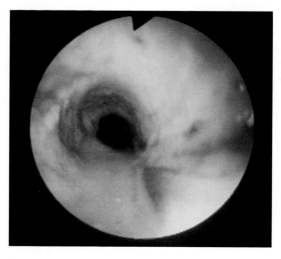

Figure 4.53 *Circumferential necrosis 4 weeks after completion of radiation therapy. The entire mucosa is abnormal.*

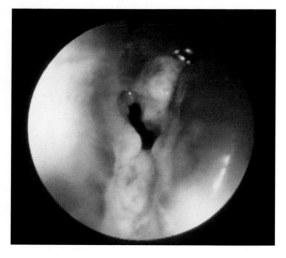

Figure 4.54 *Circumferential necrosis of esophageal wall after radiation therapy.*

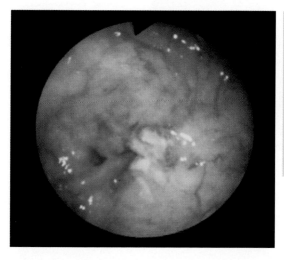

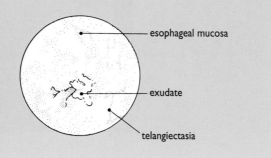

Figure 4.55 *Diffuse vascular changes can be noted in the esophageal mucosa after radiation therapy. Telangiectasias and exudates are evident.*

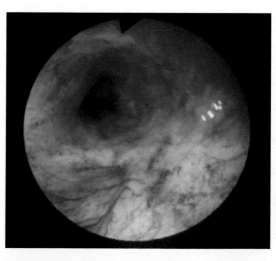

Figure 4.56 *Extensive telangiectasia after radiotherapy for esophageal cancer.*

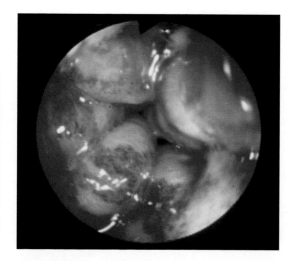

Figure 4.57 *Severe telangiectasia after radiotherapy; the esophageal wall is edematous.*

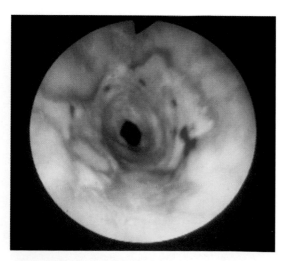

Figure 4.58 *Circumferential ulceration and necrosis causing an esophageal stricture after radiation therapy.*

endoscopy is recommended using a small-caliber endoscope, often within the first 6–12 hours. Endoscopy can determine the extent of injury to the esophagus, stomach, and duodenum, and help to guide management. Endoscopy should not be performed if there is evidence of

- Obvious signs of severe full-thickness esophageal or gastric necrosis with pleural irritation
- Mediastinal irritation
- Peritonitis
- Free air in the abdomen.

Endoscopic Examination

If exposure is confined to the mouth, the esophagus may appear normal. Stage I injury to the esophagus is mild, with minimal erythema of the mucosa (Fig. 4.62). Stage II is characterized by focal ulceration (Fig. 4.63). In stage III there is extensive necrosis of the mucosa (Fig. 4.64). The more extensive the necrosis, the greater the likelihood of serious sequelae such as stricture formation (Fig. 4.65). Strictures involve the proximal esophagus and may be long and extensive and difficult to dilate. Exposure of the stomach to noxious agents produces an acute gastritis with erythema, exudates, erosions, and ulcerations.

Long-standing strictures produced by lye are thought to be premalignant. Consequently, yearly endoscopy or exfoliative cytology may be beneficial to detect early malignancy. Irregularities of the mucosa should be biopsied and brushed for cytology. Endoscopy should be considered when such patients have a change in symptoms with a worsening of dysphagia.

INJURY BY MEDICINES

Prolonged contact with certain medicines can irritate the esophageal mucosa, causing esophagitis and ulceration. Affected patients often have motility disorders of the esophagus or abnormally narrowed esophageal segments. The

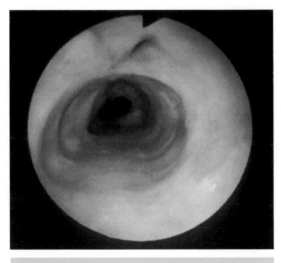
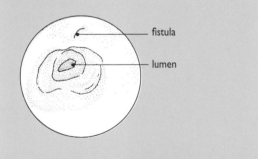

Figure 4.59 After radiation therapy for breast cancer, esophagitis resulted in a tracheoesophageal fistula. The orifice of the fistula is seen here, and the surrounding mucosa is pale.

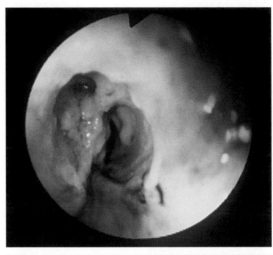

Figure 4.60 Deep ulceration with an impending tracheoesophageal fistula can be observed in this patient with severe radiation esophagitis.

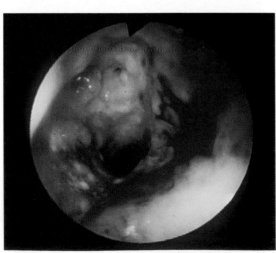
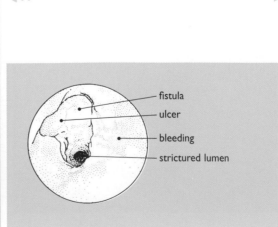
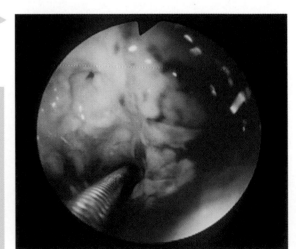

Figure 4.61 (A) Severe radiation esophagitis, with stricture, ulceration, and early fistula. **(B)** A guidewire is passed endoscopically through the stricture, reducing the chance of perforation during dilation.

problem may occur in patients with normal peristalsis if certain medications are ingested with minimal fluid right before lying down. Tetracycline taken chronically for acne is a common offender. These patients often present with severe odynophagia, dysphagia, or chest pain. The injury is often in the proximal esophagus but may occur proximal to a physiologic or pathologic narrowing, such as above the impression caused by the left atrium or by an enlarged aorta.

Endoscopic Examination

Often, a localized area of injury is seen associated with exudation and ulceration (Fig. 4.66). In other cases the esophageal mucosa may appear relatively normal, with a cleanly punched-out ulcer or, in some cases, two 'kissing' ulcers on opposite sides of the esophageal wall (Fig. 4.67). If the necrosis is severe, the mucosa may slough with bleeding (Fig. 4.68). Subsequently, a stricture may form in the area of the injury (Figs. 4.69 and 4.70). In most

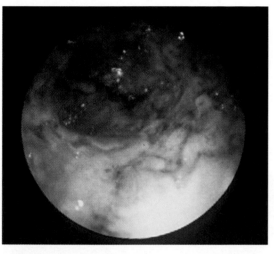

Figure 4.62 *Stage I–II esophageal injury after caustic ingestion. The patient presented with retrosternal pain and was found to have mild to moderate esophageal damage with erythema.*

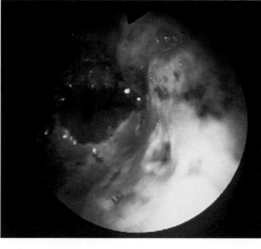

Figure 4.63 *Stage II esophageal injury. Focal ulceration is noted proximal to the esophagogastric junction.*

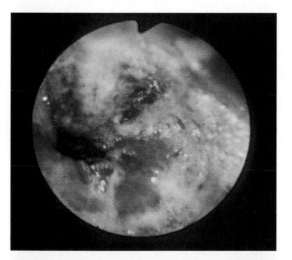

Figure 4.64 *Stage III esophageal injury. The mucosa was extensively burned by caustic ingestion and is edematous. The lumen is narrowed.*

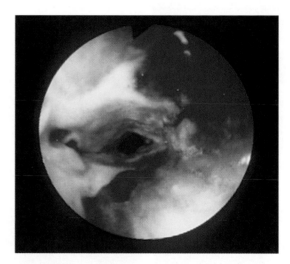

Figure 4.65 *Esophageal stricture caused by severe caustic injury. The area proximal to the stenosis is erythematous and friable.*

Figure 4.66 *Ulceration and stenosis in the proximal esophagus due to pill ingestion.*

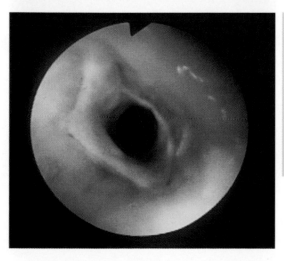

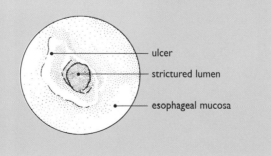

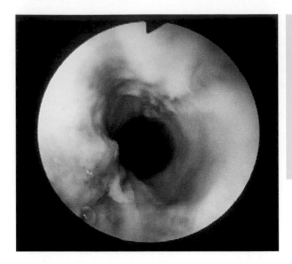

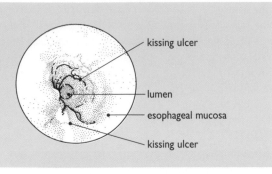

Figure 4.67 *'Kissing ulcers' in the proximal esophagus caused by the ingestion of indomethacin.*

▽ **A**

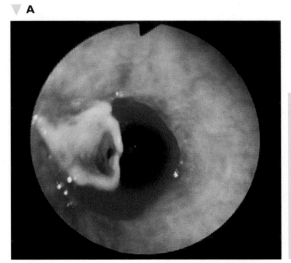

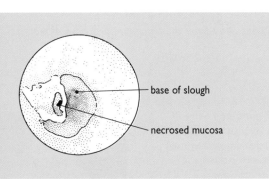

▽ **B**

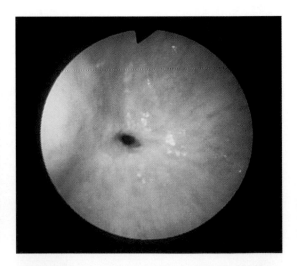

Figure 4.68 (A) *Severe, drug-induced esophageal injury. The narrowed, circumferentially injured esophageal mucosa has pulled away from the wall and is being sloughed.* **(B)** *A close-up view of the sloughed mucosa reveals raw, bleeding underlying submucosa.*

▽ **A**

▽ **B**

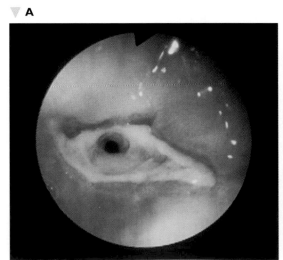

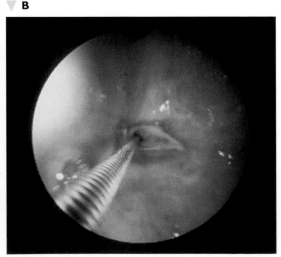

Figure 4.69 (A) *Proximal esophagitis with a stricture caused by medication ingestion.* **(B)** *A guidewire is passed endoscopically to facilitate dilation of the stricture.*

Figure 4.70 *This tight esophageal stricture resulted from medication. The mucosa down to the stricture appears normal.*

of these patients the esophageal mucosa distal to the injury is normal, which helps differentiate this type of injury from reflux injury. In the absence of Barrett's metaplasia, reflux damage is always noted distally, starting just above the squamocolumnar junction.

TRAUMATIC INJURY

Nasogastric tubes, placed postoperatively while the ileus resolves or used therapeutically for conditions such as pancreatitis, are the most common cause of traumatic injury to the esophagus. The tube interferes with swallowing, makes reflux of gastric contents into the distal esophagus more likely, and interferes with the natural acid-clearing mechanism of the distal esophagus. The likelihood of injury increases with time, with the most severe injuries occurring after more than 1 week; however, significant injury may occur sooner. Less frequently, endoscopes and Sengstaken-Blakemore tubes used to control bleeding esophageal varices may injure the wall.

Frequent and forceful vomiting may also injure the esophagus. The gastric mucosa may prolapse into the distal esophagus, tearing the esophageal or gastric mucosa. This type of mucosal injury with bleeding is called a Mallory-Weiss tear. A deeper, full-thickness tear is referred to as Boerhaave syndrome.

Endoscopic Examination

Injury from nasogastric tubes varies from red streaks with rows of submucosal petechiae to severe esophagitis with linear ulcers, erythema, and exudation (Figs. 4.71–4.73). If the injury continues, a tight stricture may result. These strictures are often short but may involve more than 10 cm of esophagus. Dilation may be difficult, especially if the stricture is long. Because of this problem, some physicians favor the placement of percutaneous gastrostomy tubes. Draining the stomach via a gastrostomy reduces the chance of reflux and obviates the need for a tube through the esophagogastric junction. The gastrostomy tube can be used to feed the patient, sometimes in conjunction with feeding jejunostomy tubes.

Injury from an endoscopic procedure has a characteristic appearance of erythema with a few scattered petechiae in a linear pattern (Fig. 4.74).

Mallory-Weiss tears cause upper gastrointestinal bleeding, and may occur in the esophagus (Figs. 4.75 and 4.76) or in the stomach (Fig. 4.77). At

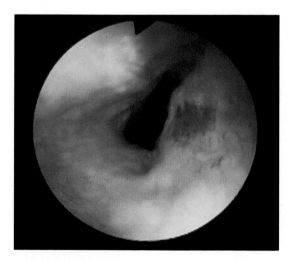
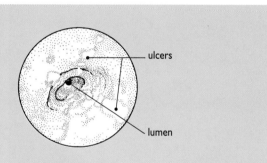

Figure 4.71 Shallow, linear esophageal ulcers caused by prolonged contact with a nasogastric tube.

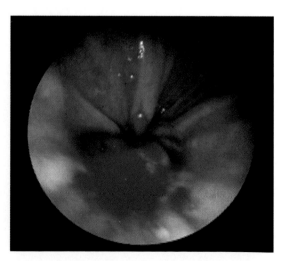

Figure 4.72 Longitudinal erosions and exudates caused by a nasogastric tube that had been in place only 24 hours.

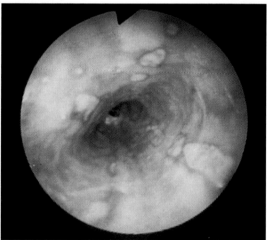

Figure 4.73 The erythematous patch in the distal esophagus is a submucosal bruise caused by suction from a nasogastric tube.

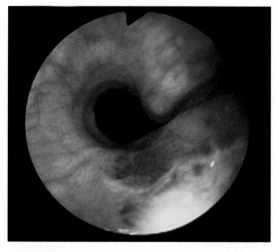

Figure 4.74 Evidence of minimal trauma to the esophagus in the form of scattered petechiae and minimal exudation resulted from endoscopy several days earlier.

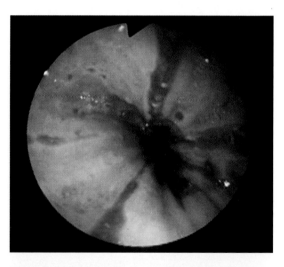

Figure 4.75 An actively bleeding Mallory-Weiss tear just above the esophagogastric junction.

endoscopy, they may appear to be actively bleeding (Fig. 4.78), show signs of recent hemorrhage with an adherent clot, or show no evidence of recent bleeding. In some cases a protruding clot may be noted (Figs. 4.79 and 4.80).

Rarely, an adjacent hematoma may be seen (Fig. 4.81). The tears in the mucosa may be superficial, or deep (Fig. 4.82), although not transmural. Patients with full-thickness tears usually show clinical signs of a perforated

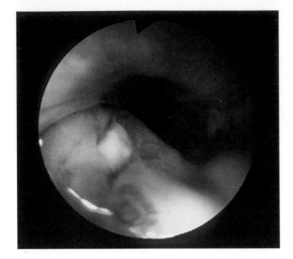

Figure 4.76 *Esophageal Mallory-Weiss tear with white base.*

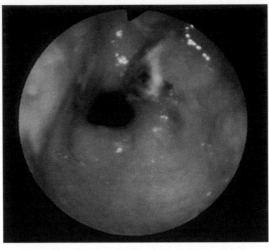

Figure 4.77 *A Mallory-Weiss tear on the gastric side of the squamocolumnar junction. The bleeding point is seen as a dot on the lesion; no active bleeding is noted.*

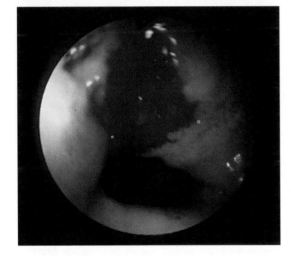

Figure 4.78 *Tear caused by overstretching with an endoscopic balloon. Bleeding is active.*

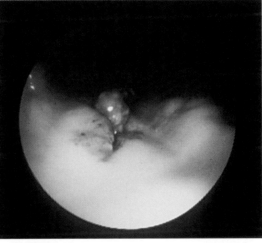

Figure 4.79 *A Mallory-Weiss tear in a patient on hemodialysis for renal failure. The patient bled severely. A protruding coagulum is seen at the base of the tear.*

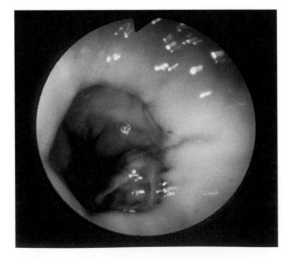

Figure 4.80 *Mallory-Weiss tear with adherent adjacent clot.*

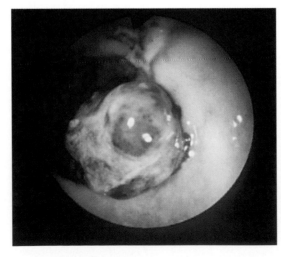

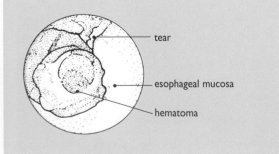

Figure 4.81 *Mallory-Weiss tear with adjacent hematoma involving the distal esophageal wall.*

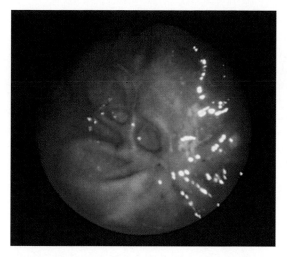

Figure 5.18 *Healed gastric ulcer on greater curvature showing scarring and retraction with converging folds.*

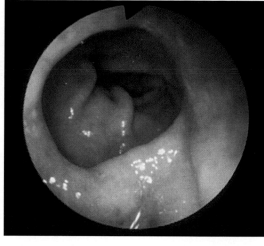

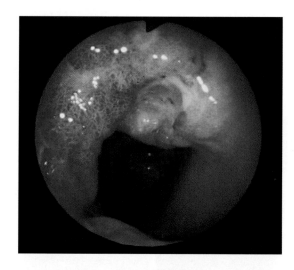

Figure 5.19 *Antral diaphragm has occurred presumably after healing of gastric ulcers.*

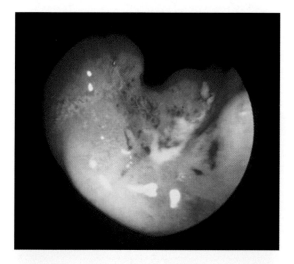

Figure 5.20 *Malignant gastric ulcer of the angularis, with irregular ulcer base and irregular erythema of the margins.*

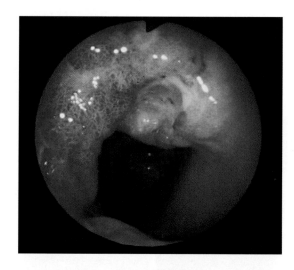

Figure 5.21 *This benign-looking gastric ulcer proved to be malignant after multiple biopsies. Note uniform erythema of the surrounding mucosa.*

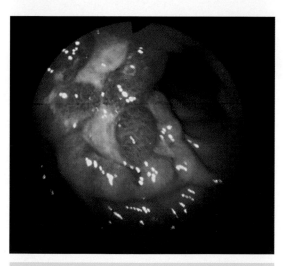

Figure 5.22 *Malignant gastric ulcer in the antrum. The nodular heaped-up margins are particularly suggestive of malignancy.*

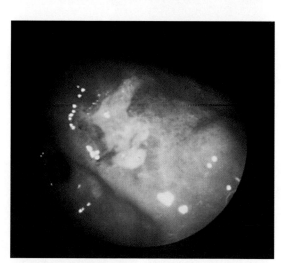

Figure 5.23 *This gastric ulcer demonstrates signs of malignancy: a depressed and discolored area, folds that do not merge with the ulcer crater, and irregularity of the crater.*

EXOGENOUS CAUSES OF GASTRIC ULCERS

Mechanical pressure on the gastric mucosa can cause significant gastric ulceration. An example is an ulcer caused by pressure necrosis resulting from an intragastric balloon used as a treatment for obesity (Fig. 5.24). Drugs can also cause gastric ulceration, similar to that noted in the esophagus. These ulcers may occur in the antrum (as is often the case with aspirin) or elsewhere in the stomach, such as the cardia.

BIOPSY

The early changes of gastric cancer are endoscopically misdiagnosed as benign disease in approximately 10% of cases. Therefore, many endoscopists feel that multiple biopsies must be obtained from any gastric ulcer. Biopsies should be taken from each quadrant of the lesion, ideally from the inner edge of the margin, and from the ulcer base if it is nodular or abnormal in appearance. Often only one or two of eight to ten biopsy specimens will reveal a focus of malignancy. Depressed areas at the erythematous margin of an ulcer should be recognized as high risk areas for a tumor and should be biopsied preferentially. Such depressed areas may appear so red that the differentiation between a neoplasm and regenerating tissue at the margin of a benign peptic ulcer may be difficult.

Healing of a gastric ulcer is no guarantee of its benign nature, because benign and malignant ulcers may have a similar healing cycle, and a seemingly healed ulcer may still contain a malignancy. Therefore, several biopsy examinations may be needed, occasionally with biopsies of the ulcer scar, to exclude malignancy.

Provided multiple biopsies are taken, a high accuracy in distinguishing benign from malignant gastric ulcers is probable. When indicated, endoscopic brush cytology should be performed before biopsy, for maximum diagnostic yield. Of value, though rarely used, is the salvage cytology technique, which uses a mucous trap between the endoscope and the suction line. The biopsy channel is aspirated between biopsy specimens and 1–5 ml fluid is collected. The fluid is diluted with alcohol or other suitable fixative and submitted for cytologic examination. This technique salvages malignant cells within the channel that have dropped off the biopsy forceps.

▼ **A**

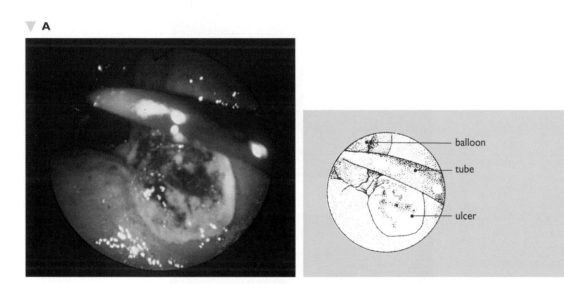

▼ **B**

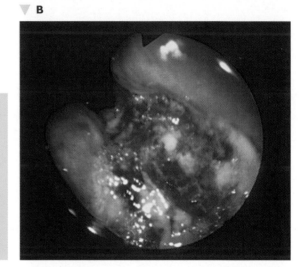

Figure 5.24 (**A**) Large ulceration along the lesser curvature due to pressure necrosis from a gastric balloon inserted for obesity. (**B**) A close-up view.

▼ **A**   ▼ **B**

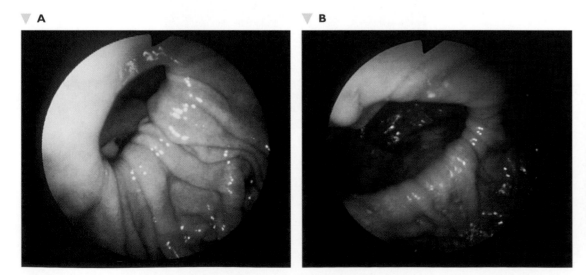

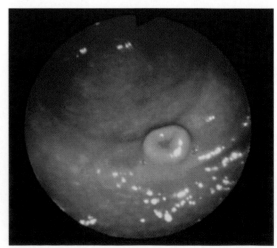

Figure 5.25 (**A**) Subcardial diverticulum, with folds entering the outpouching. (**B**) Close-up view of diverticulum.

Figure 5.26 Characteristic appearance of ectopic pancreatic tissue. Note the central dimple.

ANATOMIC ABNORMALITIES

GASTRIC DIVERTICULUM

A gastric diverticulum is an outpouching of all of the wall layers. The sub-cardial region about 2 cm distal from the cardia and 3 cm dorsal to the lesser curvature is most commonly affected (Fig. 5.25). Less common sites are the prepyloric region and, rarely, the fundus or gastric greater curvature. The mouth of the diverticulum may be round, oval or slit-like. Radial folds frequently enter the diverticular outpouching. Potential complications are ulceration, hemorrhage, and food impaction, but these are rare.

ECTOPIC PANCREATIC TISSUE

Ectopic masses of pancreatic tissue are usually encountered along the greater curvature of the antrum (Fig. 5.26). Foci of ectopic pancreas often show characteristic bridging folds. A dimple or depression may be seen on the surface, which represents the opening of the draining ectopic pancreatic tissue (Fig. 5.27).

GASTROESOPHAGEAL PROLAPSE

Discrete gastroesophageal prolapse may be observed during endoscopy. Violent vomiting or retching during endoscopy may lead to repetitive forceful gastroesophageal prolapse and subsequent traumatization of the gastric mucosa. A major part of the stomach may enter the esophagus, especially when the hiatal ring is patulous. A characteristic endoscopic finding is the presence of a knuckle of congested and sometimes bleeding mucosa that repeatedly prolapses into the esophageal lumen during retching (Fig. 5.28) and retracts into the stomach during relaxation. The resulting lesion is usually within 5 cm of the gastroesophageal junction, though not continuous with it. The damaged area is usually a well defined, relatively small, circular area of congested or hemorrhagic mucosa. The edges are usually abrupt, with normal mucosa suddenly changing to erythematous or blotchy, bright red, hyperemic mucosa. The shape and position of the lesion depends on which part of the stomach is forced through the cardiac orifice. Either a ring-like or a disk-type lesion may be produced. As a consequence of prolapse, more extensive intramural bleeding may occur, occasionally leading to sloughing of the underlying mucosa (Figs. 5.29 and 5.30).

▼ A 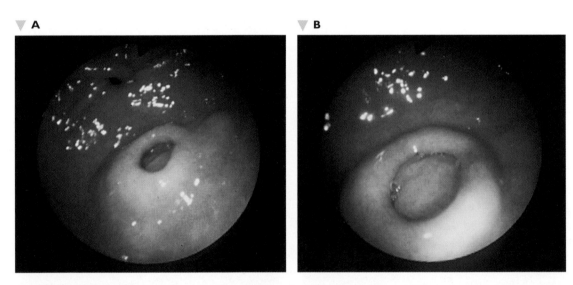 ▼ B

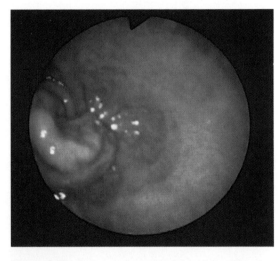

Figure 5.27 (**A**) Ectopic pancreas with central depression along the greater curvature. (**B**) A close-up view.

Figure 5.28 Gastroesophageal prolapse. A knuckle of reddened gastric mucosa is visible in the distal esophagus.

▼ A 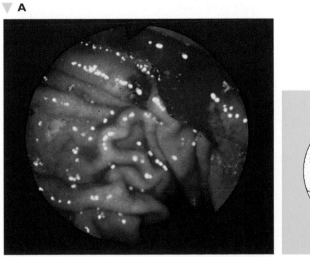 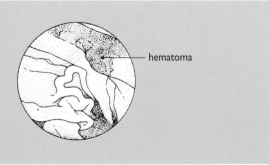 ▼ B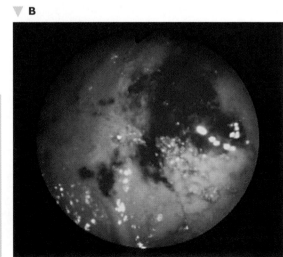

Figure 5.29 (**A**) Damage to the greater curvature area with erythema, intramural petechiae, and hematoma formation caused by gastroesophageal prolapse. (**B**) A better view of the hematoma.

MALLORY-WEISS TEAR

Mechanical laceration in the area of the gastroesophageal junction, termed a Mallory-Weiss tear, is a common cause of upper gastrointestinal bleeding. A sudden increase in intra-abdominal pressure during violent retching or vomiting is considered the main cause. Alcoholics or patients on dialysis are most susceptible. The tears are usually linear, longitudinally oriented, and occasionally star-shaped. Tears are usually only a few millimeters wide, but sometimes up to several centimeters long. They often extend up into the squamous mucosa, but more commonly involve the columnar cardiac-type mucosa. The tears may be superficial or extend into the submucosa. During the acute phase, oozing or even spurting bleeding may be seen, although most often the lesion is covered with an adherent clot. After sloughing of the clot a superficial necrotic defect remains, covered with a white base. Rapid healing usually occurs (Fig. 5.31). A visible vessel may be seen in the lesion base (Fig. 5.32). A tear may only be seen with the endoscope tip retroflexed (Fig. 5.33).

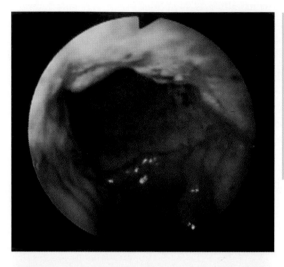

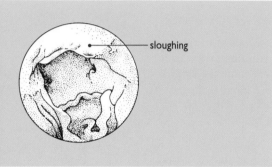

Figure 5.30 *Sloughing of the subcardial lesser curvature area after intramural bleeding secondary to prolonged violent retching.*

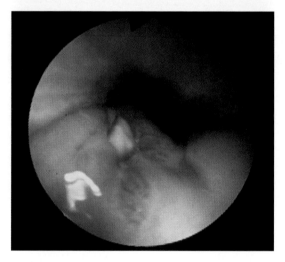

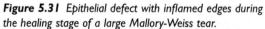

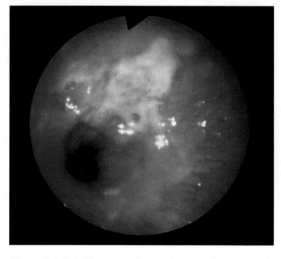

Figure 5.31 *Epithelial defect with inflamed edges during the healing stage of a large Mallory-Weiss tear.*

Figure 5.32 *A Mallory-Weiss tear is seen with a central spot thought to be a visible vessel.*

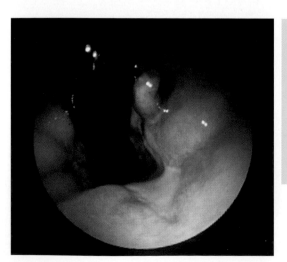

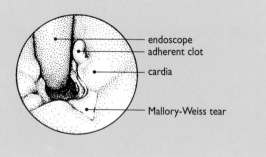

Figure 5.33 *A Mallory-Weiss tear at the cardia is best seen with the endoscope tip retroflexed in the stomach. An adherent clot is noted.*

VASCULAR ABNORMALITIES

GASTRIC TELANGIECTASES

The terminology of vascular lesions in the upper gastrointestinal tract is confusing. Vascular lesions have been described by many terms such as arteriovenous malformations, angiodysplasia, telangiectasia, hemangioma, telangiopathy, and mucosal vascular abnormalities. Although telangiectatic vessels can be seen endoscopically, it is not possible to determine the size or depth of the underlying vascular structures. This may be important when considering endoscopic treatment with a heater probe or laser.

Gastric telangiectases have been associated with von Willebrand's disease, collagen vascular disorders, Turner's syndrome, valvular heart disease, previous radiation therapy, chronic renal failure, and especially Rendu-Osler-Weber syndrome (hereditary hemorrhagic telangiectasia). The latter disorder is inherited as an autosomal dominant trait with an incidence of about 5 per 100 000. These patients have telangiectases of mucous membranes, tongue, toes, and fingers. Most bleeding telangiectases in Rendu-Osler-Weber syndrome are located in the cecum, right colon, or the posterior aspect of the gastric corpus. The duodenal bulb, the postbulbar duodenum, and the sigmoid colon are less commonly involved.

Endoscopically, telangiectases are bright cherry red, flat or slightly elevated lesions, varying in diameter from pinpoint to 10 mm. They may be single or multiple (Figs. 5.34–5.36). Small telangiectatic lesions are limited to the mucosal layer. Larger, slightly elevated, or umbilicated lesions may have extensive submucosal or transmural anastomoses. An arteriovenous malformation may be localized to the fundus (Fig. 5.37).

The differential diagnosis of small flat telangiectatic lesions includes clots or adherent blood, erosion, an endoscopic suction artifact (Fig. 5.38), and, rarely, Kaposi's sarcoma (Fig. 5.39). Petechiae and submucosal hemorrhages related to thrombocytopenia, sepsis, severe coagulopathy, or renal failure are easily distinguished by their appearance and clinical setting. Depressed, angiomatous lesions may be mistaken for ulcers or erosions, particularly if adherent clots are present.

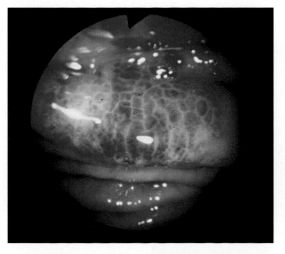

Figure 5.34 *An intensely red, slightly raised telangiectatic lesion along the posterior wall of the corpus. Note the star-like contours of the lesion.*

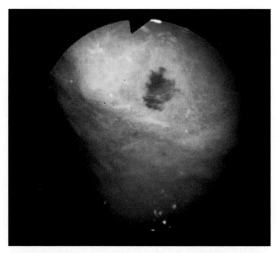

Figure 5.35 *A solitary telangiectasia in the proximal stomach. Mild inflammatory changes are visible in the surrounding mucosa.*

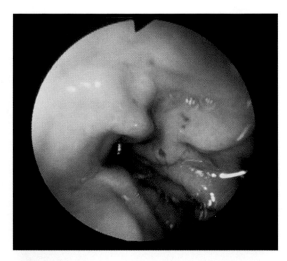

Figure 5.36 *Multiple, small, red telangiectasias in a patient with Rendu-Osler-Weber syndrome.*

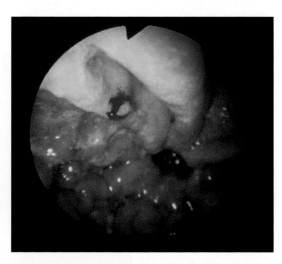

Figure 5.37 *Arteriovenous malformation localized to the gastric fundus.*

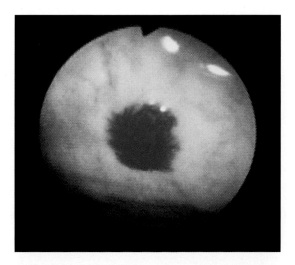

Figure 5.38 *Suction artifact in a Billroth II stomach mimics a vascular lesion.*

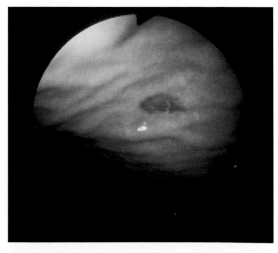

Figure 5.39 *This small focus of Kaposi's sarcoma mimics a telangiectatic lesion.*

Small, flat, discrete telangiectases measuring less than 5 mm in diameter are the easiest to treat endoscopically, using bipolar electrocoagulation, heater probe, or laser (Figs. 5.40–5.42). Larger lesions can also be treated, but they may bleed during therapy. This induced bleeding can usually be stopped with further endoscopic treatment.

More extensive telangiectatic lesions called gastric antral vascular ectasia (GAVE) occur, especially in the antrum, in patients with cirrhosis of the liver. Parallel longitudinal rugal folds are seen traversing the antrum and converging onto the pylorus, each containing a visible convoluted column of vessels. The aggregate appearance resembles the stripes on a watermelon (Figs. 5.43 and 5.44). In addition, round red spots may be observed in the surrounding mucosa (Fig. 5.45). Unlike the abnormalities seen in hemorrhagic gastritis, the red linear streaks in the antrum blanch upon pressure

with a biopsy forceps. There is a peculiar tendency for the telangiectatic lesions to cluster along the crest of the longitudinal folds. Spontaneous bleeding and bleeding on contact is frequently noted. On careful inspection, some of the red dots have a brownish discoloration suggesting prior bleeding. The mucosa is unusually mobile with a tendency to prolapse into and out of the aborally progressing contraction waves.

Histologically, capillaries are dilated with focal thrombosis and fibromuscular hyperplasia of the lamina propria. The lesion is thought to develop from intramural vascular shunts as a response to portal hypertension. Endoscopic biopsies are inadvisable because such lesions may bleed excessively. If these lesions do cause clinically significant blood loss, laser therapy may be helpful to treat the lesion and reduce bleeding.

▼ **A** ▼ **B**

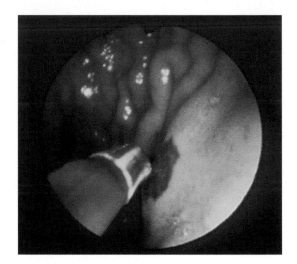

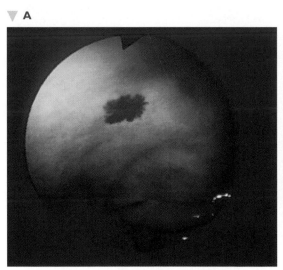

Figure 5.40 *Bipolar electrocoagulation probe in close proximity to a telangiectatic lesion.*

Figure 5.41 *(A) Gastric angiodysplastic lesion before laser therapy. (B) A small ulcer remains a few days after laser photocoagulation.*

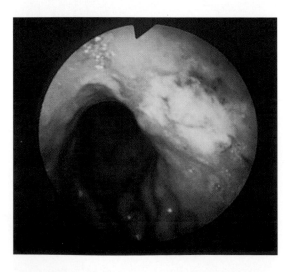

Figure 5.42 *Necrotic changes and whitish discoloration 1 day after coagulation of a large hemangioma with a heater probe.*

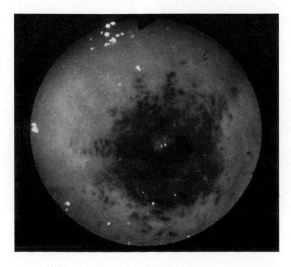

Figure 5.43 *Antral telangiectasia. Note the characteristic linear red stripes.*

PORTAL HYPERTENSIVE CONGESTIVE GASTROPATHY

Patients with portal hypertension may present with congestion of the gastric mucosa, or congestive gastroenteropathy. This type of lesion is thought to occur mainly in the body of the stomach but may also be seen in the antrum. It is characterized by congestion of the gastric mucosa and reportedly correlates to the degree of portal hypertension and the extent of mucosal congestion, as measured by reflectance spectrophotometry. The mucosa appears diffusely red; petechiae and small amounts of bleeding may be noted (Figs. 5.46 and 5.47). Gastric varices may also be found in these patients.

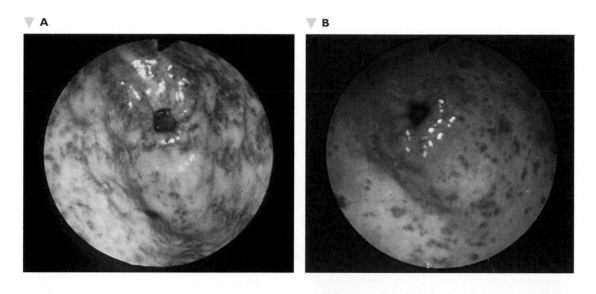

Figure 5.44 (**A** and **B**) Two cases of antral telangiectasia, with somewhat convoluted and sacculated columns of vessels.

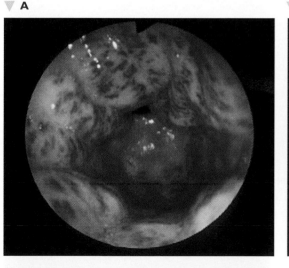

Figure 5.45 (**A** and **B**) Antral telangiectasia in two patients. (**A**) A peculiar alignment of erythematous dots along the ridges of mucosal folds. (**B**) What appears to be gastric angiomatosis of the antrum.

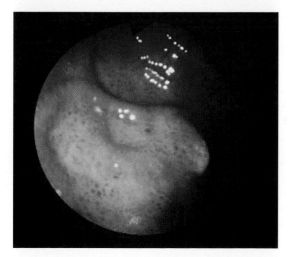

Figure 5.46 Congestive gastroenteropathy with portal hypertension. The mucosa is red and petechiae are noted.

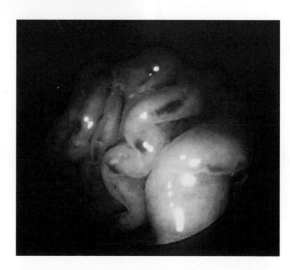

Figure 5.47 Congestive gastroenteropathy in a patient with portal hypertension. The mucosa is red and friable; a small amount of bleeding is noted.

GASTRIC VARICES

Gastric varices are seen as submucosal structures that may have a mottled appearance or even resemble clusters of grapes (Figs. 5.48–5.50). The bluish color characteristic of esophageal varices is usually absent in the stomach.

Gastric varices may be confused with enlarged folds, except when they run perpendicularly to the axis of the folds. Isolated gastric varices may develop as a consequence of pancreatic disorders that obstruct the splenic vein (Figs. 5.51 and 5.52).

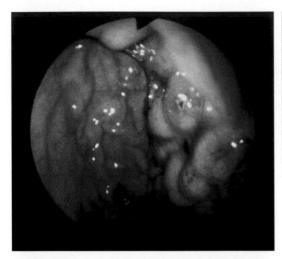

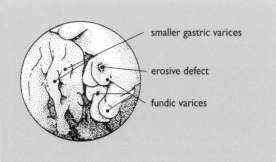

Figure 5.48 A cluster of varices in the gastric fundus, with erythematous spots on top of convex bulges.

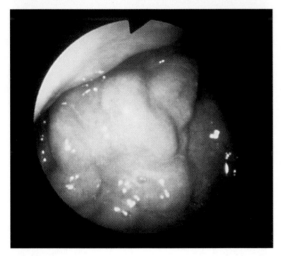

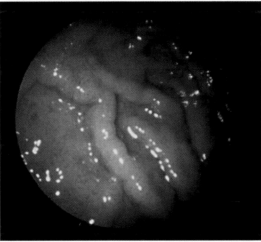

Figure 5.49 A cluster of tortuous fundic varices covered by normal-appearing mucosa, which may be confused with enlarged gastric folds.

Figure 5.50 Gastric varices mimicking gastric folds. Note the discrete nodularity.

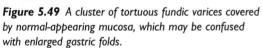

▼ **A**　　　　▼ **B**

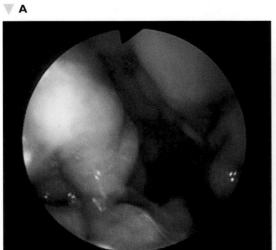

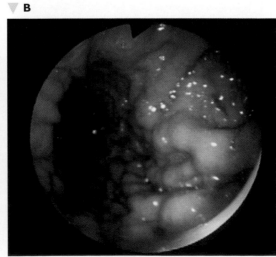

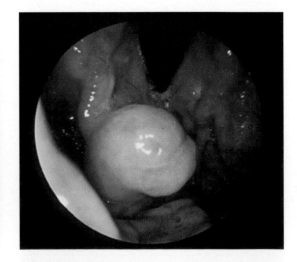

Figure 5.51 (**A** and **B**) Two views of gastric varices caused by pancreatic disease resulting in thrombosis of the splenic vein.

Figure 5.52 Gastric varix at the cardia simulates tumor. Biopsy can cause severe bleeding.

DIEULAFOY LESION

A Dieulafoy lesion is a vascular abnormality characterized by brisk bleeding caused by a protuberant artery with little or no surrounding ulceration. Endoscopically, the lesion may not be visible unless there is spurting bleeding or an adherent clot projects from the luminal surface (Fig. 5.53). It may be difficult to diagnose this lesion endoscopically. Several endoscopies may be needed and the chance that surgery will be required to control bleeding is higher than with a gastric ulcer. These lesions have been effectively treated hemostatically with endoscopic injection of epinephrine or ethoxysclerol, photocoagulation with the Nd:YAG laser or application of the heater probe. The underlying vascular anomaly is detectable with endosonography.

VASCULITIS

Vasculitis involving the stomach is rare. The changes are nonspecific and include edema, erythema, and submucosal bleeding spots. The overall appearance resembles hemorrhagic gastritis (Fig. 5.54).

OTHER GASTRIC ABNORMALITIES

GASTRIC ISCHEMIA

Rarely, ischemic necrosis of the stomach may occur if the arterial blood supply to the stomach is severely compromised as a result of obstruction of the celiac trunk and the superior and inferior mesenteric arteries. Ischemic damage is usually characterized by extensive sloughing of the superficial layers of the stomach with a sharp transition between the infarcted areas and the normal adjacent mucosa (Fig. 5.55).

FOREIGN BODIES

Foreign bodies such as coins, balls, dental drills, dental plates, blades, and knives may become lodged in the stomach (Fig. 5.56). If the object is sharp, a plastic overtube is recommended to protect the cardia and the esophagus

▼ **A**

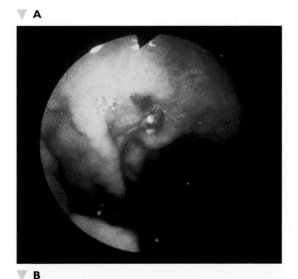

Figure 5.53 (**A**) *Dieulafoy lesion covered with an adherent clot. This lesion was responsible for recurrent massive bleeding.* (**B**) *Corresponding histology of the anomaly.*

▼ **B**

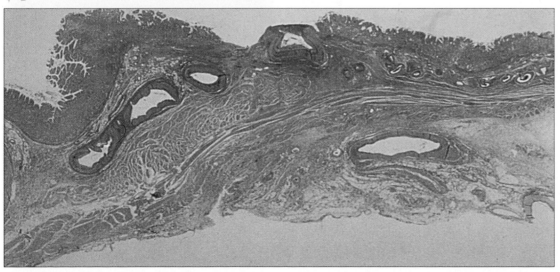

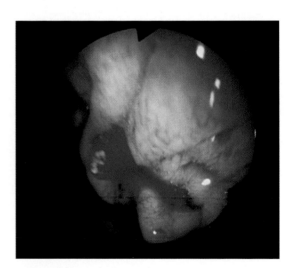

Figure 5.54 *Histologically confirmed vasculitis of the stomach mucosa, with hemorrhagic gastritis and chronic bleeding.*

during removal. An overtube protects against tracheal aspiration as the object is removed. The overtube also allows multiple passages of the endoscope into the stomach, as may be required to remove multiple foreign bodies. Strong grasping forceps or polypectomy snares are recommended for removal. If both ends of an object impact the stomach wall, a lasso may be created around the foreign object using a double-channel endoscope. The use of a

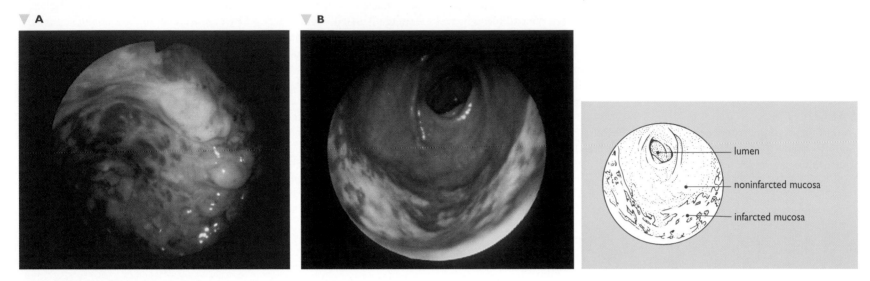

Figure 5.55 *Gastric ischemia. (**A**) Whitish necrotic slough in the proximal stomach. (**B**) In this view the sharp transition in the distal stomach between infarcted and noninfarcted mucosa can be seen.*

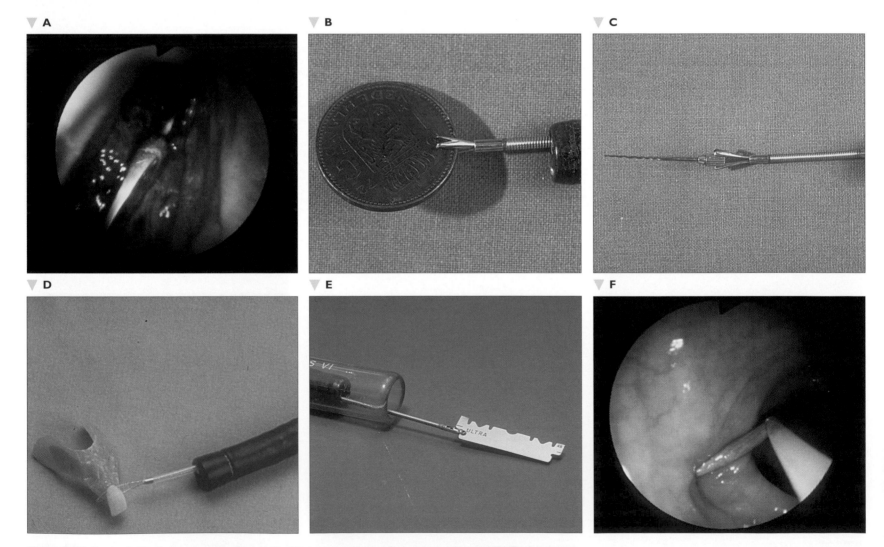

Figure 5.56 *Foreign bodies in the stomach. (**A**) A knife. (**B**) A removed coin. (**C**) A removed dental drill. (**D**) A removed dental plate. (**E**) A removed razor blade. Use of an overtube to remove the blade safely is demonstrated. (**F**) A piece of wood is grasped with a snare before endoscopic removal.*

lasso enables the endoscopist to retrieve the foreign object, usually with minimal difficulty, provided the object is flexible enough to pass the cardia and upper esophageal sphincter while being held (Fig. 5.57).

THE POSTOPERATIVE STOMACH

The stomach is a site of various surgical procedures. The endoscopist should be aware of the different features that develop as a consequence of surgical manipulation.

SURGICAL ARTIFACTS
Pyloroplasty

After truncal vagotomy, a concomitant pyloroplasty is often carried out. The defect created by a Heineke-Mikulicz procedure is typified by an open pylorus through which another ring may be seen. This type of pyloroplasty can be difficult to examine. The endoscopist must be concerned about the occurrence of an ulcer in the deformed area. Therefore it is important to examine the areas of both rings and the mucosa between the rings carefully

(Fig. 5.58). The Jaboulay pyloroplasty is actually an anastomosis between the antrum and the duodenum created adjacent to the stenosed pylorus. When a deep ulcer results in a fistulous tract between the antrum and duodenal bulb, a double pylorus is noted, similar to the defect after a surgical gastroduodenostomy (Fig. 5.59).

Partial Gastrectomy

In a Billroth I partial gastrectomy, the rugal folds terminate abruptly and circumferentially around the stoma, occasionally creating a nodular appearance. The mucosa covering these nodules is identical to that surrounding the stoma. The width of the nodules, however, may exceed that of the more proximal rugal folds. Within the stoma, erythematous gastric mucosa joins the grayish-pink flat duodenal mucosa (Fig. 5.60).

In a Billroth II operation, the stoma is usually 15–20 cm below the gastroesophageal junction. The transition between the orange–red gastric mucosa and the more yellow–gray jejunal mucosa is easily identified within the stomal opening. Some nodular folding may be observed along the lesser curvature as a result of the surgical procedure. A carina-like structure or fold

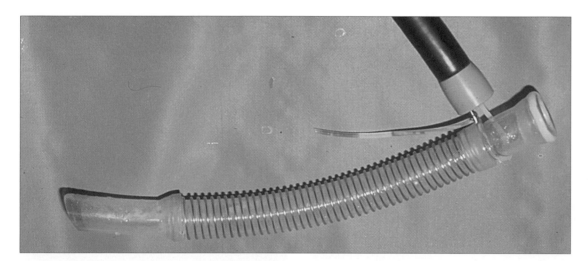

Figure 5.57 *This endoprosthesis was removed from the stomach using a double-channel endoscope.*

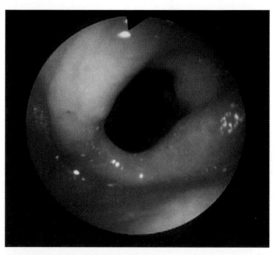

Figure 5.58 *Heineke-Mikulicz pyloroplasty, with a gaping pylorus and a concentric second ring.*

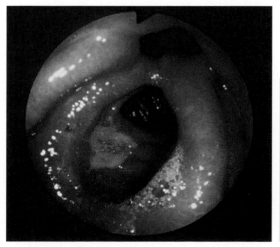

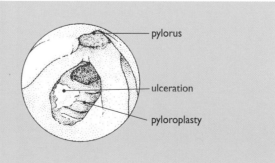

Figure 5.59 *Jaboulay-type pyloroplasty with recurrent ulceration. Note the bridge between the pylorus and the gastroduodenostomy.*

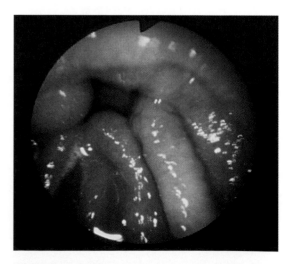

Figure 5.60 *A Billroth I partial gastrectomy produced this anastomosis with a somewhat nodular enlargement of the folds of the stoma. Erythema can also be noted.*

may be noted just beyond the gastrojejunostomy, on either side of which one may see the efferent and afferent loops (Fig. 5.61). The opening of the efferent loop is generally larger and connects more directly with the gastric lumen than does the afferent loop.

Both loops may be entered and inspected endoscopically. The afferent loop ends proximally at the duodenal bulb closure. The latter can terminate in a characteristic mass-like polyp-simulating deformity (Fig. 5.62). The papilla of Vater can often be identified. If retained antral mucosa is suspected, biop-

sies should be taken of the blind end of this afferent loop to detect the presence of gastric mucosa. The efferent loop can also be entered and traversed for 30 cm or more. Close apposition of the openings of the afferent and efferent loops at the same level is termed a double-barrel stoma. Both loops communicate directly with the gastric remnant (Fig. 5.63). The surgical deformity from a Billroth II (BII) procedure may manifest itself as abnormal-appearing gastric folds (Fig. 5.64). A granulation polyp may be noted at the level of a Billroth II anastomosis (Fig. 5.65). The presence of only one

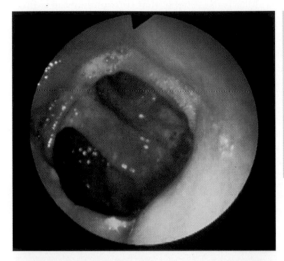

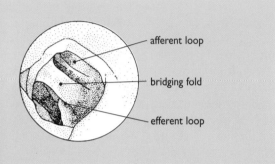

Figure 5.61 A Billroth II partial gastrectomy produced this anastomosis with a bridging fold separating the openings of the afferent and efferent loops.

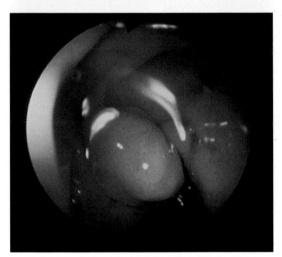

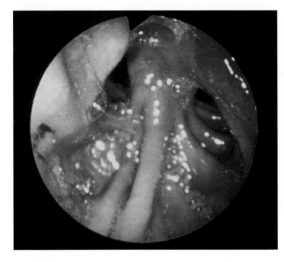

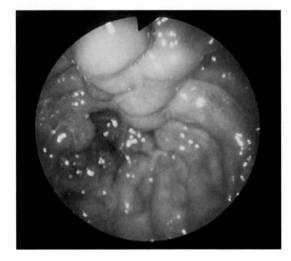

Figure 5.62 Afferent loop with an inverted duodenal bulb suture line, which may simulate a polyp.

Figure 5.63 Double-barrel stoma. Both loops are seen communicating directly with the gastric remnant.

Figure 5.64 This surgical artifact of the lesser curvature area creates the appearance of thick bulging folds covered with normal-appearing mucosa.

▼ **A**

▼ **B**

Figure 5.65 (**A** and **B**) Two views of granulation polyps at the gastric side of a Billroth II anastomosis.

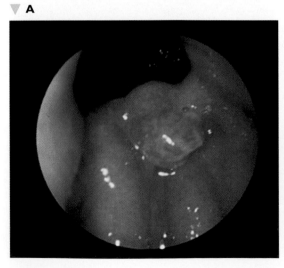

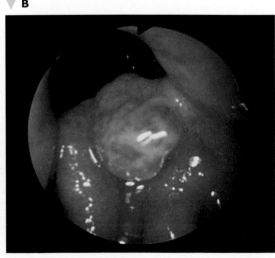

loop at the stoma suggests a Roux-en-Y anastomosis (Fig. 5.66). If the fluid in the stomach is clear and colorless, this suggests the surgery was a diversion of the Roux-en-Y type, which reduces reflux of bile into the stomach.

in the area of the anastomosis may lead to the development of an esophagus with columnar metaplasia. In the Nakayama-type anastomosis, both limbs create a reservoir pouch that can be entered and examined.

Total Gastrectomy

After total gastrectomy, the esophagus is anastomosed to the small intestine in one of three ways: end to end, end to side, or with a Nakayama-type anastomosis (Figs. 5.67–5.71). Depending upon the type of anastomosis, bile

Gastric Partition

After gastric partition or gastroplasty for obesity, the lower and upper gastric pouches are separated by a lumen that can be passed with a small caliber endoscope. Occasionally, this stoma may have to be gently dilated with a

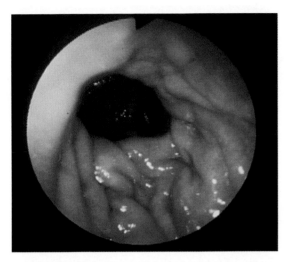

Figure 5.66 Partial gastrectomy with Roux-en-Y anastomosis. Note the normal-appearing remnant and the absence of bile.

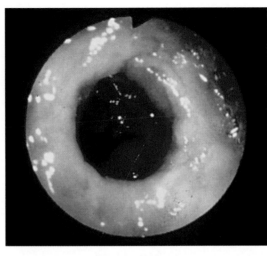

Figure 5.67 Esophagojejunostomy after total gastrectomy. Note the obvious difference in color and fold pattern between the esophagus and the small intestine.

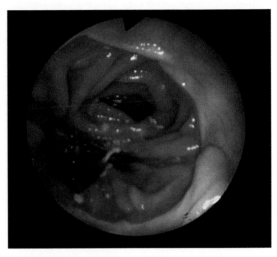

Figure 5.68 Esophagojejunal anastomosis after total gastrectomy. A pouch with two limbs can be seen just beyond the anastomosis.

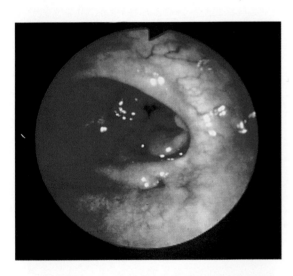

Figure 5.69 Esophagojejunostomy, with development of an endobrachy esophagus due to alkaline biliary reflux.

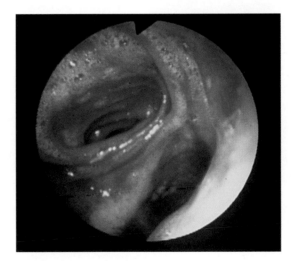

Figure 5.70 Endoscopic view of a Nakayama-type anastomosis with two lumina at the level of the anastomosis of esophagus and small intestine.

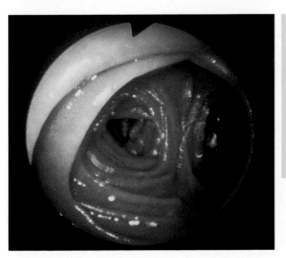

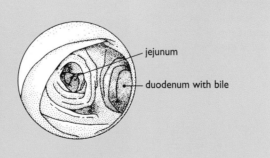

jejunum

duodenum with bile

Figure 5.71 Roux-en-Y anastomosis, with duodenal loop entering the jejunum.

dilating bougie, metal olive, or balloon catheter (Figs. 5.72 and 5.73). Care must be taken not to enlarge the stoma much over 1 cm or the purpose of the surgery will be defeated.

Gastrojejunostomy

A gastroenterostomy or jejunostomy is recognized endoscopically by the presence of a communication between the stomach and jejunum, usually along the greater curvature of the posterior wall of the distal corpus (Fig. 5.74). The distinction between gastric and small intestinal mucosa is easily recognized. Often, bile mixed with air bubbles refluxes from the small intestine into the stomach. Both the afferent and efferent sides of the anastomosis can usually be entered and examined. Gastrojejunostomy is prone to ulceration in response to copious acid secretion in the stomach.

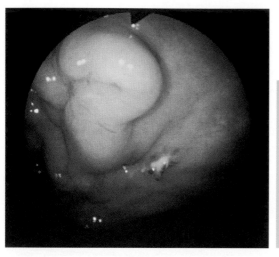

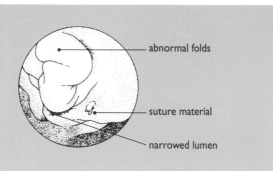

Figure 5.72 *Gastric partition, with abnormal folds along the lesser curvature and the narrowed stoma.*

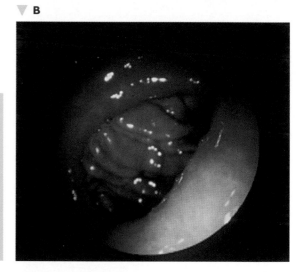

Figure 5.73 *After gastroplasty, a guidewire is inserted through the excessively narrowed lumen to guide dilation.*

▼ **A**

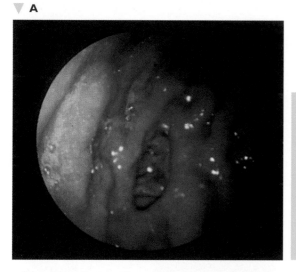

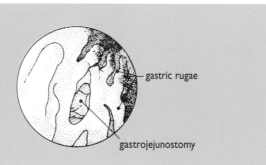

▼ **B**

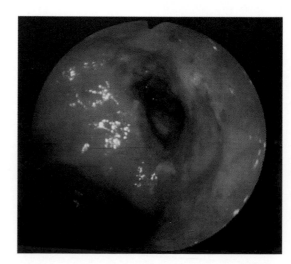

Figure 5.74 *(A) Gastrojejunostomy. (B) A close-up view of the opening.*

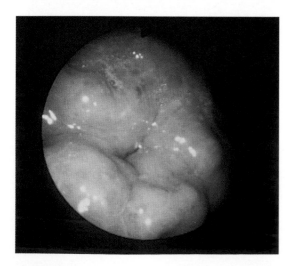

Figure 5.75 *An incompletely closed gastrostomy defect created this small fistula.*

Figure 5.76 *A gastric posterior wall defect after marsupialization of a pancreatic pseudocyst.*

Other Surgical Procedures

Rare surgical artifacts in the stomach are the consequence of previous gastrostomy (Fig. 5.75) or prior marsupialization of a pancreatic pseudocyst (Fig. 5.76).

ABNORMALITIES OF THE GASTRIC REMNANT

After partial gastrectomy, several types of abnormalities may be detectable in the gastric remnant. Slight, nonspecific erythema of the stoma is a common finding (Fig. 5.77). Such erythema is made up of innumerable reddish spots, presumably representing the areae gastricae, separated by the interconnecting lineae gastricae. Because of the mucosal capillary ectasia, there often is some degree of mucosal friability as the endoscope passes across the stomal area. Not uncommonly, the stomal area has a somewhat nodular aspect, which is usually due to the presence of prominent folds. Nodular deformity may also be caused by polypoid lesions. Such lesions may appear quite erythematous and manifest some superficial erosions (Fig. 5.78).

Protruding sutures may be observed around an area of anastomosis, even years after the previous surgery. Characteristically, retained sutures will occur as small suture granulomas. These nodules may appear discolored, and it may be possible to see the actual suture material. Exudation and inflammation may be present (Fig. 5.79). If the inflammation is severe, an ulcer may be found. Suture granulomas are submucosal masses that result from marked inflammation around suture material. They tend to deform the stoma in an asymmetrical fashion and occasionally mimic gastric neoplasm. Sutures rarely cause symptoms and need not be removed. By contrast, suture ulcers may produce symptoms and removal of such sutures may initiate healing. This is done by extracting them with a biopsy forceps or cutting with a suture-cutting forceps (Fig. 5.80).

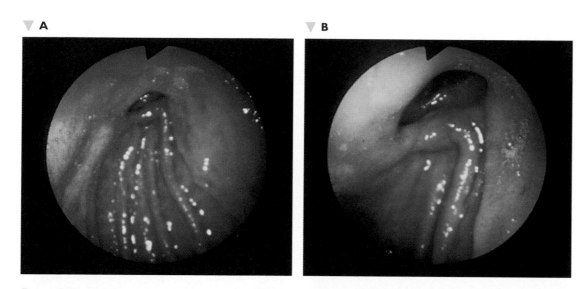

Figure 5.77 (A) Billroth II stoma with nonspecific erythema. (B) A close-up view of the stoma.

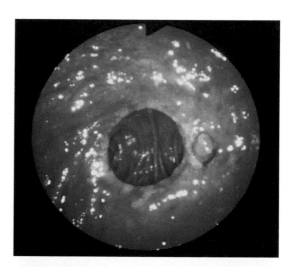

Figure 5.78 Billroth II stoma with small, polypoid excrescence and white discoloration at the anastomotic rim. This is an example of endoscopic enterogastric reflux gastritis.

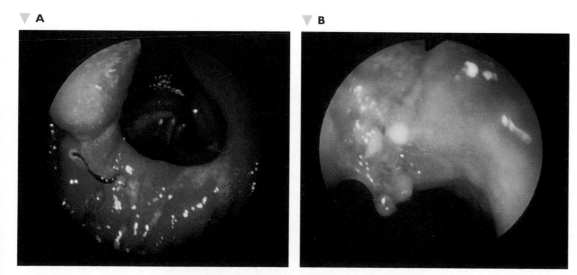

Figure 5.79 Protruding sutures. (A) Old Billroth II sutures. Note the stomal erythema. (B) Billroth II anastomosis with protruding sutures surrounded by mild inflammatory changes.

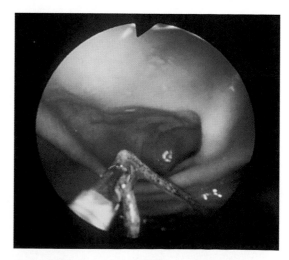

Figure 5.80 A 15-year-old Billroth II anastomosis with persistent suture material being removed with a biopsy forceps because of ongoing ulceration.

ALKALINE REFLUX GASTRITIS

Diffuse mucosal erythema and bile staining is common after partial gastrectomy. Termed endoscopic enterogastric reflux gastritis, this condition produces a burning epigastric pain (mainly postprandially), early satiety after meals, frequent bilious vomiting, nausea, and anorexia. Bile salts and lysolecithin are well known disrupters of the epithelial barrier against acid reflux, causing back-diffusion of acid in the stomach and the resulting inflammation.

The characteristic endoscopic appearance is that of severe erythema and swelling of the mucosa stained with refluxed biliary fluid. The intensely red discoloration is usually striking (Fig. 5.81). The folds are markedly swollen (Figs. 5.82), especially in the area of the stoma, and can take on a pseudopolypoid aspect. This erythema may be dramatic in patients with reflux gastritis, and is a clue to the underlying nature of the patient's illness (Fig. 5.83). There is usually friability, easily noticeable upon endoscopic manipulation. Superficial erosive defects may also be present. Histologically,

the erythema usually represents marked capillary dilation. In addition, there may be evidence of nonspecific inflammation with alteration of the epithelial layer and decreased mucus production.

STOMAL ULCER

Stomal ulceration or ulcus jejuni pepticum is common after partial gastrectomy. Erosive or ulcerative defects can best be evaluated endoscopically, although it may require considerable effort to identify ulcerative defects hidden between gastric folds or inside the jejunal edge of the stoma. Stomal ulcers are usually located within 2 cm of the anastamosis on either side of the stoma. Mucus on the mucosa may simulate an ulcer; endoscopically guided lavage using a wash catheter will clarify this issue.

A jejunal ulcer is similar in appearance to a bulbar ulcer, with a fibrinoid, whitish-gray crater and inflamed edges (Figs. 5.84 and 5.85). Occasionally, they may be large or multiple (Fig. 5.86). If the ulcer is in the stomach it is

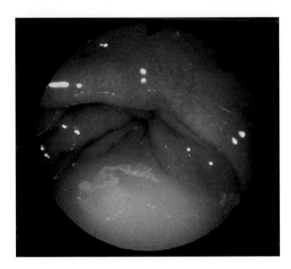

Figure 5.81 *Alkaline reflux gastritis, with intense erythema and copious amounts of bile refluxed into the stomach remnant.*

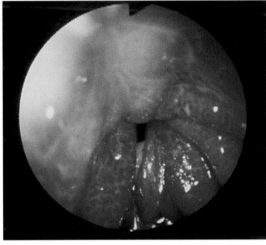

Figure 5.82 *Alkaline reflux gastritis, with heavy folds and conspicuous erythematous changes of the mucosa.*

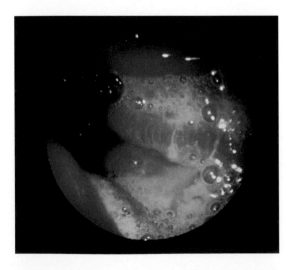

Figure 5.83 *Alkaline reflux gastritis, with intense erythema and swollen folds.*

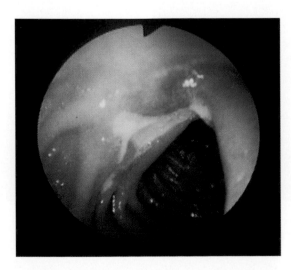

Figure 5.84 *Ulcus jejuni pepticum in the efferent loop after a Billroth II partial gastrectomy.*

considered a gastric ulcer. Bleeding may be a complication (Fig. 5.87). Rarely, a jejunal ulcer may perforate into the colon, creating a gastrojejunal colonic fistula. Gastroenteric fistula may also occur (Fig. 5.88). If the ulcer is entirely within the intestinal mucosa, gastric hypersecretion may be present (Fig. 5.89). Hypergastrinemia must always be excluded with recurrent stomal ulceration.

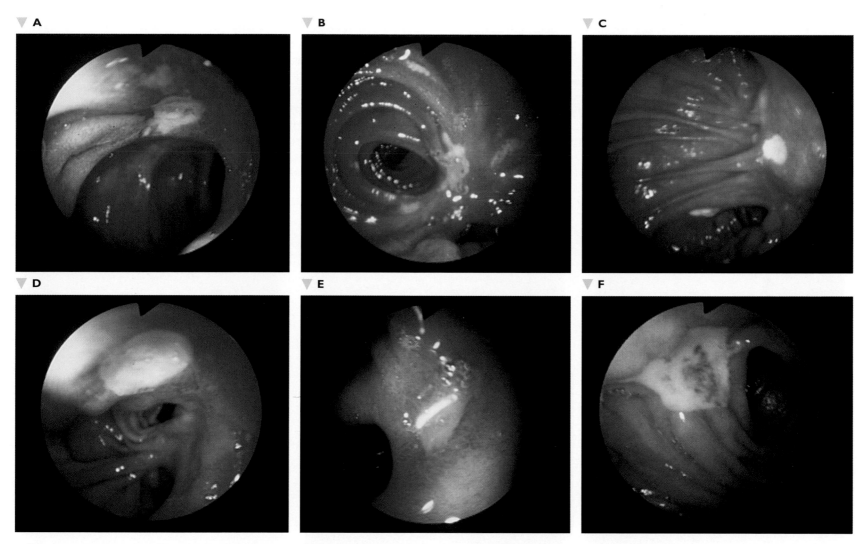

Figure 5.85 (A–F) Six examples of ulcus jejuni pepticum, showing clear ulceration on the jejunal side of the anastomosis. The ulcer base is white or bile-stained.

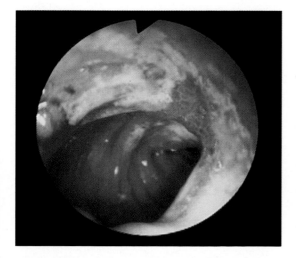

Figure 5.86 Multiple superficial ulcus jejuni pepticum.

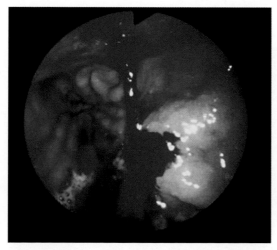

Figure 5.87 Spurting bleeding from an ulcus jejuni pepticum.

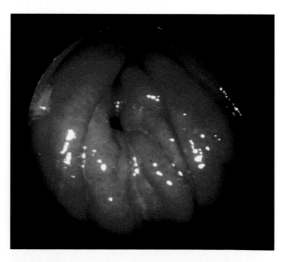

Figure 5.88 Gastroenteric fistula in a Billroth II stomach, presumed to be caused by postoperative ulceration.

STOMAL NARROWING

Stomal narrowing or stricturing may be a result of surgical technique (peristomal leak or hematoma) or secondary to stomal ulceration. Inability to pass a 10 mm endoscope across the stomal area suggests stenosis, except when the stoma is constructed with an unusual angle. To exclude obstruction confidently, both loops should be inspected for at least 5 cm. The endoscopic appearance of stricturing is that of a narrowed, fibrotic opening at the stomal area that resists passage of the endoscope. Often there is concomitant evidence of food residue or bezoar formation indicative of gastric stasis (Figs. 5.90 and 5.91).

STOMAL INTUSSUSCEPTION

Stomal intussusception is a rare, serious complication that may involve the efferent or afferent loop, or both. Endoscopically, an erythematous mass made up of jejunal folds is seen projecting through the stoma into the lumen (Fig. 5.92). The mass may prolapse intermittently through the stomal opening into the gastric lumen during episodes of vomiting or retching during endoscopy. Sometimes, conspicuous erythema are seen in the upper segment of the efferent or afferent loop, indicating previous intussusception.

BEZOAR FORMATION

A gastric bezoar is a mass of solidified food that persists in the stomach. It is a common complication after surgery for peptic ulcer disease. Bezoars may be a clinical problem in patients who have had a gastrectomy. The cause of the abnormality is not known. Various types of vegetable matter may form a mass that cannot be passed from the stomach (Fig 5.93). This mass may actually produce obstruction of the gastric outlet. There may be obstruction at the level of the stoma, but usually the stoma is wide open, indicating that bezoar formation is related to dysmotility of the gastric remnant, presumably secondary to damage of the gastric pacemaker area.

Usually a bezoar is loosely constructed and has an irregular appearance. Fragmentation may be attempted endoscopically using a wash jet technique. An overtube can be inserted for repeated passage of the endoscope as pieces of the bezoar are removed. The overtube also protects the patient's airway as the objects are removed. Endoscopic removal is followed by a combination of dietary restriction of fiber, instruction in proper mastication, and occasionally the use of an oral preparation of cellulase.

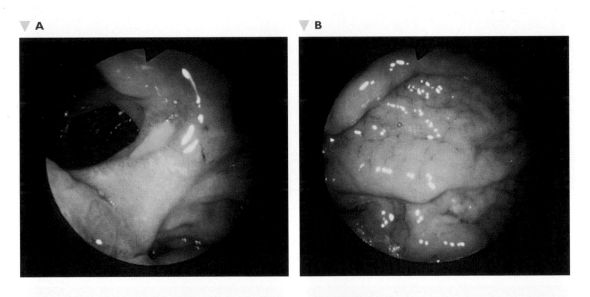

▼ A ▼ B

Figure 5.89 (A) Ulcus jejuni pepticum located at the barrel between efferent and afferent loops. This ulcer was resistant to H$_2$-receptor blockade therapy. (B) Prominent areae gastricae pattern compatible with acid hypersecretion.

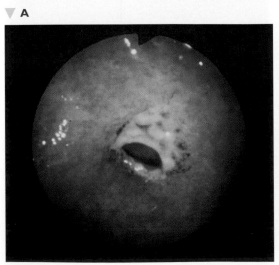
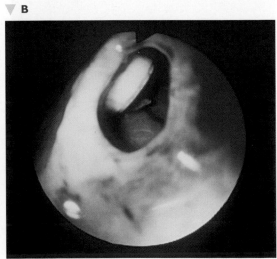

▼ A ▼ B

Figure 5.90 (A) Billroth I stomach with stromal stricture. (B) Retained tablet just beyond the stricture.

Bezoars may also form in an intact stomach as result of motility disturbances or diabetes, and also in postvagotomy pyloric stenosis (Fig. 5.94). In certain geographical areas, persimmon bezoars are the most common form of post-operative phytobezoar.

MUCOSAL ALTERATIONS

Endoscopic atrophic gastritis and chronic gastritis with atrophy are common after partial gastrectomy (Fig. 5.95). Development of xanthelasma or xan-thoma is not uncommon in such atrophic mucosa. These xanthelasmas are tiny plaque-like lesions measuring up to a few millimeters in diameter. They

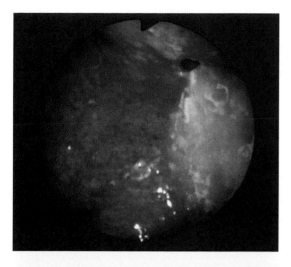

Figure 5.91 Billroth II stomach with stomal stricturing and biliary reflux.

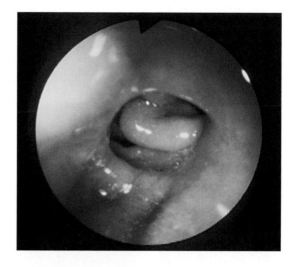

Figure 5.92 Receding intussuscepting folds through a Billroth II stoma.

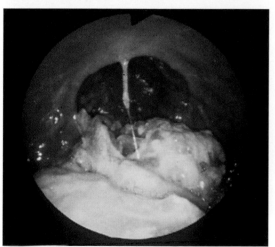

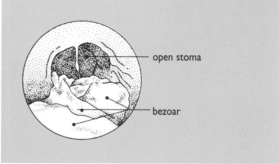

Figure 5.93 Bezoar in a Billroth II stomach. The stoma is wide open.

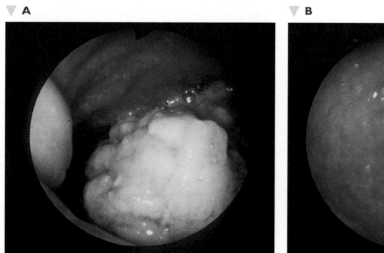

Figure 5.94 **(A)** Bezoar formation caused by pyloric stenosis after esophageal transection for bleeding varices. **(B)** Pyloric stenosis.

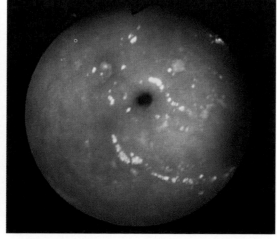

Figure 5.95 Atrophic gastritis in a partially resected stomach.

are composed of foamy lipid-laden macrophages, may be single or multiple, and are yellow in color (Fig. 5.96). Xanthoma may also develop in the intact stomach in the absence of atrophic gastritis. Such xanthomatous lesions may be flat or raised (Fig. 5.97). Intestinal metaplasia is also common in the resected stomach. This may be seen as tiny whitish patches usually in the area of the anastomosis (Figs. 5.98–5.100).

POSTGASTRECTOMY NEOPLASIA

Patients who have had partial gastrectomies are at a somewhat increased risk of gastric cancer after 10–20 years, although this risk varies by geographical region (high in Scandinavia and low in the USA). Before development of invasive cancer, severe dysplasia may be detectable in routine biopsies (Figs. 5.101 and 5.102). Early malignancies are not associated with symptoms and in asymptomatic patients are usually only found upon routine screening. The most common appearance is that of a small polypoid mass, an area of mucosal discoloration or a minor erosive-ulcerative defect (Fig. 5.103). Such lesions may arise anywhere within the remnant and may be multifocal, but the mucosa within 2 cm the stoma and anastomosis is by far the most common location. The vast majority of the gastric remnant cancers are seen as advanced lesions and look like polypoid masses or infiltrating lesions. Such cancers usually involve the stoma and extend for variable distances into the remnant (Fig. 5.104). Some of these malignancies have a linitis plastica appearance, involving the entire remnant and spreading submucosally above the gastroesophageal junction (Fig. 5.105).

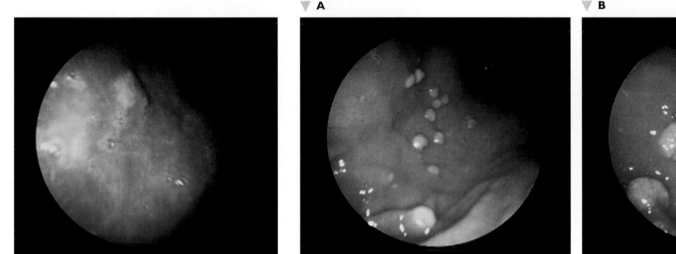

Figure 5.96 *Xanthelasma in atrophic Billroth II mucosa.*

Figure 5.97 *(A and B) Two examples of a raised xanthoma in an intact stomach.*

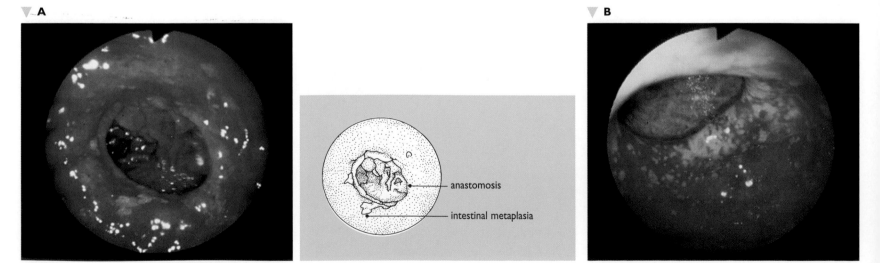

Figure 5.98 *(A) Whitish discolored areas at the anastomosis due to intestinal metaplasia. The bright white spots are endoscopic light reflections from the mucosal surface. (B) More extensive intestinal metaplasia.*

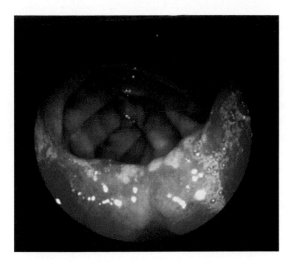

Figure 5.99 White mucosal spots at level of anastomosis after gastric resection. The surrounding mucosa is red. The spots are areas of intestinal metaplasia.

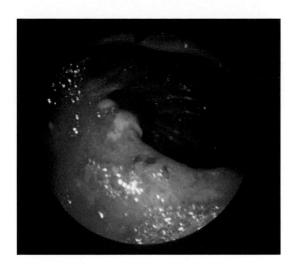

Figure 5.100 Billroth II anastomosis with white raised areas at the anastomosis, which were found on biopsy to be intestinal metaplasia.

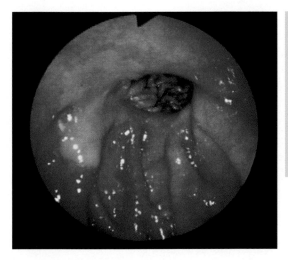

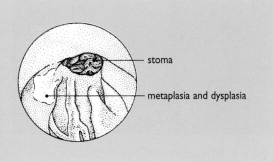

Figure 5.101 Stomal area 20 years after a Billroth II resection shows evidence of severe dysplasia.

Figure 5.102 Intestinal metaplasia and dysplasia in other areas of stoma.

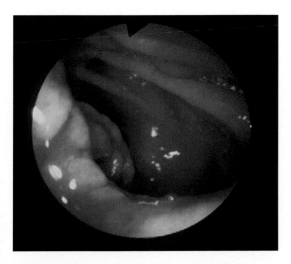

Figure 5.103 A small, polypoid Billroth II stump cancer.

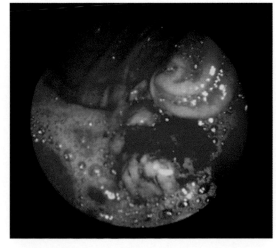

Figure 5.104 Malignancy spreading along the lesser curvature, seen with the endoscope retroflexed.

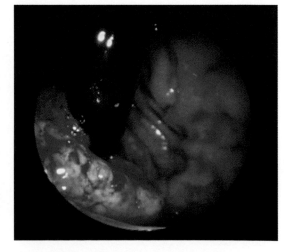

As the prognosis of advanced cancer is dismal, some investigators advocate periodic endoscopic screening of all postgastrectomy patients. When there is evidence of severe dysplasia, more frequent examinations are indicated. Others feel that the risk is too low to justify screening. The decision must be based partly on the incidence of cancer in the specific country. If screening is done, multiple biopsies from all quadrants of the stomal area and of the lesser and greater curve must be obtained because even severe dysplasia may be invisible to the naked eye. Because of friability and atrophic changes, there is an increased chance of bleeding after multiple biopsies (Fig. 5.106).

GASTRIC ULCER IN AIDS PATIENTS

In a patient with AIDS and upper gastrointestinal symptoms, endoscopy may be indicated for several reasons. Esophagitis caused by cytomegalovirus (CMV), herpes, or *Candida* can cause abdominal pain, chest pain, nausea and vomiting. Gastric ulcer may also be caused by CMV (Figs. 5.107 and 5.108). Biopsy of the ulcer margin and often also of the base are necessary to see the classic cytopathic changes of CMV. In contrast to ulcers of the esophagus (in which the base must be biopsied), in the stomach the columnar epithelium surrounding an ulcer often also contains the virus. Viral cultures, including a specimen for a Shell vial culture, should be obtained, when appropriate, to identify CMV in cases of gastric ulcer.

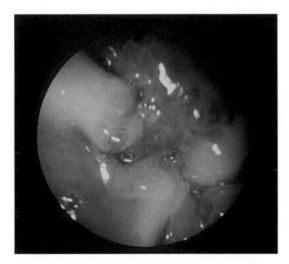

Figure 5.105 Stump cancer spreading into the distal esophagus.

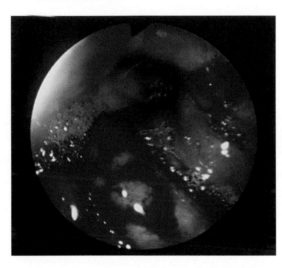

Figure 5.106 Long-standing Billroth II remnant with alkaline reflux gastritis after biopsy. Note the abundant blood loss.

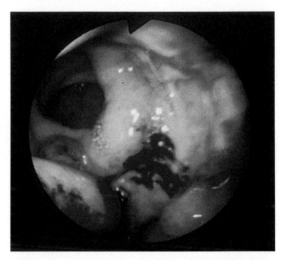

Figure 5.107 Deep gastric ulcer in an AIDS patient. The ulcer is white based, friable and somewhat irregular. Biopsies are indicated to diagnose CMV by pathology and viral culture. This was a CMV ulcer.

Figure 5.108 CMV gastric ulcer.

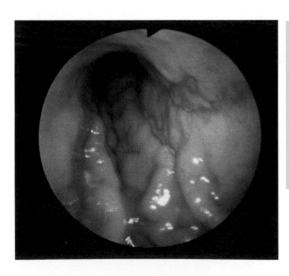

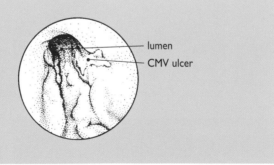

lumen
CMV ulcer

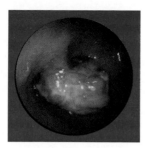

6

Stomach II: Tumors and Polyps

In this chapter we consider the differential diagnosis of gastric lesions, including early and advanced adenocarcinoma, less common gastric malignancies, such as Kaposi's sarcoma in AIDS, the endoscopic ultrasound appearance of neoplasia, and gastric polyps.

ADENOCARCINOMA

Even though the incidence of gastric carcinoma has decreased over the past several decades, it is still the third most common gastrointestinal malignancy after colonic and pancreatic cancer. The disease usually occurs in patients over 50 years old. Japan, Chile, Finland, parts of the former USSR, and Colombia have especially high incidences of gastric carcinoma. Of the gastric malignant lesions, adenocarcinoma accounts for about 85–90%. The cause of gastric adenocarcinoma is not known, but both genetic and environmental factors may be involved. There is currently increasing interest in studying the role of *Helicobacter pylori* in gastric cancer. A sequence has been suggested starting with inflammation leading to atrophy, intestinal metaplasia, dysplasia and finally adenocarcinoma. Up to 70% or more of gastric cancer may be related to *H. pylori* infection. The odds ratio of an increase in malignancy associated with positive tests for *H. pylori* may be as high as 7:1. The risk of developing cancer seems to be higher with acquisition of the infection at an early age. Obviously, complex multiple factors are thought to be involved with gastric carcinogenesis. The disease tends to run in some families. There are geographic areas in which the disease is highly prevalent. People who relocate from these areas reduce the risk by about 25%, and their descendants have a further 25% reduction in risk.

RISK FACTORS

Conditions associated with an increased incidence of gastric cancer include previous gastric surgery, adenomatous gastric polyps, autoimmune gastritis with pernicious anemia, and atrophic gastritis with intestinal metaplasia. The association with gastric surgery was noted several decades ago and re-examined recently. In some countries the incidence of gastric carcinoma 20 years after a Billroth II gastrectomy is as high as 8%. The relative risk is thought on average to be between 1 and 2 and therefore not sufficiently high to recommend screening. The presence of adenomatous polyps is associated with an increased incidence of cancer of the stomach. The association with

atrophic gastritis occurs mainly with gastritis involving the antrum, focal changes in the rest of the stomach, no parietal cell antibodies, and a moderate decrease in acid production.

PROGNOSIS

Survival rates are high if gastric cancer is diagnosed early, with 5-year survival rates of over 90%. In the later stages, 5-year survival is only about 10%. In most countries only 5–8% of cases are diagnosed at an early stage, compared with 30% in Japan, where endoscopic screening programs are used widely. Screening programs of this type may not be practical in areas in which gastric cancer is less prevalent. New diagnostic techniques using tumor markers or endoscopic ultrasound may make screening programs more practical in the future.

SITES OF DISEASE

Although figures vary, approximately 40% of gastric carcinomas occur in the body, 35% in the antrum, 20% in the cardia or fundal area, and 5–10% are diffuse. Adenocarcinoma of the cardia can extend into the distal esophagus, causing dysphagia. A barium esophagram will confirm the diagnosis by showing a narrowed esophagogastric junction. Endoscopy and biopsy are necessary to establish the diagnosis. Occasionally the tumor invades submucosally and can appear with an achalasia-like radiographic picture. This may also be found with metastatic lesions to this area.

ADVANCED GASTRIC ADENOCARCINOMA
Classification and Endoscopic Appearance

The TNM system is commonly used to classify gastric adenocarcinoma. *T* refers to the extent of tumor invasion (T_1–T_4); *N* refers to nodal involvement (N_0–N_3); and *M* refers to the presence of metastases (M_0 or M_1).

The Borrmann method is applicable to endoscopy. In this classification, advanced gastric cancer is divided into four stages (Fig. 6.1).

Type I: Nonulcerated, exophytic polypoid masses growing into the lumen.

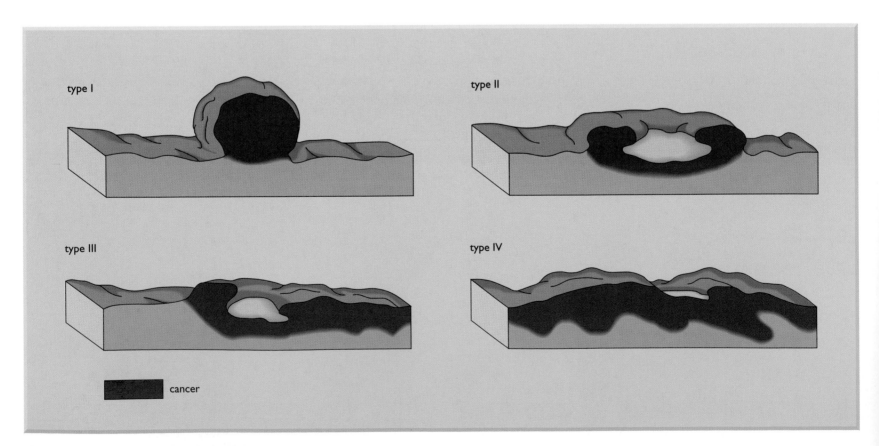

type I

type II

type III

type IV

cancer

Figure 6.1 *Borrmann classification of advanced gastric cancer.*

Type II: Circumscribed masses with sharp margins and a central ulceration.
Type III: Less well circumscribed, infiltrating masses, with ulceration. Ulcer margin blends into the surrounding mucosa. The base is infiltrated with cancer.
Type IV: Diffusely infiltrating masses that are mainly submucosal. Local areas of ulceration may occur. Submucosal spread makes endoscopic recognition and histologic verification difficult. Very diffuse tumors, referred to as linitis plastica, characteristically are associated with poor gastric distensibility and little peristalsis.

Type I Carcinoma

These represent 3–20% of gastric cancers, depending on the series. Of 5-year survivors, 30% have type I carcinomas. The tumors present as polypoid masses without ulceration. They are commonly (60%) located in the gastric body (Fig. 6.2) but also occur in the cardia and antrum (Figs. 6.3 and 6.4). The lesions are well demarcated from the surrounding mucosa. The surface is irregular and grayish (Fig. 6.5). As malignant cells are at the surface of the lesion, biopsy is often positive. The mass may be friable and bleed (Fig. 6.6), and may narrow the lumen.

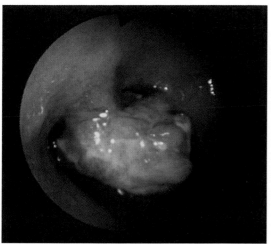

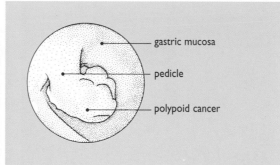

Figure 6.2 Type I adenocarcinoma of body of stomach appears polypoid and pedunculated.

▼ **A**

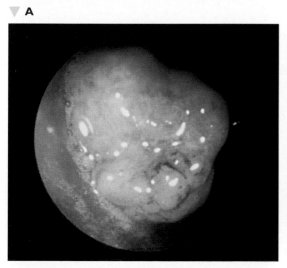

▼ **B**

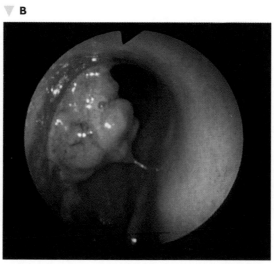

Figure 6.3 (**A** and **B**) Two views of polypoid adenocarcinoma of the antrum.

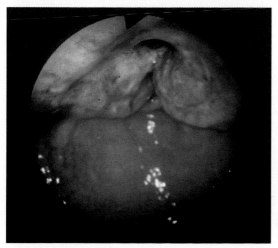

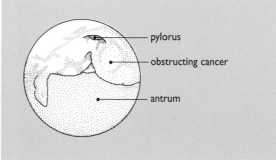

Figure 6.4 Type I adenocarcinoma of the antrum, occluding the gastric outlet.

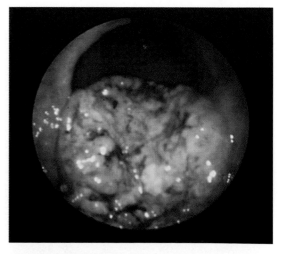

Figure 6.5 Type I gastric adenocarcinoma with a friable, irregular and nodular surface, and typical gray exudate.

Type II Carcinoma

Of gastric carcinomas, 20–40% have the configuration of an ulcerated mass. About 60% of 5-year survivors have this type of lesion. The lesion is usually a clear mass, well demarcated from the surrounding mucosa. Rugal folds terminate at the edge of the mass, separated from the ulcer base by tumor nodules and infiltrated tissue (Fig. 6.7). The base of the ulcerated lesion is necrotic tumor and granulation tissue, often with tumor nodules (Fig. 6.8).

The tissue over the mass, surrounding the ulcer, is often abnormal with erythema (Fig. 6.9). The lesions are usually easily distinguished from benign gastric ulcers because of the associated mass. Biopsy of the irregular nodular margins or nodules in the base of the ulcer is usually positive for cancer.

Gastric adenocarcinoma can also sometimes resemble a benign gastric ulcer and this type of cancer must be detected by taking multiple, four-quadrant

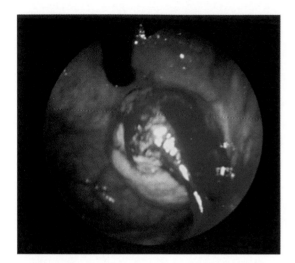
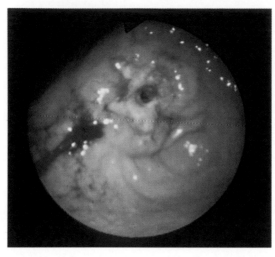

Figure 6.6 Bleeding polypoid type I adenocarcinoma of the cardia.

Figure 6.7 Type II adenocarcinoma of the distal antrum. A central ulcer is separated from the surrounding mucosa by tumor nodules and infiltrated folds.

A 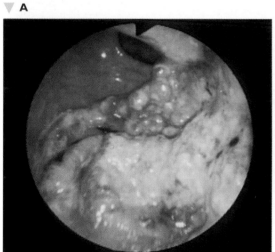 **B**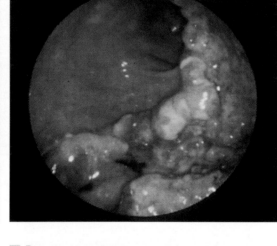

Figure 6.8 (**A**) Type II adenocarcinoma with a large central ulcer. The base of the ulcer is necrotic tumor, granulation tissue, and tumor nodules. (**B**) In this view, tumor nodules can be clearly seen at the distal rim of the ulcer. This would be an appropriate area for biopsy.

A 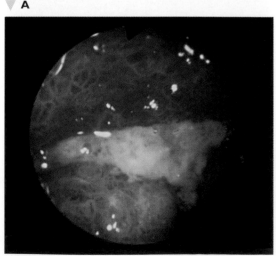 **B**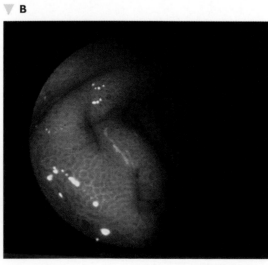

Figure 6.9 Two examples of erythematous mucosa surrounding the central ulcer of a type II adenocarcinoma: (**A**) a large ulcer (**B**) a small linear ulcer.

biopsies of the ulcer. However, there may be clues to the malignant nature of the ulcer. Surrounding folds that end in nodules at the periphery of the ulcer rather than at the margin itself (Fig. 6.10) and an irregular margin with nodularity and erythema of the surrounding mucosa (Fig. 6.11) are both signs of malignancy. The malignant ulcer often appears as a large, deep ulcer with slightly nodular and erythematous margins (Fig. 6.12).

Type III Carcinoma

This pattern account for 10–15% of gastric cancers. The lesions may be confused with benign gastric ulcers. Only 10–15% of 5-year survivors have type III lesions. There is infiltration of the wall with associated central ulceration. The infiltration of the tumor may appear as heavy folds rather than a clear mass (Figs. 6.13 and 6.14). The central ulceration may be large, often over

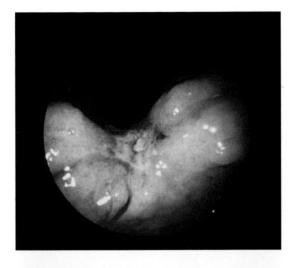

Figure 6.10 Malignant gastric ulcer. The ulcer is irregular and the folds surrounding the tumor are nodular and heaped up.

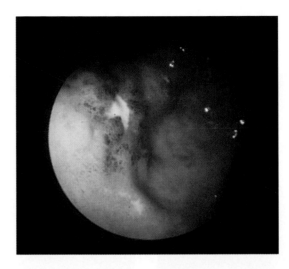

Figure 6.11 Malignant gastric ulcer. The ulcer is fairly small but the surrounding mucosa is red and slightly nodular.

▼ **A**

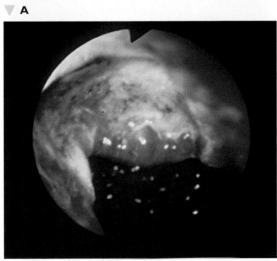

▼ **B**

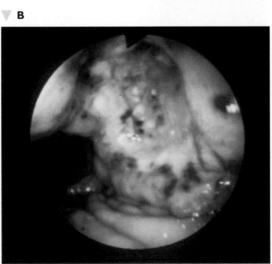

▼ **C**

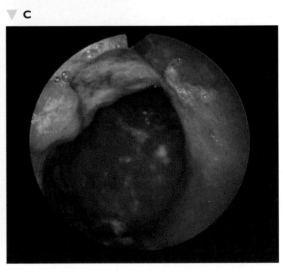

Figure 6.12 (**A–C**) Three cases of malignant gastric ulcers. The ulcers are large and deep. The surrounding mucosa is erythematous and slightly nodular. Eight to ten biopsies taken from the margin of each ulcer are indicated to establish that these are adenocarcinomas.

◄ **A**

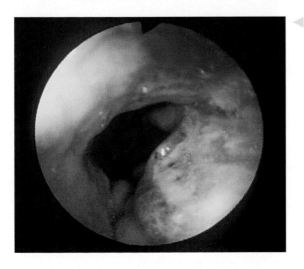

◄ **B**

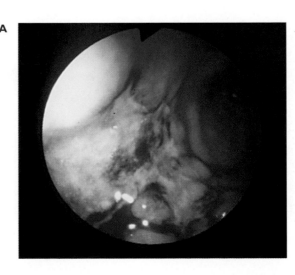

Figure 6.13 (**A** and **B**) Type III adenocarcinoma. The tumor is diffusely infiltrating with associated ulcers and friability seen in **B**.

3 cm in diameter (Fig. 6.15). Often the ulcer, even if infiltrated, may be surrounded by normal mucosa, making accurate biopsy difficult (Fig. 6.16). Biopsy is most productive if taken at the margin of the ulcer with the surrounding mucosa. Biopsies should also be taken of distorted areas of the base of the ulcer and nodules, or irregular areas at the margin.

Retroflexion of the endoscope may be necessary to view the entire margin of the ulcer to determine whether abnormal mucosa is present, suggesting a gastric cancer (Fig. 6.17). Retroflexion is also frequently necessary to permit biopsy and cytology of the abnormal area. Sometimes the tumor may occur as a large ulcerated infiltrating lesion with exudation and friability, making identification of the margins difficult (Fig. 6.18).

Type IV Carcinoma

This diffuse infiltrating pattern accounts for 30–50% of gastric cancers. People with this pattern do not usually survive 5 years. These tumors may be localized (70%) or diffuse (30%) even to the extent of involving the entire

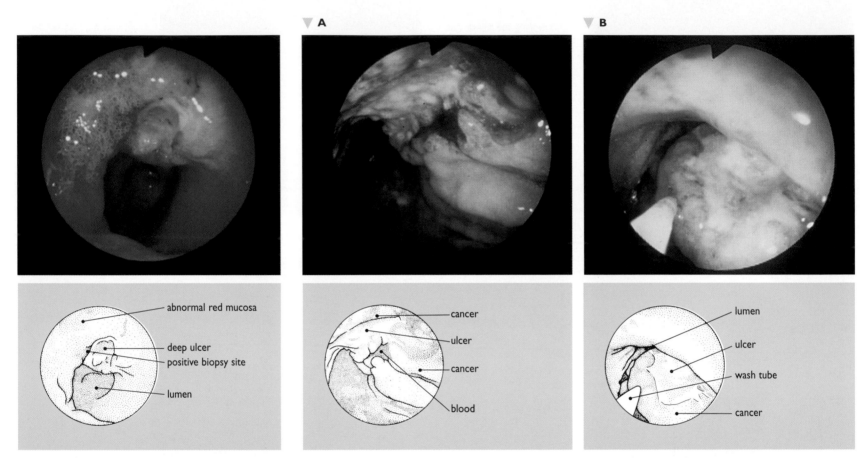

Figure 6.14 *This deep ulcer is seen in association with a type III adenocarcinoma. The folds adjacent to the ulcer are indurated and positive on biopsy for carcinoma.*

Figure 6.15 *Large ulcerations associated with type III gastric cancers. (**A**) The mucosa surrounding the ulcer is infiltrated. (**B**) A wash tube is seen in preparation for obtaining a jet cytology.*

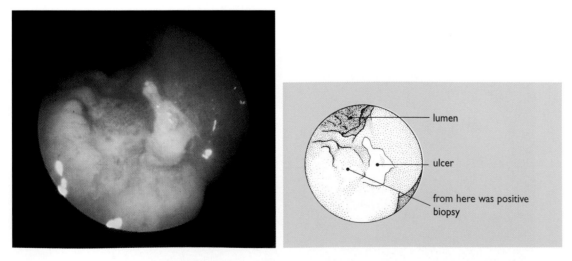

Figure 6.16 *Although this is a malignant gastric cancer, the surrounding mucosa appears relatively normal. Note, however, that the mucosa to the left of the ulcer is irregular and depressed. Biopsy taken from this area was positive for cancer.*

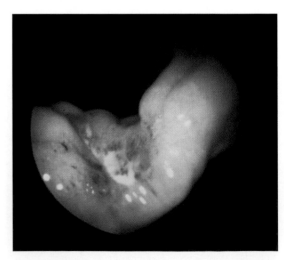

Figure 6.17 *Malignant ulcer of the angularis. The tumor can only be visualized, brushed for cytology, and biopsied with the endoscope retroflexed.*

stomach. Many of the localized tumors involve the proximal stomach (cardia or fundus). The diffuse type is called linitis plastica. The tumor growth pattern is submucosal. The gastric lumen is narrowed by areas infiltrated with tumor and is less distensible than is normal with air insufflation (Fig. 6.19). The covering mucosa may appear relatively normal (Fig. 6.20) or red and inflamed, mimicking gastritis (Figs. 6.21 and 6.22). Visible nodules seen at

▼ **A**   ▼ **B**   ▼ **C**

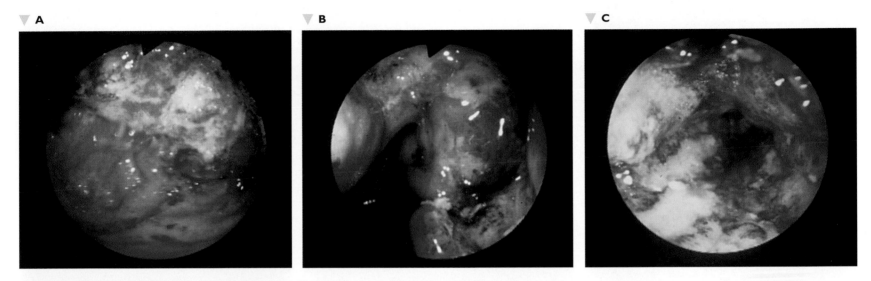

Figure 6.18 *(A–C)* *Examples of large, poorly defined type III adenocarcinomas. Exudation and friability make identification of the margins difficult.*

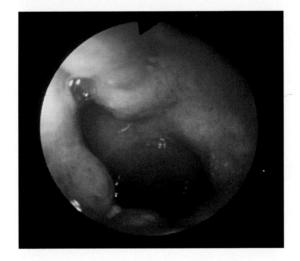

Figure 6.19 *Type IV adenocarcinoma of the stomach (linitis plastica). The lumen is narrowed and the walls less distensible because of the infiltrating tumor.*

▼ **A**   ▼ **B**   ▼ **C**

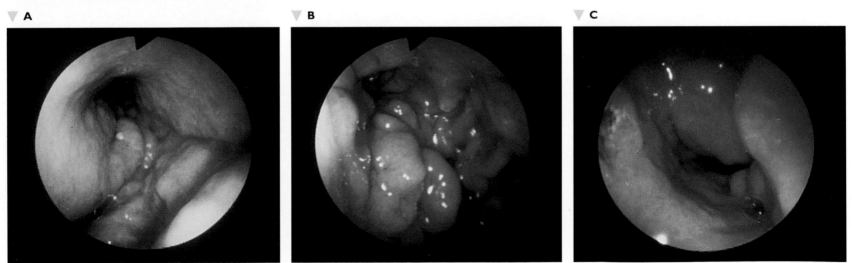

Figure 6.20 *(A–C)* *Three cases of type IV adenocarcinoma (linitis plastica). The mucosa covering the diffusely infiltrating tumor appears normal.*

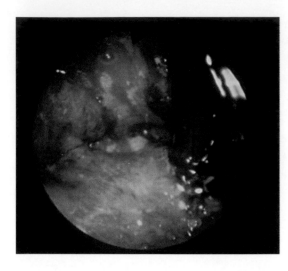

Figure 6.21 *The heavy, indurated folds of linitis plastica are covered with abnormal mucosa, seen with the endoscope retroflexed.*

endoscopy may be covered with normal mucosa (Fig. 6.20) or abnormal erythematous mucosa (Fig. 6.23). Sixty percent of these lesions are reported to have areas of tumor breakthrough. These areas are red with roughened mucosa and a dull appearance (Figs. 6.24 and 6.25), distinct from the normal appearance of the gastric mucosa. The rugal folds are infiltrated or replaced by tumor. These irregular areas of mucosa should be biopsied to increase the likelihood of sampling malignant tissue. One should also biopsy masses or nodules. Limited areas of ulceration may be noted in association with diffuse inflammation, and these may be difficult to differentiate from a type III lesion (Fig. 6.26).

Other Endoscopic Considerations

Adenocarcinoma of the cardia can be seen as the endoscope is passed down the esophagus (Fig. 6.27) or with a U-turn to retroflex the endoscope tip. If the tumor is mainly infiltrative, the endoscopic view may be of heavy irregular folds covered with normal mucosa (Fig. 6.28). However, ulceration and obvious tumor breakthrough may be noted (Fig. 6.29).

▼ A ▼ B ▼ C

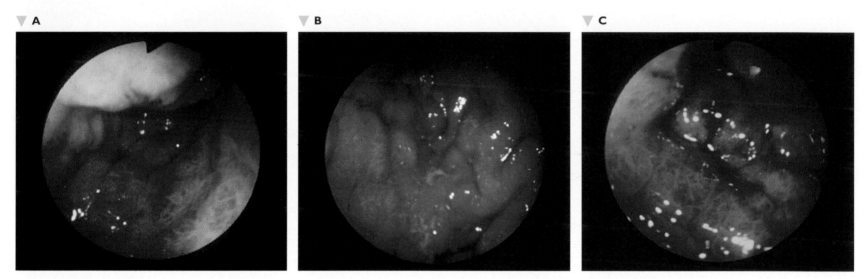

Figure 6.22 *(A) Linitis plastica mimicking gastritis, with red inflamed edematous mucosa. Diagnosis is only possible with deep biopsy. (B) A second case of linitis plastica mimicking gastritis. (C) A close-up view of the mucosa reveals edema, erythema, and friability.*

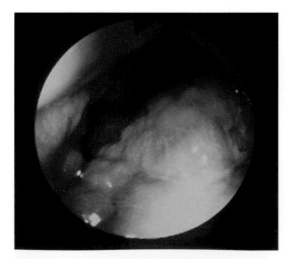

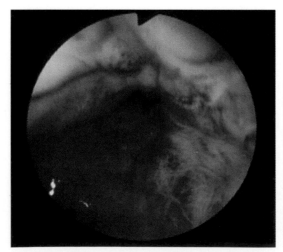

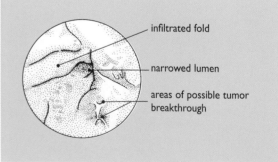

Figure 6.23 *Nodules in a patient with linitis plastica. The mucosa over the nodules appears mildy erythematous.*

Figure 6.24 *Linitis plastica with erythematous mucosa. The lumen is narrowed by the infiltrating tumor. The stellate, red areas may represent tumor breakthrough.*

▼ A

▼ B

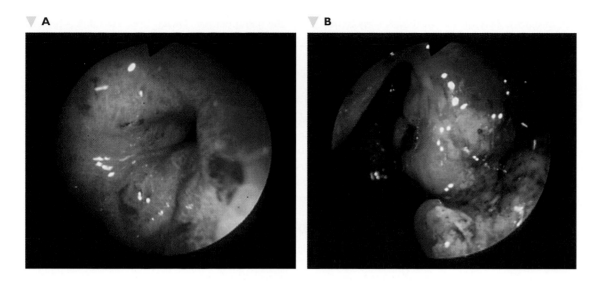

Figure 6.25 (**A**) Linitis plastica with diffusely red covering mucosa and darker red areas of possible tumor breakthrough. (**B**) Linitis plastica with diffused abnormal mucosa and possible tumor breakthrough nodules.

▼ A

▼ B

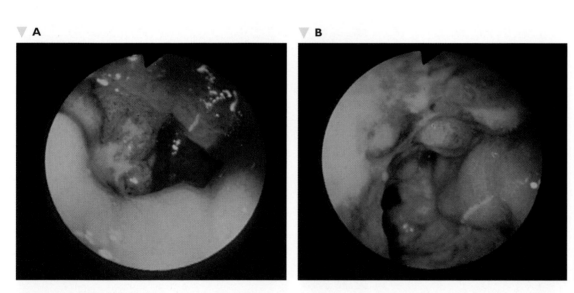

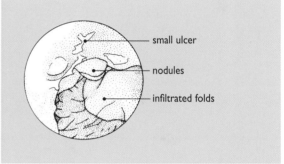

small ulcer

nodules

infiltrated folds

Figure 6.26 (**A** and **B**) Extensive linitis plastica with nodules and ulcerations. These appearances may lead to confusion with type III lesions.

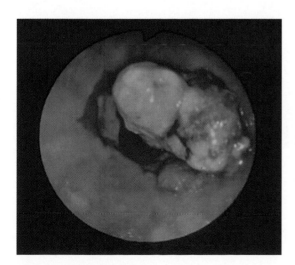

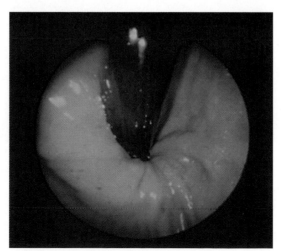

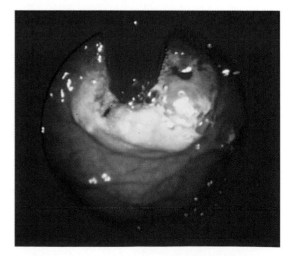

Figure 6.27 Adenocarcinoma of the cardia extending into the distal esophagus.

Figure 6.28 Adenocarcinoma of the cardia. The tumor cannot be seen with the endoscope retroflexed, but the indurated mucosa and the impression of a mass surrounding the endoscope can be noted.

Figure 6.29 Adenocarcinoma of the cardia seen with the endoscope retroflexed. The mucosa over the tumor is abnormal, with nodularity and ulceration.

Especially with infiltrating tumors (types III and IV), the diagnosis may not be easy because the covering mucosa appears relatively normal. Other clues must be used to detect the presence of an abnormal gastric wall. The folds of the stomach may appear rigid and fixed. If the mucosa over these folds is pulled with a forceps out into the lumen, it may not 'tent' as it would normally because the mucosa is adherent to the firm, infiltrating tumor underneath. This fixation suggests a tumor, but in some cases tumor may be present without the loss of tenting.

Another clue to the presence of a tumor is an area of abrupt change. At the junction of a tumor and the normal wall adjacent to the tumor, there may be a sharp margin or shelf-like effect. Endoscopic ultrasound is an ideal method of studying areas of suspected submucosal masses or diffuse infiltrating adenocarcinomas.

Biopsy

Many endoscopists favor the use of a large-particle biopsy forceps, which yields a larger tissue specimen than routine endoscopic forceps. The number of biopsies taken influences the true-positive rate. If three are taken, the rate of positivity is roughly 60%. If six or more are taken, the accuracy is over 90%. Several studies have demonstrated that multiple biopsies are associated with a higher true-positive rate (10 biopsies = 99%).

New Diagnostic and Therapeutic Techniques

New technology may aid in diagnosis. Endoscopic ultrasound permits high-resolution imaging of the intestinal wall and adjacent structures. Computed tomography and magnetic resonance imaging may also play a role in determining the extent of gastric tumors. Endoscopic laser photocoagulation using the Nd:YAG laser may be useful for recurrent tumors or in patients who are not candidates for the surgical removal of their tumor (Fig. 6.30).

EARLY GASTRIC ADENOCARCINOMA

Early endoscopic diagnosis of gastric cancer obviously makes a difference to outcome, since the 5-year survival rate for early cancer is so much better than for advanced cancer. By definition, the lesion in early gastric cancer involves

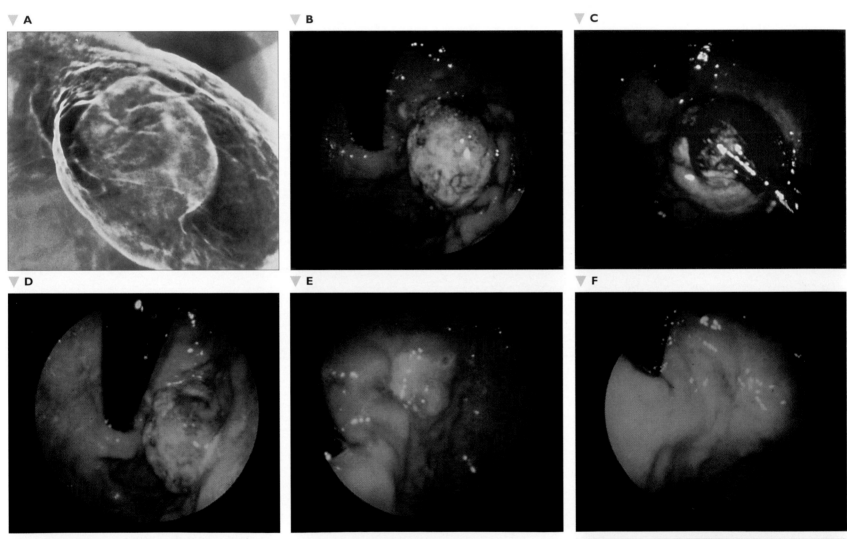

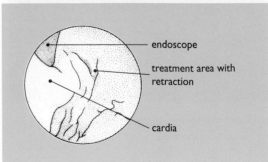

Figure 6.30 *Endoscopic laser photocoagulation.* (**A**) *X-ray of gastric carcinoma in an elderly woman who presented with gastrointestinal bleeding.* (**B**) *Endoscopy reveals a large polypoid cancer in the cardia. The tumor is best seen on retroflexion.* (**C**) *The tumor begins to bleed while being inspected endoscopically.* (**D**) *After partial Nd:YAG laser therapy, the tumor is smaller and there is no evidence of bleeding.* (**E**) *Several weeks later after more laser therapy, no cancer is seen. Only a small ulcer is noted in the area of treatment.* (**F**) *Finally, the area is completely healed. Biopsy of the area is negative for residual tumor. The only abnormality is a slight retraction in the treated area.*

the mucosa and submucosa but does not extend to the muscularis propria of the stomach wall. In some cases, lesions followed for 2–3 years remain localized without evidence of extension into the muscle layer. Some early cancers spread on the gastric mucosa and submucosa without involvement of the muscularis propria. This superficial spreading type may be a variant of early gastric cancer or may be a separate entity.

Classification and Endoscopic Appearance

The Japanese Endoscopy Society formulated a widely used classification of this tumor. There are three types and three subtypes (Fig. 6.31). In addition there are combinations of lesions that incorporate more than one classification. In these combined lesions the predominant pattern is listed first.

Type I: Polypoid lesion of mucosa protruding into lumen.

Type II: Subtle tumor of mucosa. Not as prominent as type I (polyp) or type III (ulcer). Type II is divided into three subtypes:

IIa, area of focal mucosal elevation, less marked than in type I;

IIb, flat area of abnormal mucosa;

IIc, depressed tumor with cancer at base of depression.

Type III: Gastric ulcer with cancer at the margin.

Lesions combining type III and subtype IIc account for about one-half of all cases of early gastric cancers. About 20% of early cancers are the raised types (I and IIa). The flat or depressed types are found in approximately 30% of cases.

For the most part, symptoms of early gastric cancer are similar to those of advanced cancers. Dyspepsia and epigastric pain occur in early and advanced cases in 65–80% of patients. Hematemesis or melena are seen marginally more often in early than in advanced cancer, and early cancer has a marginally lower incidence of weight loss. Diagnosis is made endoscopically. Lesions of early gastric cancer are relatively subtle and in many instances difficult to distinguish from normal mucosa or nonmalignant gastric lesions.

Type I Carcinoma

The surface of type I polypoid lesions is usually nodular or irregular, more so than is found with typical hyperplastic polyps, adenomatous polyps, and submucosal lesions such as a leiomyoma. The surface may appear erythematous (Fig. 6.32).

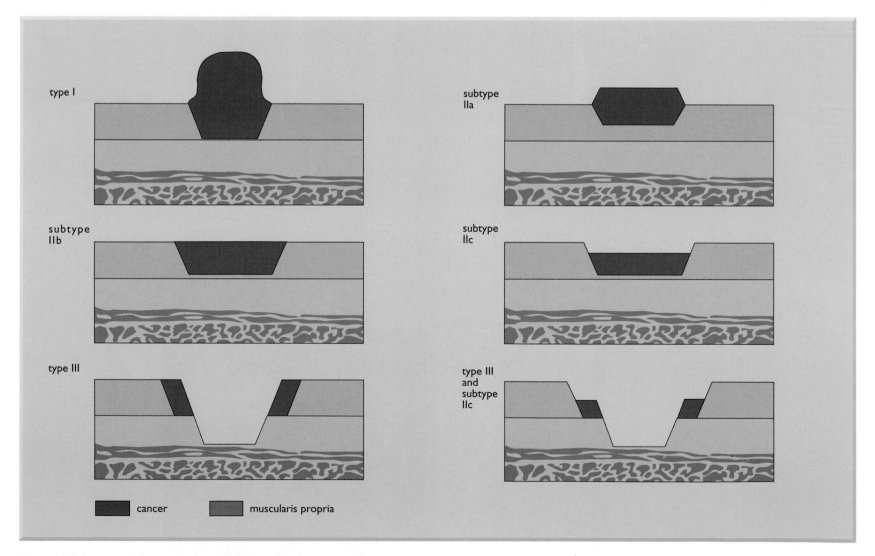

type I

subtype IIa

subtype IIb

subtype IIc

type III

type III and subtype IIc

cancer   muscularis propria

Figure 6.31 *Japanese Endoscopy Society classification of early gastric cancer.*

A

B

C

D

E

F

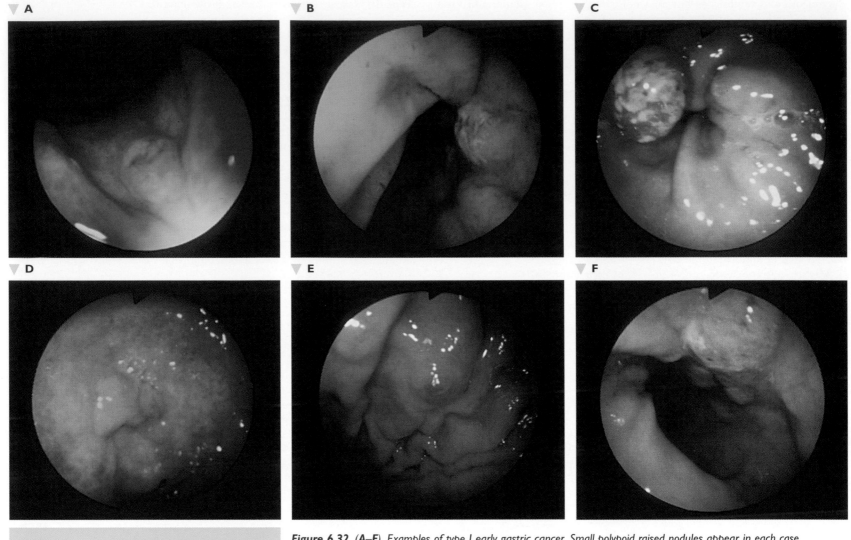

Figure 6.32 (**A–F**) Examples of type I early gastric cancer. Small polypoid raised nodules appear in each case, sometimes with signs of erythema.

— raised early cancer

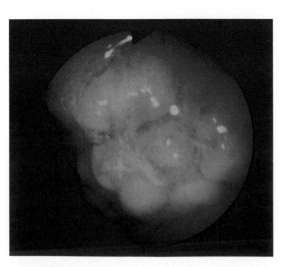

Figure 6.33 Subtype IIa early gastric cancer. The tumor is slightly raised but not polypoid.

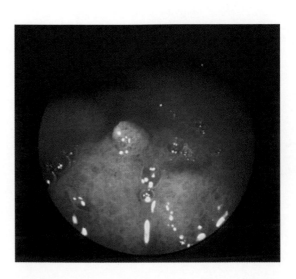

Figure 6.34 Subtype IIa early gastric cancer.

Type II Carcinoma

In subtype IIa, lesions appear as slightly raised – but not polypoid – irregular areas of gastric mucosa (Figs. 6.33 and 6.34).

Subtype IIb may be difficult to diagnose. The mucosa is neither raised nor depressed (Fig. 6.35). The color may appear abnormal with white or gray areas (Fig. 6.36), or uniformly red, in contrast to the lacy reticulated erythematous appearance of regenerative mucosa adjacent to a benign gastric ulcer.

In subtype IIc, lesions are slightly depressed areas of abnormal mucosa (Figs. 6.37 and 6.38).

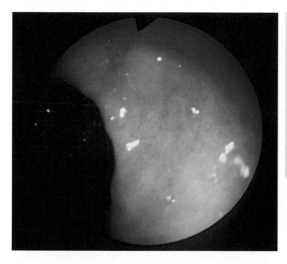

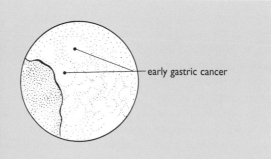

Figure 6.35 *Early gastric cancer subtype IIb. The mucosal abnormality is very subtle. The mucosa is slightly red.*

▽ **A**

▽ **B**

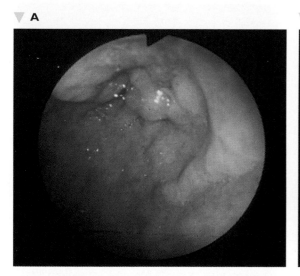

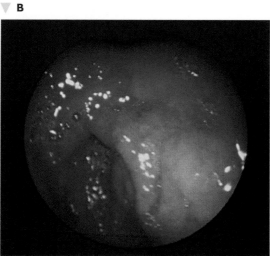

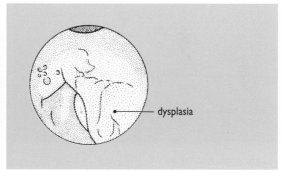

Figure 6.36 *(A and B) Examples of subtype IIb early gastric cancer. The mucosa demonstrates subtle changes such as slight discoloration and a roughened, irregular appearance.*

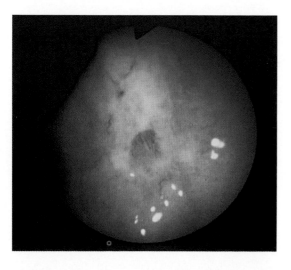

Figure 6.37 *Subtype IIc early gastric cancer. A slightly depressed white area can be noted.*

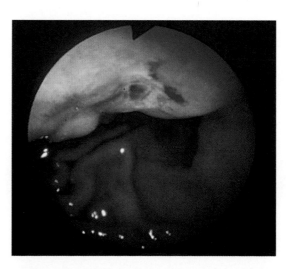

Figure 6.38 *Early gastric cancer subtype IIc. A slightly depressed area surrounded by minimal mucosal abnormality is seen.*

Subtypes IIb and IIc may have an appearance similar to a healing gastric ulcer. However, benign ulcers have smooth, tapered rugal folds that end at the healing area, whereas early cancers have abnormal fold terminations with clubbing or nodules. The color of the mucosa surrounding a healing ulcer has the red lacy appearance of the areae gastricae. In early cancer the mucosa is either intensely red or irregular with red and gray–white areas. These areas are typically sharply demarcated from the surrounding gastric mucosa and, in IIc lesions, slightly depressed.

Type III Carcinoma

A type III lesion is also difficult to diagnose. It may appear adjacent to a benign-appearing gastric ulcer with the tumor in the tissue at the margin of the ulcer crater (Figs. 6.39 and 6.40). The cancer may be in only one quadrant and therefore can be missed if the entire margin of a gastric ulcer is not inspected and biopsied. This inspection may require a retroflexed view of the ulcer. The base of the ulcer may be free of tumor. Signs of tumor include depressed and discolored areas. One should also look for abnormalities of the surrounding folds. In the combination lesions (IIc and III, or III and IIc, where the first symbol of each pair designates the primary morphologic pattern), distinct ulcers are associated with abnormal adjacent mucosa, often with irregular, depressed, and erythematous areas.

Biopsy

The lesions of early gastric cancer may respond to standard antiulcer therapy and may heal and recur in a cycle similar to benign gastric ulcers. For this reason many endoscopists biopsy all gastric ulcers and repeat biopsies until the lesion is completely healed. If at least two biopsies are taken from each of the four quadrants of the ulcer (total eight), there is better than a 90% chance of detecting cancer if present. For ulcers, the margin of each quadrant is biopsied; the base is less productive. For polyps and for flat and depressed areas (types I, IIa, IIb, and IIc), the base or center of the lesion should be sampled. Cytology is not as helpful in early cancer as in other tumors. Brushing for cytology is done under endoscopic guidance and should include the red irregular depressed mucosa or the margin of the ulcer in the areas of abnormal mucosa.

Endosonography of the Stomach in Gastric Adenocarcinoma

Endosonography is a valuable aid to the complete evaluation of gastric neoplasia. Ultrasound is considered to be the most accurate imaging method for staging the depth of tumor involvement (Fig. 6.41), and the use of endosonography in the diagnosis of early gastric cancer is attracting considerable interest. Currently, only patients who are not surgical candidates are considered for mucosal resections or for Nd:YAG laser endoscopic therapy of these early,

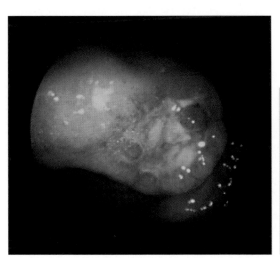
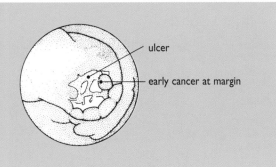

Figure 6.39 *Type III early gastric cancer. Gastric ulceration as well as early cancer at the margin are evident.*

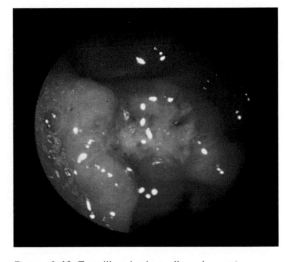

Figure 6.40 *Type III and subtype IIc early gastric cancer appearing as an ulcer with abnormal, red and depressed surrounding mucosa. The surrounding folds are not normal, they appear nodular.*

Figure 6.41 *Early gastric carcinoma located in the mucosa with a small area of penetration into the submucosa. This is a T_1 lesion. (Courtesy of Dr T.L. Tio)*

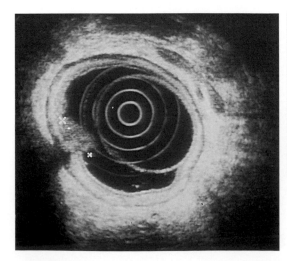
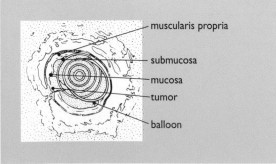

limited lesions. In the future, however, ultrasound may be used routinely to identify patients whose lesions are suitable for primary endoscopic therapy. Thus endosonography may prove to be the imaging technique of choice for guiding the application of therapy, following regression of the lesion, and monitoring to detect recurrence (Fig. 6.42).

The endosonographic image can often clearly delineate the extent of wall involvement and that of adjacent structures, the presence of abnormal lymph nodes, and other features of gastric cancer not apparent with endoscopy (Figs. 6.43–6.46).

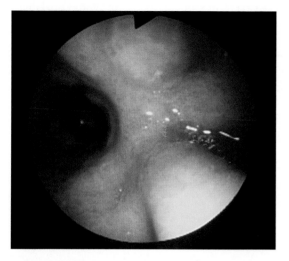

Figure 6.42 *Early gastric cancer after therapy with Nd:YAG laser in a patient who was not a surgical candidate. The tumor is no longer evident. The mucosa in the treated area is retracted and radiating folds are present.*

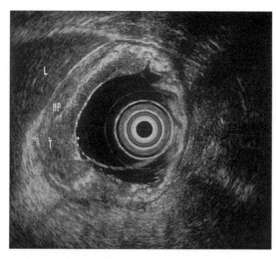
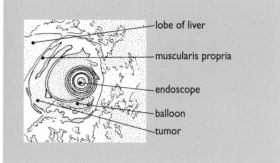

Figure 6.43 *Gastric carcinoma with tumor infiltration into the muscularis propria. This was a T_2 gastric cancer. (Courtesy of Dr T.L. Tio)*

lobe of liver
muscularis propria
endoscope
balloon
tumor

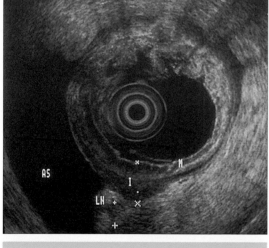
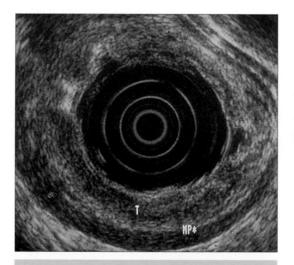
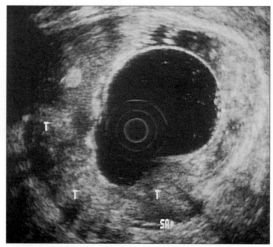

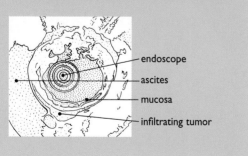

endoscope
ascites
mucosa
infiltrating tumor

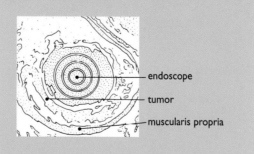

endoscope
tumor
muscularis propria

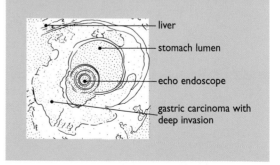

liver
stomach lumen
echo endoscope
gastric carcinoma with deep invasion

Figure 6.44 *Gastric cancer with deep infiltration through the muscularis propria and through the serosa. This was a T_3 tumor. (Courtesy of Dr T.L. Tio)*

Figure 6.45 *This gastric cancer is infiltrating the mucosa and the submucosa and penetrating into the muscularis propria. The muscularis propria is markedly thickened. This is linitis plastica staged as T_2. (Courtesy of Dr T.L. Tio)*

Figure 6.46 *T_4 gastric carcinoma with deep extension into the tissues adjacent to the stomach walls. (Courtesy of Dr T.L. Tio)*

OTHER GASTRIC MALIGNANCIES

The next most common tumor after adenocarcinoma is lymphoma, followed by leiomyosarcoma. Other less common tumors are Kaposi's sarcoma and metastatic gastric disease.

GASTRIC LYMPHOMA

About 4–8% of gastric tumors are lymphomas. Unlike advanced adenocarcinoma, lymphoma often responds well to therapy, especially if diagnosed at an early stage. Stage I (stomach wall only) has an 80% 5-year survival rate; stage IV (widespread disease) rarely survives 5 years.

Primary gastric lymphoma includes non-Hodgkin's lymphoma and less commonly Hodgkin's lymphoma. The gastric tumors are more often diffuse than nodular. The nodular lymphocytic types have the best 5-year survival rates. Precise diagnosis is essential to guide treatment. Diagnosis of gastric involvement with generalized abdominal lymphoma is important because knowledge of gastric involvement can affect decisions regarding therapy.

An interesting recent association is the high percentage of *H. pylori* infection in mucosa associated lymphoid tissue (MALT)-type gastric lymphoma. This lymphoma appears to be an *H. pylori* antigen driven malignancy. Partial and even complete regression of these lymphomas has been described after cure of the *H. pylori* infection.

Endoscopic Appearance

Gastric lymphoma may be difficult to differentiate from adenocarcinoma or a benign ulcer. Endoscopy in gastric lymphoma is associated with visual diagnosis of a suspected neoplasm in 75% of cases; in the rest, a diagnosis of a benign ulcer or other disease is suspected. Biopsies are always necessary to distinguish between benign disease and tumor.

Characteristically, gastric lymphoma occurs as an infiltrating lesion of the gastric mucosa, often associated with ulceration (Figs. 6.47 and 6.48). There may also be polypoid aspects to the appearance of the tumor (Fig. 6.49). Occasionally it may resemble an infiltrative adenocarcinoma (linitis plastica) (Figs. 6.50 and 6.51). Single or multiple ulcers may be seen in association

▼ **A**

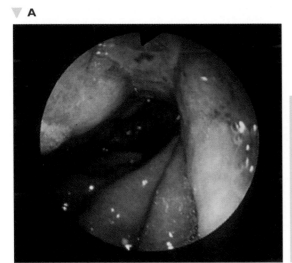

▼ **B**

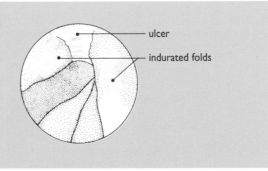

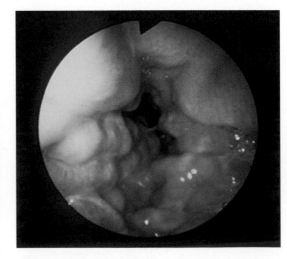

Figure 6.47 *A large ulcer in a patient with non-Hodgkin's lymphoma. The folds surrounding the ulcer are indurated and infiltrated (A). A different view of the ulcer (B) reveals friability and narrowing of the lumen caused by the indurated folds.*

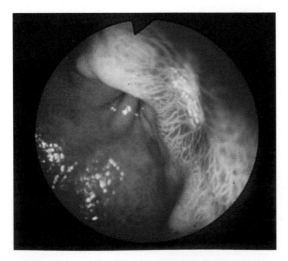

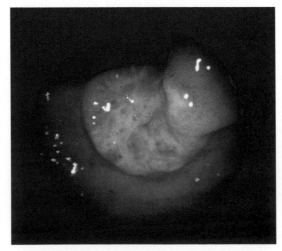

Figure 6.48 *Gastric lymphoma appearing as an atypical ulcer with very erythematous surrounding mucosa.*

Figure 6.49 *Non-Hodgkin's gastric lymphoma demonstrates a polypoid appearance.*

Figure 6.50 *In this lymphoma the gastric rugae are infiltrated and may be confused with linitis plastica.*

with the infiltration (Figs. 6.52 and 6.53). A single ulcer may be deep with a raised margin (Figs. 6.54 and 6.55). The ulcers may also have an irregular margin, which increases the suspicion of a tumor being present. The appearance is often that of infiltrated folds with diffuse ulceration and a very irregular nodular margin (Figs. 6.56 and 6.57). The tumor may be anywhere in the stomach, but often occurs in the body or antrum and may narrow the lumen (Fig. 6.58).

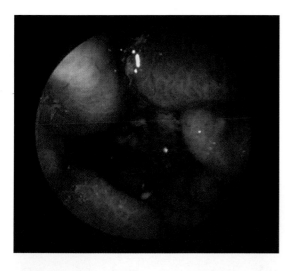

Figure 6.51 *Gastric lymphoma with infiltrated rugae narrowing the lumen. The covering mucosa is erythematous.*

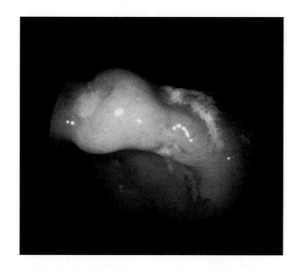

Figure 6.52 *Non-Hodgkin's lymphoma of the stomach with two ulcers involving the angularis. The surrounding mucosa is nodular.*

▼ **A**

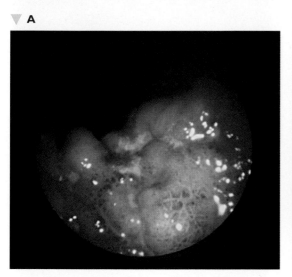

▼ **B**

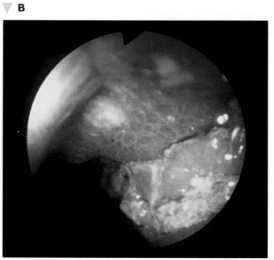

Figure 6.53 (*A and B*) *Hodgkin's disease involving the stomach. There are multiple ulcers with nodular, irregular erythematous intervening mucosa.*

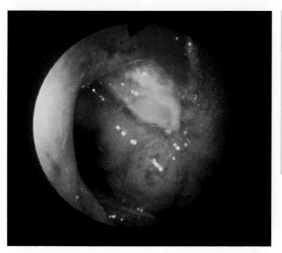

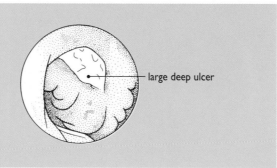

large deep ulcer

Figure 6.54 *A large deep ulcer associated with gastric lymphoma.*

▼ **A**

▼ **B**

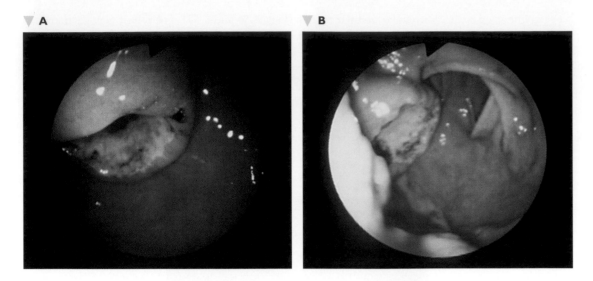

Figure 6.55 (A and B) Two examples of gastric lymphoma appearing as deep ulcers with a raised margin.

▼ **A**

▼ **B**

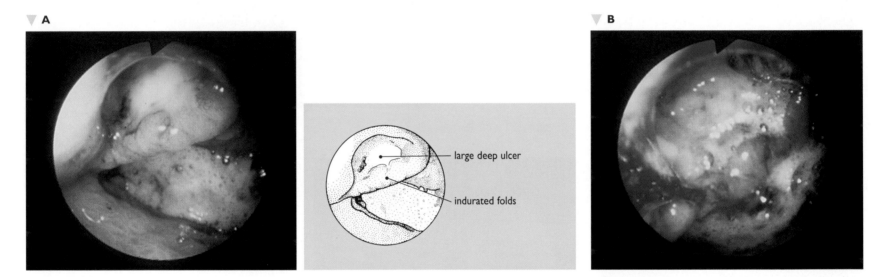

large deep ulcer

indurated folds

Figure 6.56 (A) Recurrent, diffuse non-Hodgkin's lymphoma involving an extensive area of the stomach. The ulcer is large, and the surrounding mucosa is friable, nodular, and clearly infiltrated. (B) In this view the nodularity at the ulcer margin is seen.

▼ **A**

▼ **B**

▼ **C**

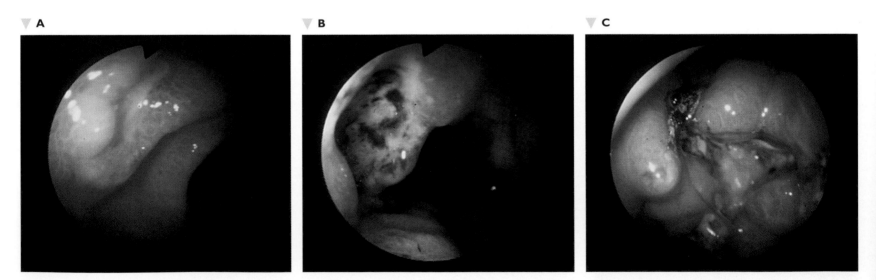

Figure 6.57 (A–C) Three cases of non-Hodgkin's lymphoma with a central ulcer and thick surrounding folds.

Lymphomas of the stomach may also appear as single or multiple mass lesions. They are often firm and covered with relatively normal-appearing mucosa. Lesions may be large sessile polypoid masses or smaller lesions (as small as 1–2 cm). Large lesions may be associated with protein-losing enteropathy (Fig. 6.59). Burkitt's lymphoma may appear as a polypoid mass with a deep central ulceration (Fig. 6.60).

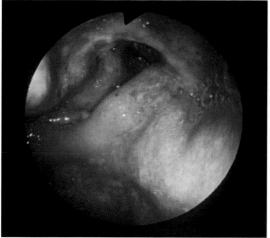

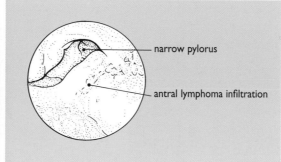

Figure 6.58 Gastric lymphoma involving the distal antrum and the pylorus, producing pyloric narrowing.

▼ **A**

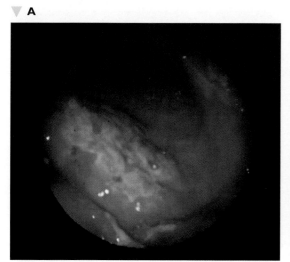

▼ **B**

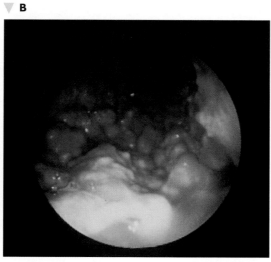

Figure 6.59 (**A**) Extensive non-Hodgkin's lymphoma with nodular involvement of the gastric wall. This lesion was associated with protein-losing enteropathy. (**B**) The diffuse nodular involvement is better seen in this slightly different view.

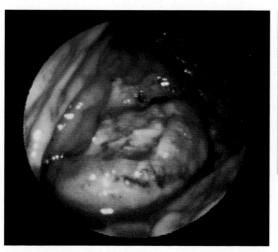

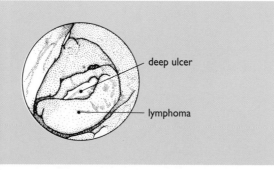

Figure 6.60 Burkitt's lymphoma of the gastric body, with a central ulceration. (Courtesy of Dr Michael Priebe)

Biopsy and other Diagnostic Techniques

Diagnosis of lymphoma of the stomach is accomplished with endoscopic examination, biopsy, and cytology. The yield of biopsy in this lesion is 70–80% and may be as high as 90%. This is slightly better than is seen with infiltrating adenocarcinoma, perhaps because the tumor is more accessible because of the diffuse associated ulceration. Lymphoma is not often as totally submucosal as adenocarcinoma; however, it is still important to biopsy areas with the highest potential yield of positivity (i.e. ulcers, nodules, and areas of abnormal mucosa) and to perform multiple biopsies (Fig. 6.61). Some recommend 10–15 biopsies if lymphoma is suspected. Endoscopically guided sheathed brush cytology may help in the diagnosis. In some instances lymphocytes in the brushing provide a clue. Sometimes deeper biopsies may be necessary, either using endoscopic techniques or at surgery. Endoscopic needle cytology may be helpful in making a diagnosis.

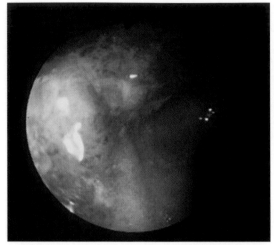
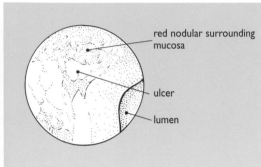

Figure 6.61 *Gastric lymphoma occurring with red, nodular mucosa and a small central ulcer. The abnormal mucosa would be an excellent place to biopsy.*

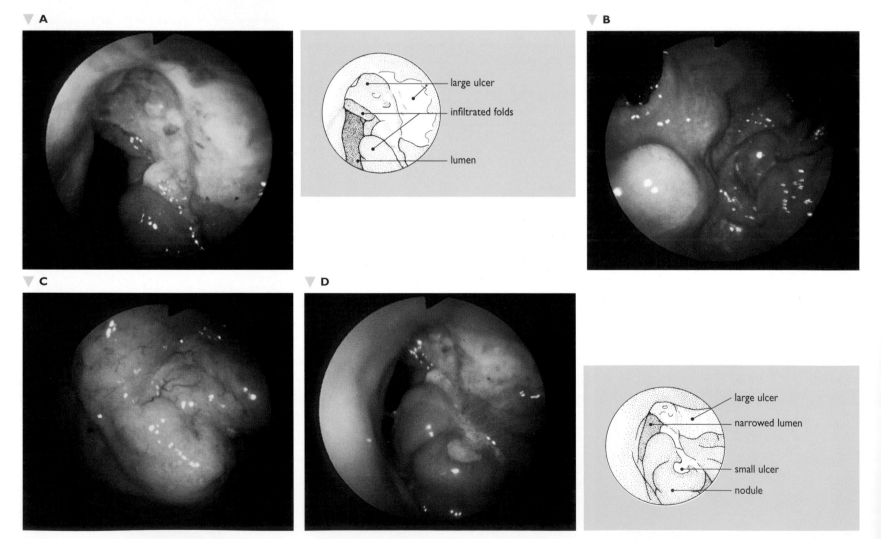

Figure 6.62 *Radiation therapy. (**A**) A large, irregular ulcer in the body of the stomach, caused by gastric lymphoma. (**B**) With the endoscope retroflexed, large nodules can be seen in the fundus. (**C**) In the area of the junction of the corpus and fundus the mucosa appears abnormal with nodules and an irregular, coarse fold pattern caused by the infiltration of the lymphoma. (**D**) Multiple lymphomatous ulcers of varying sizes can be seen in the midcorpus.*

Endoscopy may also be useful to monitor the effect of radiation therapy (Fig. 6.62) or chemotherapy (Figs. 6.63 and 6.64). Ulcers resolve and the thickened, infiltrated mucosa returns to normal.

Cross-sectional imaging techniques such as computed tomography may help in the diagnosis of gastric lymphoma by demonstrating a mass, a thickened gastric wall, or involvement of adjacent lymph nodes. Endosonography is an excellent method for determining the depth of wall invasion and involvement of adjacent organs (Fig. 6.65). High-resolution ultrasound can also be used to follow the response to therapy, seen as a reduction in the size of the mass and the thickness of the wall.

▼ E ▼ F ▼ G

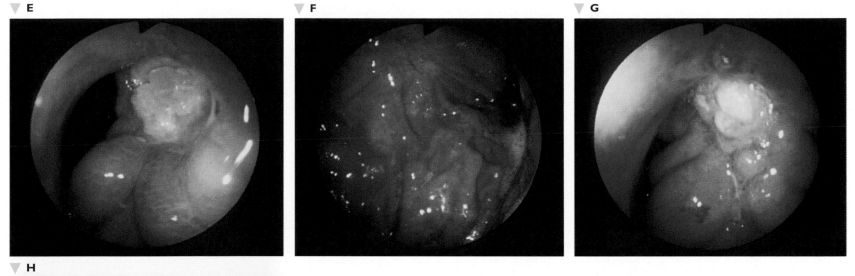

▼ H

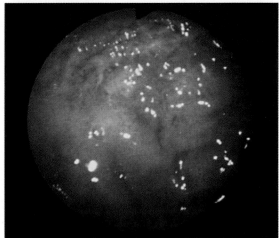

(E) Two weeks after radiation therapy, the small ulcers are gone, the folds converge, and the large ulcer is somewhat smaller. The mucosa is still abnormal, with indurated folds and erythematous mucosa surrounding the ulcer. (F) Five weeks after radiation therapy, the nodules and coarse folds are returning to normal, abnormal vessels can still be seen on the mucosa; (G) the small ulcers are gone, and the large ulcer is smaller. Biopsy of the ulcer was negative for tumor; (H) the fundus appears more normal with a less nodular appearance and nearly normal folds.

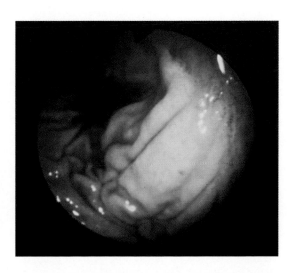

Figure 6.63 Chemotherapy. This patient had been treated with chemotherapy for gastric lymphoma. The stomach now appears normal except for the suggestion of slightly heavy folds.

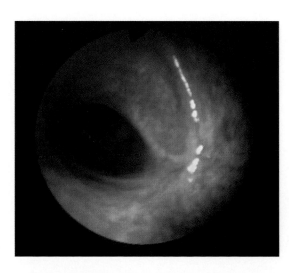

Figure 6.64 Gastric lymphoma after chemotherapy. There is no evidence of residual tumor, just a retracted area where tumor had been present.

GASTRIC SARCOMA

Sarcomas account for approximately 2% of gastric malignancies. These mesenchymal lesions are characteristically large masses (4–5 cm) with primarily submucosal extension (Fig. 6.66). The mass frequently extends outside of the stomach. In approximately 20% of patients there is a central depression in the surface of the mass caused by necrosis (Figs. 6.67–6.69). These

lesions may cause gastrointestinal bleeding (Fig. 6.70). Smaller lesions may appear similar to leiomyomas (submucosal polyps). Leiomyosarcoma is the most common tumor of this type. The differential diagnosis may be a problem even with tissue obtained at biopsy. Histologic examination by biopsy is not often as positive as with other tumors because of the largely submu-

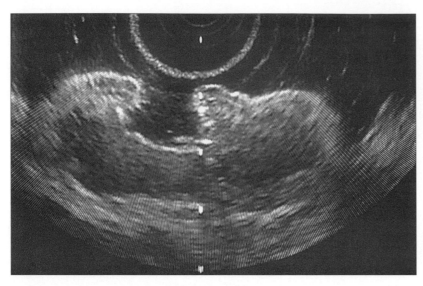

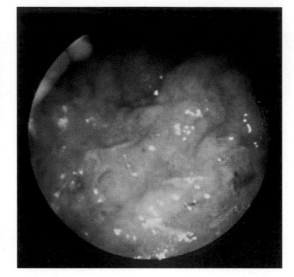

Figure 6.66 *Generalized lymphosarcoma involving the stomach with multiple enlarged folds and superficial ulcers. The submucosal nature of the tumor is suggested by the diffuse nodularity.*

Figure 6.65 *Endoscopic ultrasound image shows a deep ulcer with a tumor mass at the base and margin. This mass proved to be a lymphoma.*

▼ **A**

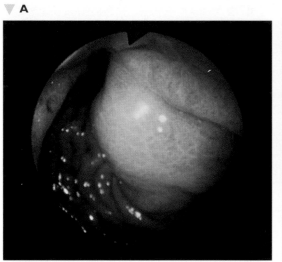

▼ **B**

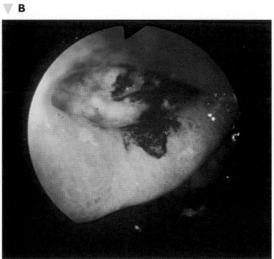

Figure 6.67 *(A) A large mesenchymal tumor is protruding into the proximal gastric lumen. (B) With further insertion of the endoscope it is possible to see the necrosis in the center of the mass, presenting as a deep depression or ulcer. The ulcer is friable.*

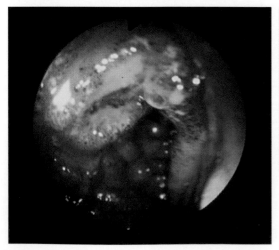

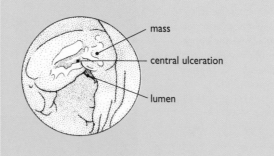

Figure 6.68 *Leiomyosarcoma of the stomach, covered with abnormal mucosa; there is a central ulceration.*

cosal growth pattern. Cytology is of little use in these tumors. The characteristic finding on biopsy is spindle cells with evidence of increased mitotic activity. Less commonly seen sarcomas include liposarcomas, rhabdomyosarcoma, and other spindle cell sarcomas. The different types of sarcoma cannot be distinguished endoscopically.

KAPOSI'S SARCOMA

Kaposi's sarcoma is a systemic disease that involves the skin (especially the soles of the feet and the nose) and may involve the gastrointestinal tract, especially the stomach and colon. Typically, the lesion is seen in patients with AIDS and, rarely, in the elderly. About one-half of patients with AIDS and cutaneous Kaposi's sarcoma have involvement of the gasatrointestinal tract.

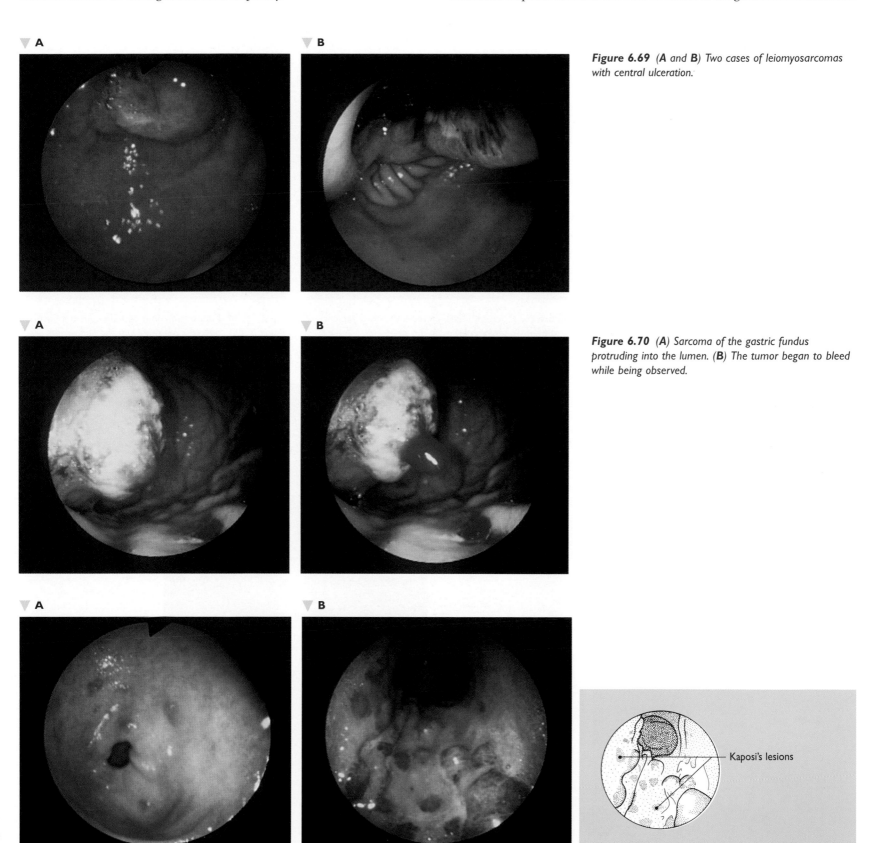

Figure 6.69 (**A** and **B**) *Two cases of leiomyosarcomas with central ulceration.*

Figure 6.70 (**A**) *Sarcoma of the gastric fundus protruding into the lumen.* (**B**) *The tumor began to bleed while being observed.*

Kaposi's lesions

Figure 6.71 *Examples of multiple lesions of Kaposi's sarcoma in two patients with AIDS.* (**A**) *Small early lesions.* (**B**) *Larger later lesions.*

There are three endoscopic appearances of this tumor: single or multiple (Fig. 6.71) maculopapular lesions (Fig. 6.72), polypoid lesions (Fig. 6.73), and ulcerating lesions. Kaposi's sarcoma can also appear in a diffuse form rather than as an isolated maculopapular lesion (Fig. 6.74). Characteristically the lesions are intensely red because of the underlying histopathology, which is that of a capillary hemangiosarcoma with endothelial proliferation. One may see a sessile polyp with red mucosa (Figs. 6.75 and 6.76) and occasionally an ulcerated center (Fig. 6.77). Biopsy is not always diagnostic unless the tumor is on the surface of the lesion. Characteristic findings at biopsy are mesenchymal-type tissue with vascular spaces and endothelial cells among spindle cells.

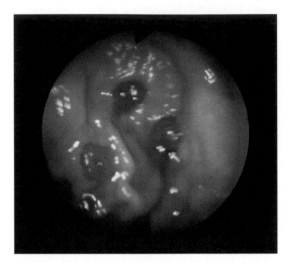

Figure 6.72 *Gastric Kaposi's sarcoma. Lesions appear as red raised maculopapular lesions.*

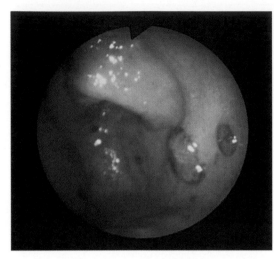

Figure 6.73 *Several sessile polypoid lesions in patient with Kaposi's sarcoma involving the stomach.*

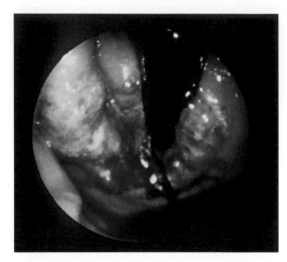

Figure 6.74 *Kaposi's sarcoma appearing as a diffuse lesion of the cardia region, seen with the endoscope retroflexed in the stomach.*

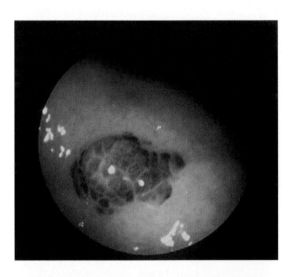

Figure 6.75 *Lesion of Kaposi's sarcoma in a patient with AIDS. The lesion could be confused with a polyp, but the covering mucosa has the characteristic striking red appearance.*

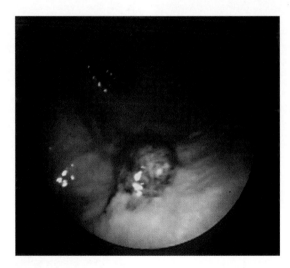

Figure 6.76 *Kaposi's sarcoma in the antrum occurring as a raised red mass. The pylorus is in the background.*

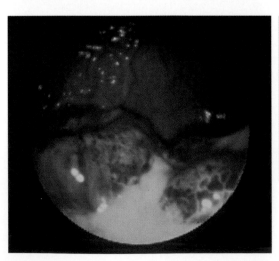

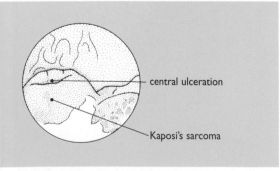

central ulceration

Kaposi's sarcoma

Figure 6.77 *Central ulceration in the larger of two Kaposi's sarcoma lesions in a patient with AIDS. (Courtesy of Dr Fred Weinstein)*

METASTATIC GASTRIC DISEASE

Cancer of the lung and breast and melanoma may metastasize to the stomach. More rarely, tumors of the pancreas, testis, thyroid, and female genital tract may metastasize to the stomach. The finding of a gastric lesion may be the first indication of metastatic spread. These patients may present with pain or bleeding and are then diagnosed at endoscopy to have lesions suggestive of metastases.

These lesions may present as small (1–2 cm), multiple submucosal lesions (Fig. 6.78) or as tumors that project into the lumen with a central ulceration thought to result from outgrowth of the blood supply. This ulceration may be the cause of a presenting symptom of gastrointestinal hemorrhage. Characteristic pigmentation may be noted in melanoma although larger lesions may be amelanotic or contain limited pigment (Figs. 6.79 and 6.80). Other cancers, such as metastatic breast cancer, may appear as diffuse infiltrative growths (Figs. 6.81 and 6.82) or sessile, polypoid masses (Fig. 6.83).

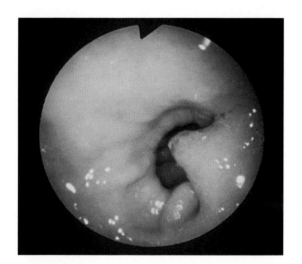

Figure 6.78 Intramural metastasis in the antral wall of the stomach in a patient with squamous cell carcinoma of the esophagus.

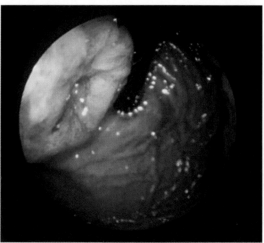

Figure 6.79 Gastric metastasis of an amelanotic melanosarcoma, seen as an umbilicated lesion adjacent to the endoscope, and observed as the endoscope tip is retroflexed.

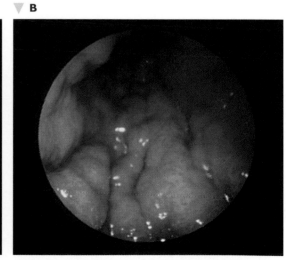

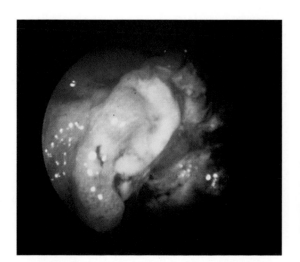

Figure 6.80 Large metastasis of melanosarcoma to the stomach. The folds are distorted and there is a suggestion of pigment in the upper right part of the lesion.

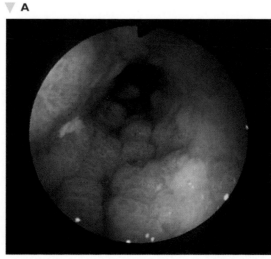

▼ A   ▼ B

Figure 6.81 (**A and B**) Two examples of metastatic lesions to the stomach from breast carcinoma. The gastric mucosa appears nodular and friable. These tumors infiltrated diffusely. Biopsy was positive for breast carcinoma in each case.

GASTRIC POLYPS

Gastric polyps are detected in 2–3% of upper gastrointestinal endoscopic examinations, often incidentally. They are usually small, with a diameter of less than 1–2 cm. Occasionally a polyp is seen on barium x-ray and is the reason for a referral for endoscopy. With larger polyps, patients may complain of vague abdominal discomfort, bleeding may occur, and rarely a prolapsing antral polyp may obstruct the gastric outlet.

Polyps may be neoplastic or nonneoplastic. Neoplastic lesions that may occur as polyps of the stomach include adenoma (relatively rare), carcinoma (the most common polypoid neoplastic lesion), and some unusual lesions such as carcinoids. Any gastric neoplasm may appear as a polyp. Gastric adenocarcinomas appearing as polyps are discussed earlier in this chapter.

About 80–90% of gastric polyps are nonneoplastic. They can be divided into epithelial and nonepithelial types. The epithelial lesions include hyperplastic polyps (the most common polyp seen in the stomach) and polyps seen with a variety of polyposis conditions of the gastrointestinal tract including juvenile polyposis, Peutz-Jeghers syndrome, and Cronkhite-Canada syndrome.

These three types of polyps can be difficult to distinguish histologically with the exception of the Peutz-Jeghers polyp, which can be differentiated if the entire polyp is available for examination. Endoscopically, these polyps may appear similar except that the Peutz-Jeghers polyp is usually larger than the others (Fig. 6.84). All three of these polyps are characteristically larger than the typical hyperplastic polyp (3–4 cm compared with 1–2 cm).

The other type of epithelial polyp in the stomach is the fundal gland polyp seen in patients with and without familial polyposis coli (FPC) syndrome. These fundal gland polyps consist of dilated foveolae and glandular structures. Patients with FPC have an increased incidence both of adenomas of the stomach and fundal gland polyps. Adenomatous polyps are considered a risk factor for the development of gastric carcinoma, whereas fundal gland polyps are not. Patients with Gardner's syndrome may also develop multiple adenomas.

Patients may present with multiple gastric polyps. If the polyps are adenomatous there is considered to be an increased risk of malignancy. If the polyps are hyperplastic there is no risk of the polyps themselves becoming malignant, but the surrounding atrophic gastritis may be a fertile soil for the development of malignancy. The fundal gland polyps are not considered to be premalignant.

▼ **A**   ▼ **B**

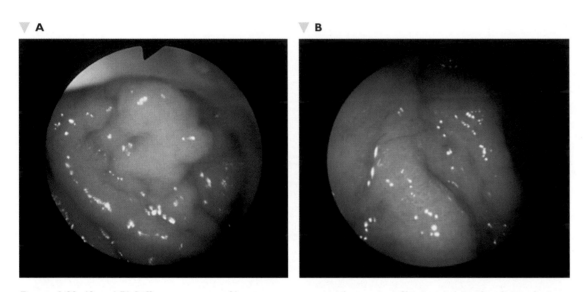

Figure 6.82 (**A** and **B**) Diffuse metastases of breast cancer to stomach appears infiltrative and simulate linitis plastica.

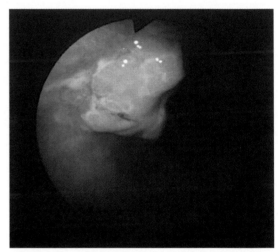

Figure 6.83 Intragastric metastasis of carcinoma of the breast. The lesion appears sessile and polypoid, covered with irregular nodular mucosa.

▼ **A**   ▼ **B**

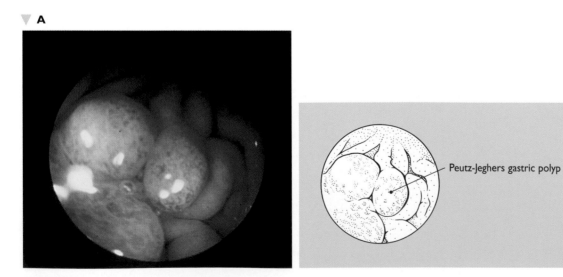

Peutz-Jeghers gastric polyp

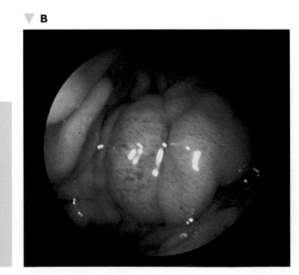

Figure 6.84 (**A** and **B**) Two views of Peutz-Jeghers gastric polyp. The polyp surface is multilobed and erythematous. The base or stalk is not seen in these photographs.

Nonneoplastic nonepithelial polyps of mesenchymal origin include leiomyomas, adenomyomas, hamartomas, and lipomas. They are discussed separately under *Submucosal Masses* towards the end of this chapter.

NEOPLASTIC POLYPS
Adenomatous Polyps

Adenomas are uncommon, accounting for only 5–10% of polypoid lesions in the stomach. Up to 40% contain a focus of carcinoma, especially the larger villous lesions (greater than 2 cm). These polyps may become malignant with time. The risk of cancer in the adjacent stomach tissue may be as high as 30%. These polyps are usually larger than hyperplastic polyps when first detected (over 1 cm in two-thirds of patients). The average size of gastric adenomas is 3–4 cm. These polyps are associated with atrophic gastritis and FPC, although the majority of the gastric polyps in FPC are nonadenomatous with glandular cysts. When adenomas occur in FPC, there is disagreement as to the risk of gastric cancer. The risk of malignant degeneration may vary in different countries.

Adenomas of the stomach have three histologic configurations, similar to adenomas of the colon: tubular, villous, and mixed or tubulovillous. The latter two are associated with the highest risk of developing cancer in the polyp. Villous tumors are often large, antral, sessile, superficially eroded, associated with blood loss, and may obstruct the gastric outlet.

There is disagreement about whether hyperplastic polyps can develop into adenomatous polyps of the stomach. The confusion stems from the rare case in which a polyp contains elements of both adenoma and hyperplastic polyp.

Endoscopic Appearance

Adenomatous polyps are reddish in color, often with a multilobed surface (Fig. 6.85). The surface may be smooth or superficially eroded (Fig. 6.86). The presence of erosion or ulceration is thought to correlate with an increased risk of cancer in the polyp. Similarly, superficial erosion and atypia may increase the likelihood of a gastric cancer being present (Figs. 6.87 and 6.88). Adenomatous polyps are usually sessile but may have a pedicle

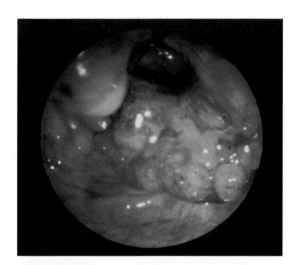

Figure 6.85 Adenoma of the stomach. The polyp is multilobed.

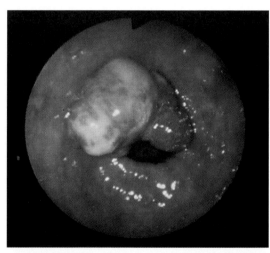

Figure 6.86 Adenoma of the antrum. The surface is eroded and covered with exudate.

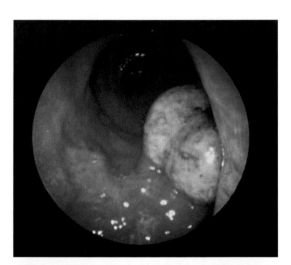

Figure 6.87 Adenomatous polyp of the antrum. The surface is slightly atypical and eroded. In fact, this was associated with a diffuse gastric adenocarcinoma proximally.

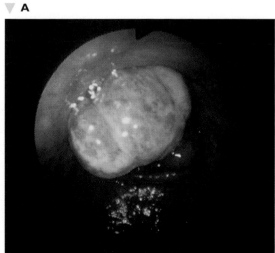

▼ A

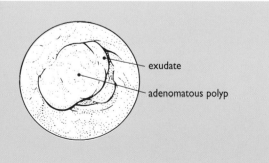

exudate

adenomatous polyp

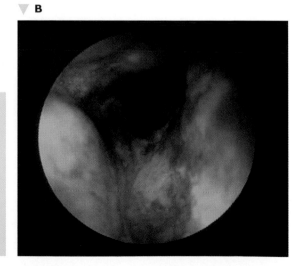

▼ B

Figure 6.88 (A) Adenomatous polyp with superficial erosion and exudation. Histologically, atypia was noted. (B) Circumferential cancer was found to be present along the entire proximal stomach.

similar to a hyperplastic polyp. They occur in the antrum and, less frequently, in the body of the stomach. Adenomas occur singly in 60% of cases. The surrounding mucosa often shows atrophic changes (Fig. 6.89).

NON-NEOPLASTIC EPITHELIAL POLYPS
Hyperplastic Polyps

Hyperplastic polyps are the most common polypoid lesions of the stomach, far more common than adenomatous polyps. They do not seem to enlarge with time as do adenomatous polyps. The histology is that of hyperplasia of foveolar elements. These polyps may also be seen in the stump after gastrectomy. Rarely, hyperplastic polyps are associated with a carcinoma or an adenoma in the same lesion.

Hyperplastic polyps and adenomas are both associated with chronic gastritis with varying degrees of atrophy. The likelihood that hyperplastic polyps are associated with atrophic gastritis is proportional to the number of polyps. If there are more than 10 polyps, the chance of associated atrophic gastritis is as high as 30%. These polyps probably never become cancerous, but there is a slightly increased risk of cancer elsewhere in the atrophic stomach.

Endoscopic Appearance

Hyperplastic polyps can occur throughout the stomach. They are usually less than 1.5 cm in diameter (Fig. 6.90), may be single or multiple, and may be sessile (Fig. 6.91) or pedunculated. A long stalk may be seen (Fig. 6.92). The mucosa covering a small polyp may appear normal. With larger polyps, the overlying mucosa is often red and friable, and there may be a small erosion or ulceration on the tip of the polyp. The mucosa in which these polyps occur may be atrophic or show evidence of gastritis. The 10–20% of polyps that are larger than 2 cm may be confused with adenomatous or carcinomatous lesions.

The lesions seen in endoscopic raised erosive gastritis (varioliform gastritis) may resemble hyperplastic polyps histologically because of the foveolar hyperplasia. Both may represent a response of the gastric mucosa to injury. In raised erosive gastritis, the injury induces an erosion with hyperplasia of the surrounding mucosa (Fig. 6.93), whereas with a hyperplastic polyp there is hyperplasia without an erosion in most cases (Fig. 6.94).

Fundal Gland Polyps

Fundal gland polyps are seen as single, multiple, or as a carpet of polyps in the gastric fundus (Figs. 6.95–6.98). The polyps are bumps with dilated gas-

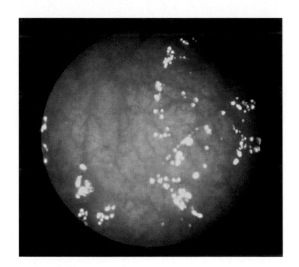

Figure 6.89 *Atrophic gastric mucosa in a patient with an adenomatous polyp. Blood vessels are visible through the mucosa. The polyp is not visible.*

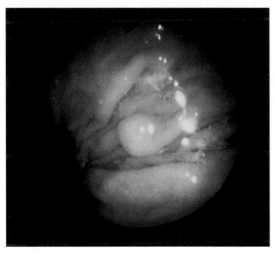

Figure 6.90 *A small gastric hyperplastic polyp in a patient with atrophic gastritis.*

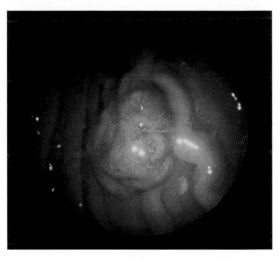

Figure 6.91 *Sessile hyperplastic polyp in the stomach.*

▼ A

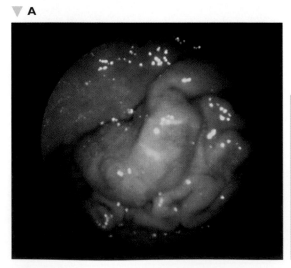

▼ B

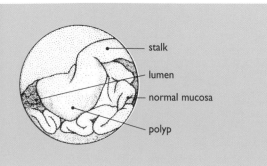

stalk
lumen
normal mucosa
polyp

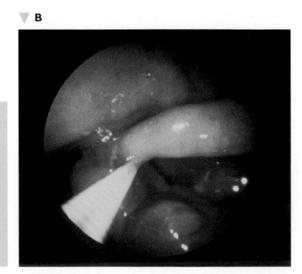

Figure 6.92 *(A and B) Hyperplastic polyps in the stomach. With manipulation, the long stalk of the polyp can be seen.*

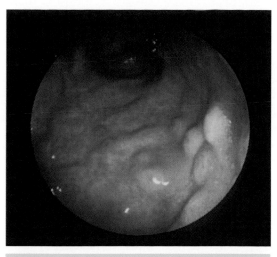

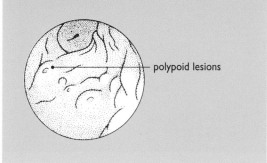

Figure 6.93 *Varioliform gastritis in the antrum of a patient with gastric cancer (relationship between gastritis and cancer unknown). Typical polypoid lesions with a central dimple are seen.*

polypoid lesions

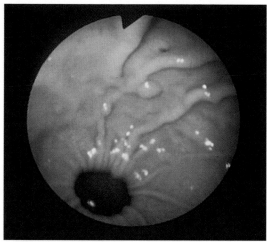

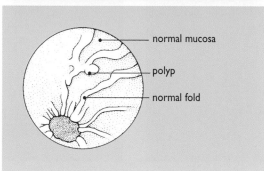

Figure 6.94 *Hyperplastic polyp in the antrum. The surrounding mucosa is normal. The polyp differs histologically from the lesion in varioliform gastritis.*

normal mucosa

polyp

normal fold

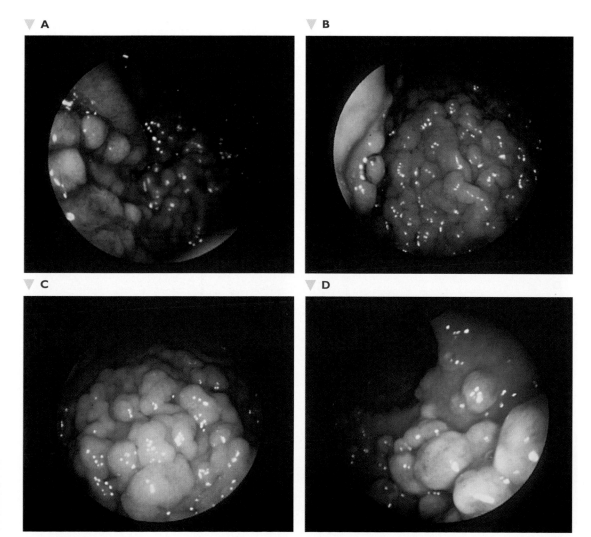

▼ A ▼ B ▼ C ▼ D

Figure 6.95 *(A–D) Multiple small fundal gland polyps of the cystic glandularis type in patients with FPC.*

tric fundal glands and foveolar cells. They occur in patients with or without FPC, and they may occur in Peutz-Jeghers syndrome. These lesions are not normally associated with gastric cancer either in the polyp or in the rest of the stomach.

MANAGEMENT OF POLYPS

Neoplastic and nonneoplastic polyps cannot be distinguished endoscopically. Forceps biopsy alone is not sufficient as the entire polyp is often needed to establish histologic type. In many instances the polyp can be removed using

standard polypectomy techniques (Fig. 6.99). However, there is a risk of hemorrhage especially after removal of large polyps. In the future it may prove useful to study the large polyp and stalk with the ultrasound endoscope to determine the vascular anatomy of the stalk before making a decision about endoscopic polypectomy. For polyps larger than 1–2 cm, the safest course is to snare off a piece or use a large biopsy forceps rather than attempt total snare resection. If the polyp proves to be hyperplastic it need not be removed, but periodic endoscopic surveillance is recommended because of the risk of carcinoma elsewhere in the stomach. If the polyp is an adenoma, especially

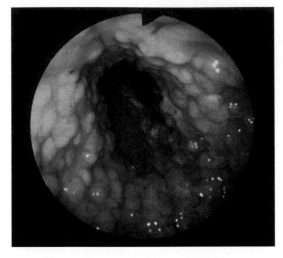

Figure 6.96 *A carpet of cystic-type fundal gland polyps in a patient with FPC.*

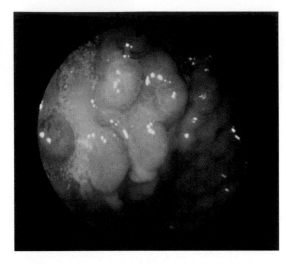

Figure 6.97 *Cystic gastric polyposis in a patient without FPC.*

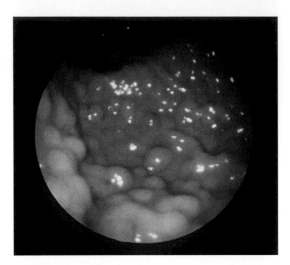

Figure 6.98 *Carpet of gastric polyps in a patient with Peutz-Jeghers syndrome.*

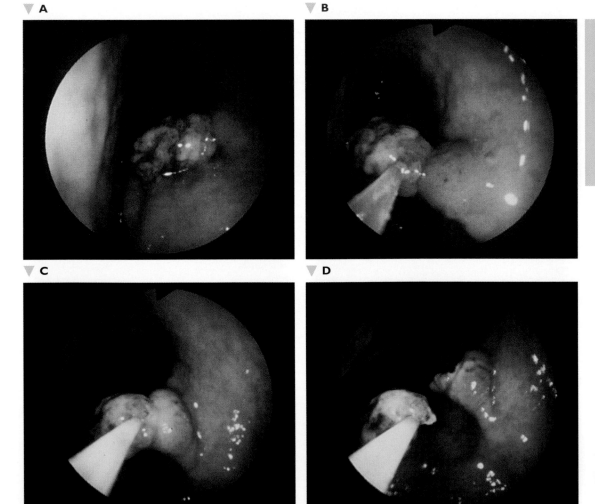

Figure 6.99 *Polypectomy. (A) A patient presented with an adenomatous gastric polyp. The surface is friable, and there is a stalk that is not well seen here. (B) The polyp is snared. (C) The stalk turns white as the wire is closed and electrosurgical coagulating current is applied. (D) The polyp is resected.*

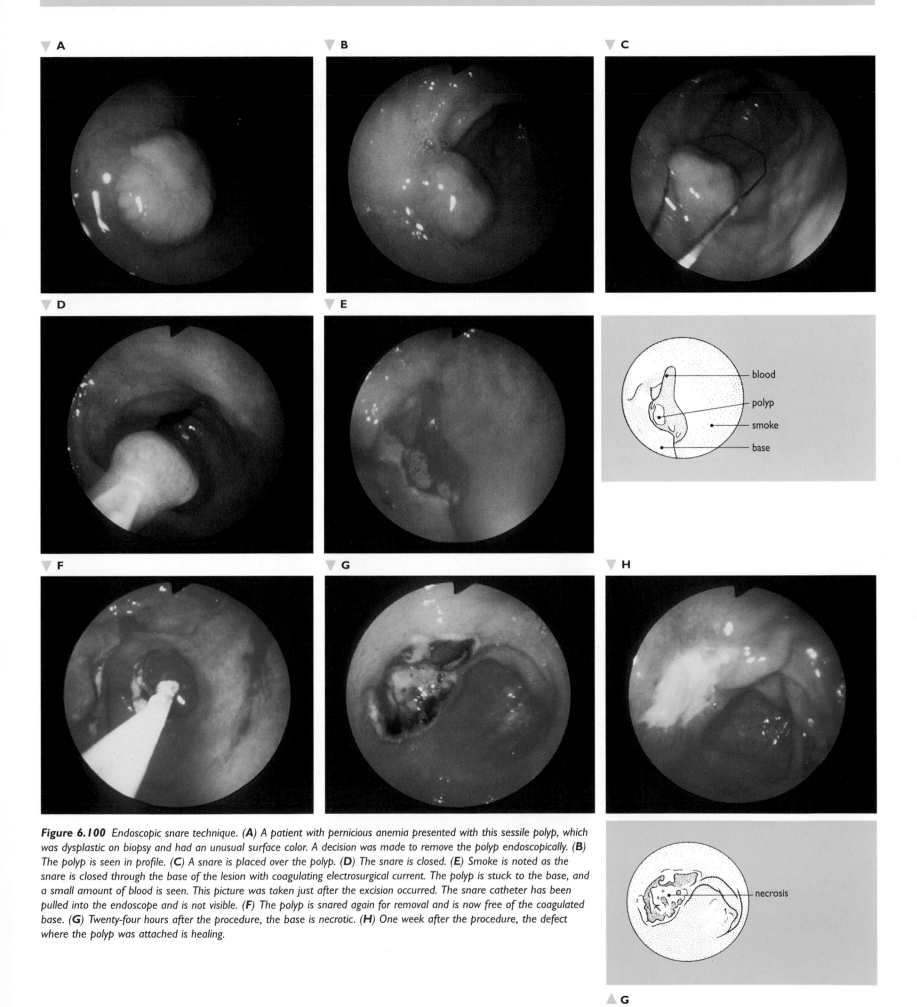

Figure 6.100 *Endoscopic snare technique.* **(A)** *A patient with pernicious anemia presented with this sessile polyp, which was dysplastic on biopsy and had an unusual surface color. A decision was made to remove the polyp endoscopically.* **(B)** *The polyp is seen in profile.* **(C)** *A snare is placed over the polyp.* **(D)** *The snare is closed.* **(E)** *Smoke is noted as the snare is closed through the base of the lesion with coagulating electrosurgical current. The polyp is stuck to the base, and a small amount of blood is seen. This picture was taken just after the excision occurred. The snare catheter has been pulled into the endoscope and is not visible.* **(F)** *The polyp is snared again for removal and is now free of the coagulated base.* **(G)** *Twenty-four hours after the procedure, the base is necrotic.* **(H)** *One week after the procedure, the defect where the polyp was attached is healing.*

if it is sessile, large, and villous or mixed tubulovillous, resection should be considered. Endoscopic snare techniques can be used (Fig. 6.100). Submucosal injection of saline or adrenaline 1:10 000 may improve the efficacy and safety of endoscopic removal by piecemeal snare polypectomy. Surgical resection may be required in some cases with large, sessile polyps. These patients should also be surveyed periodically for the development of additional polyps and cancer in the stomach. There is a 2–3% risk of developing cancer in the stomach after removal of an adenoma.

SUBMUCOSAL MASSES

There is a variety of lesions in the stomach that are occasionally symptomatic (bleeding) but are usually found incidentally at endoscopy. These include carcinoids, pancreatic rests, leiomyomas, adenomyomas, hamartomas, and lipomas. As a group these lesions are small and difficult to distinguish from hyperplastic or adenomatous polyps. A common finding is a central depression surrounded by normal mucosa. This contrasts with the eroded area that may be seen on adenomatous or hyperplastic polyps in which the erosion often covers the surface of the polyp. With a submucosal mass the ulcer is usually sharply delineated from the surrounding normal mucosa. The cause of the depression may be necrosis as a result of the tumor outgrowing its blood supply. Because of the submucosal location of these masses, there are often bridging folds on either side of the mass.

Histologic diagnosis is made using a polypectomy specimen or by performing repeated biopsies in the same area to sample progressively deeper tissue. Pedunculated lesions may be safely removed with a snare. Sessile sub-

mucosal lesions are either left or removed surgically. Once this type of lesion is recognized, patients are usually just kept under observation. If the tumor is large or bleeding, it may be necessary to remove it surgically.

ENDOSONOGRAPHY OF SUBMUCOSAL MASSES

Endoscopic ultrasound can be used to examine masses beneath the mucosal surface. With ultrasound it is possible to image the lesion, determine its size, determine whether it is limited to the wall itself or extends beyond the wall, and in some cases determine the layer of origin of the masses. This information is useful diagnostically and to direct therapy. Endoscopic ultrasound can be used to guide needle puncture for biopsy and cytology.

CARCINOIDS

Carcinoids are rarely encountered in the stomach: 1 or 2% of gastric polyps are carcinoids. The tumor is usually sessile with a small ulcer at the tip. The lesions may be multiple with small polyps or may appear as flat, occasionally ulcerated lesions. Multiple carcinoids, or enterochromaffin-like (ECL)-omas, occur in patients with gastrinoma and the multiple endocrine neoplasia, type 1 (MEN-I) syndrome. Presumably the excessive gastrin drive leads to proliferation and micronodule formation of the ECL cells. Few patients experience symptoms of the carcinoid syndrome. As the tumor grows larger than 2.0–2.5 cm the likelihood of metastases increases. Smaller lesions are less likely to metastasize. Small lesions are occasionally removed endoscopically, but large sessile lesions and malignant lesions should be removed surgically. After removal, periodic surveillance is indicated to detect the occurrence of new lesions.

▼ **A**

▼ **B**

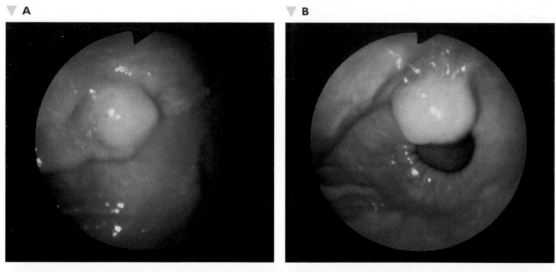

*Figure 6.101 (**A** and **B**) Small submucosal tumor, typical of a leiomyoma. There is a suggestion of bridging folds.*

▼ **A**

▼ **B**

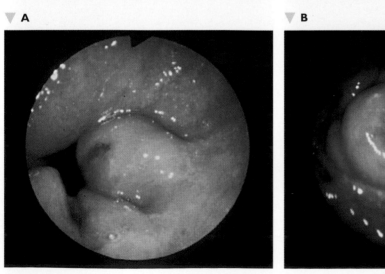
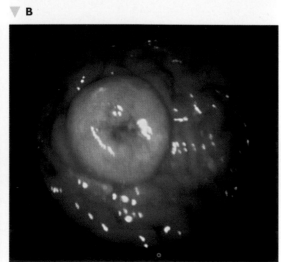

*Figure 6.102 Two leiomyomas of the stomach. (**A**) Note a small dimple on the tip of the mass. (**B**) A deeper depression in the mass is seen.*

LEIOMYOMAS

Leiomyomas are one of the more common types of submucosal tumors. They are usually small (less than 1–2 cm) (Fig. 6.101), proximal in the stomach (Fig. 6.102), and are attached firmly to the underlying gastric wall. Rarely, these tumors may be 15–20 cm and extend outside the gastric wall and into the gastric lumen (Fig. 6.103). The surface mucosa is not attached to the tumor and may be smooth or have a central depression, especially in large lesions (Figs. 6.102 and 6.103). This depression may actually be an ulcer that can bleed (Fig. 6.104). Bridging folds may be observed (Figs. 6.105 and 6.106). Histologically, the tissue consists of spindle-shaped cells. The differential diagnosis includes leiomyoblastoma, a tumor of similar appearance with a higher degree of mitotic activity and an increased risk of malignancy compared with leiomyomas.

Endosonography can be used to help differentiate a localized leiomyoma from a malignant leiomyoblastoma. The initial distinction is usually based on size; lesions of over 5 cm are more likely to be malignant than smaller lesions.

▼ A

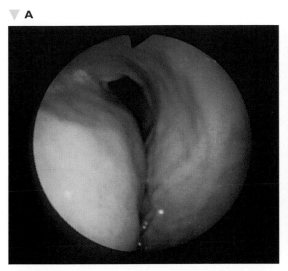

▼ B

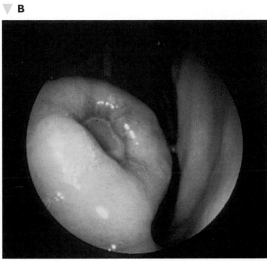

Figure 6.103 (**A**) A large submucosal leiomyoma is seen bulging into the lumen. This patient presented with gastrointestinal bleeding. (**B**) With repositioning of the endoscope, an ulcer can be seen at the tip of the mass.

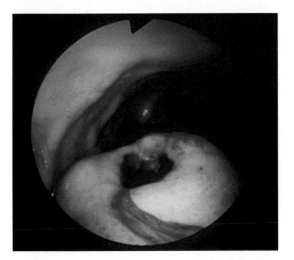

Figure 6.104 Gastric leiomyoma with central ulcerated depression and active gastrointestinal bleeding from the ulcer.

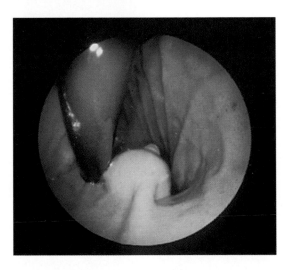

Figure 6.105 A gastric leiomyoma of the fundus with bridging folds.

▼ A

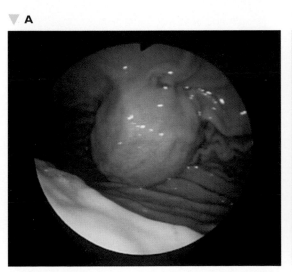

▼ B

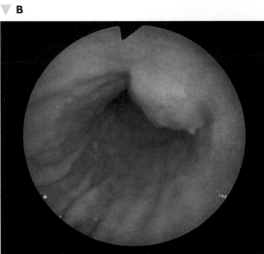

▼ C

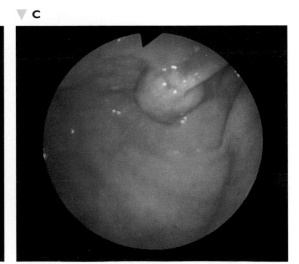

Figure 6.106 (**A–C**) Three cases of gastric leiomyoma covered with normal-appearing mucosa, with bridging folds.

ADENOMYOMAS AND HAMARTOMAS

Adenomyomas and hamartomas lesions cannot be distinguished endoscopically from other types of gastric polyps. They are the typical size for gastric polyps (1–2 cm), sessile or pedunculated, and the covering mucosa may be

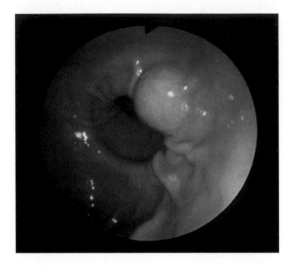

Figure 6.107 *Gastric lipoma presents a soft, yellowish-appearing submucosal mass.*

normal or show superficial erosion. Lesions that at histologic examination contain pancreatic ductal tissue and smooth muscle are called adenomyomas. These rarely contain acinar tissue as do pancreatic rests. Adenomyomas are located in the antrum on the greater curvature side, in the same area of the stomach as pancreatic rests. Without the pancreatic component to the tissue, they are called hamartomas. Hamartomas occur in patients with Peutz-Jeghers syndrome. Some gastric polyps in juvenile polyposis are hamartomas. These are not premalignant and there is no increased risk of cancer in the residual stomach.

OTHER TUMORS

Several other types of tumors involve the gastric wall, such as vascular tumors, lipomas, and neurofibromas. Firm lesions are characteristically vascular tumors of the glomus type, gastric fibromas, and neurofibromas. Lipomas are typically yellow, are often associated with lipomas elsewhere in the gastrointestinal tract, and may be pedunculated or sessile (Fig. 6.107). They are occasionally very large and seem soft when touched with a biopsy forceps. Eosinophilic granuloma is also in the differential diagnosis of a polyp. This lesion has a characteristic histology that includes infiltration by many eosinophilic leukocytes in addition to fibroblasts and histiocytes.

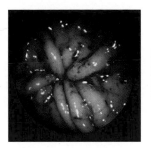

7

Stomach III: Gastritis and Upper Gastrointestinal Bleeding

In this chapter we consider a variety of inflammatory lesions of the gastric mucosa, referred to collectively as gastritis. We review the general aspects of gastritis, acute and chronic gastritis, the role of *Helicobacter pylori*, atrophic gastritis, erosive gastritis, drug-induced gastritis, hemorrhagic gastritis, stress-induced gastritis, and gastritis associated with giant folds and radiation. We also consider gastric manifestations of Crohn's disease and caustic gastric injury. A brief review of endoscopic techniques in the diagnosis of upper gastrointestinal bleeding is presented.

GASTRITIS

Normal gastric mucosa is smooth and has a brownish-red shiny appearance. The folds are regular and easily disappear upon insufflation. In gastritis, inflammatory changes take place that may be difficult to interpret because of their variability.

Several diagnostic features are characteristic of gastritis. Mucosal reddening or erythema probably reflects superficial mucosal hyperemia, which is often undetectable histologically. Patches of focal mucosal thickening and whitish discoloration are seen between reddish areas, especially in the antrum. The mucosa may look dull and granular (Fig. 7.1), and the areae gastricae pattern may be especially pronounced and irregular. Mucosal folds can be either reduced or excessively pronounced and tortuous. The mucosa may be covered with excessive amountsof mucus-like gray–yellow, brown or green material (Fig. 7.2). There may be excessive bile staining the gastric juice or smearing the mucosa. The vascular pattern, especially of the submucosa, may become visible. There may be punctate intramucosal or submucosal hemorrhages (petechiae) or larger hemorrhagic spots. Necrosis of the epithelial layer is visible as flat or raised erosive defects. The severity and distribution of these changes may vary in different parts of the stomach. In general, there is poor correlation between endoscopic findings and underlying histologic changes.

ACUTE GASTRITIS

Patients with acute gastritis experience sudden upper gastric pain, nausea, and vomiting. Many episodes are associated with excessive food or alcohol intake, but in other cases no cause of the gastritis is found. Undoubtedly some cases are due to the initial phases of infection with *Helicobacter pylori*. Symptoms are fleeting, which explains why only a few such patients are examined endoscopically.

There are three types of acute gastritis. Type 1 is the mildest form and is characterized by generalized mucosal edema, narrowing of the antrum, and a velvet-like appearance of the mucosa without erosions or other changes. Type 2, the hemorrhagic type, is characterized by swollen folds and diminished distensibility, with diffuse hemorrhagic spots and erosive defects. Type 3, the ulcerative type, is characterized by extensive erosions or ulcers accompanied by hemorrhage. After the bleeding stops, irregularly shaped ulcers may become more distinct, especially on the posterior wall of the antrum.

CHRONIC GASTRITIS

Chronic gastritis when the patient is examined in the endoscopy room, the acute phase of gastritis has subsided and the endoscopist may be faced with one of the many variants of chronic inflammation.

Endoscopic Erythematous Exudative Gastritis

Erythema of the gastric mucosa is the principal endoscopic finding in chronic erythematous exudative gastritis. The mucosa may be involved diffusely, focally, or in a linear fashion. The changes may be noted in the body, antrum, or both, and characteristically are found along the crests of the gastric folds. In addition to erythema, patchy edematous areas and, occasionally, some coarsening of the fold pattern may be noted (Figs. 7.3–7.6). Accentuation and irregularity of the areae gastricae pattern are also common (Fig. 7.7). In the antrum, patchy opalescent areas may be visible between foci of more reddened mucosa. There may be a granular unevenness to the mucosa and a loss of luster or shininess. Occasionally, reddish streaks are seen in the antrum, which run radially towards the pylorus. (These are not to be confused with gastric antral vascular ectasia). They may be secondary to damage from duodenal gastric reflux. Such gastric changes with edema and erythema are commonly observed in patients with gastric stasis, as in diabetic gastroenteropathy (Fig. 7.8).

Histologic findings are variable. Most commonly, capillaries are dilated. There is also evidence of epithelial mucin depletion. Evidence of chronic gastritis with variable degrees of activity and atrophy is frequently encountered histologically. This form of chronic gastritis is located primarily in the antrum and less often appears diffusely over the stomach or in isolated areas of the corpus or fundus.

Our understanding of the pathophysiological aspects of gastritis remains somewhat limited. However, in recent years there has been an increasing interest in the role *H. pylori* plays in its development. This bacillus is thought to be a major predisposing or causative factor in gastritis and also possibly in gastric and duodenal ulcer. Formerly known as *Campylobacter pylori*, *H. pylori* is a Gram-negative bacillus that can be identified from biopsies of the mucosa by staining and histological examination. Preferred stains include Giemsa, Genta, Warthin-Starry and monoclonal antibody stains. *H. pylori* produces high concentrations of urease and this characteristic can be used to identify the bacillus, either by analysis of biopsy tissue or by using a urea breath test. In addition, serum antibody tests capable of detecting antibodies to *H. pylori* are now available.

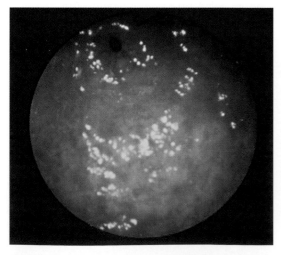

Figure 7.1 *Endoscopic features of gastritis. Antrum with mild inflammatory changes shows patchy reddening and discrete unevenness, as evidenced by irregular highlighting.*

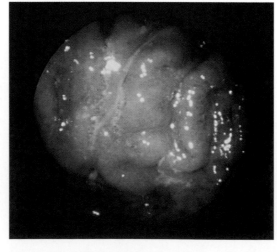
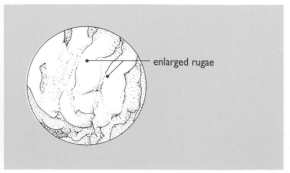

Figure 7.2 *Endoscopic features of gastritis. Mucosa covered with mucus-like material. Rugae are slightly enlarged and show an irregular pattern.*

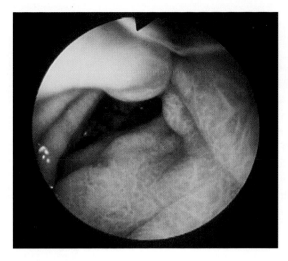

Figure 7.3 *Erythematous gastritic changes in the corpus and fundus in a patient with renal insufficiency.*

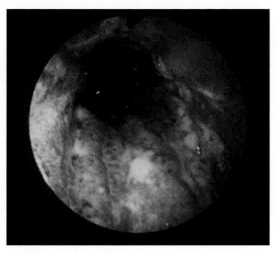

Figure 7.4 *Severe swelling and erythema of the corpus and fundus. These changes are presumably caused by portal vein thrombosis in a patient diagnosed with severe ulcerative colitis.*

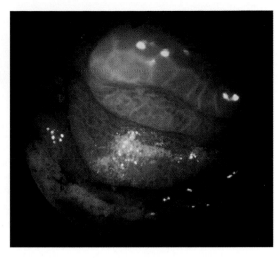

Figure 7.5 *More severe, erythematous gastritis with marked erythema, swelling, and coarsening of fold pattern.*

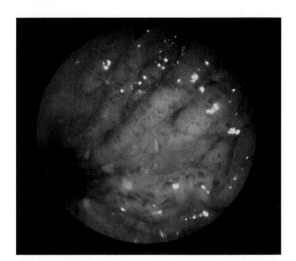

Figure 7.6 *Severe erythematous, exudative gastritis of the corpus and fundus. Coarsening of fold pattern, erythema, and mucopurulent exudate accumulation may be noted.*

▼ **A**

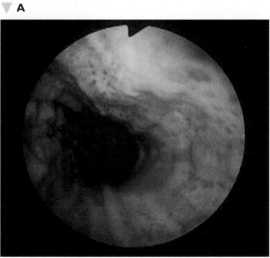

▼ **B**

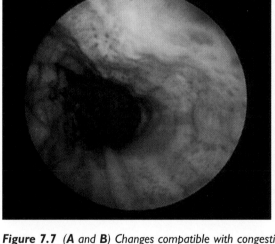

Figure 7.7 *(A and B) Changes compatible with congestive gastroenteropathy of the corpus and fundus areas include erythema and accentuation of the areae gastricae. The condition is commonly seen in cirrhosis with esophageal varices, presumably due to portal hypertension.*

▼ **A** ▼ **B**

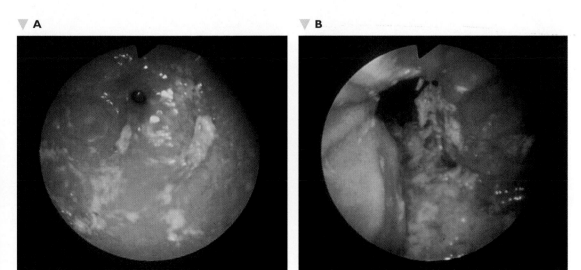

Figure 7.8 *(A and B) Diabetic gastroparesis causing food stagnation and gastric changes in the corpus. These changes are commonly observed in patients with gastric stasis (stagnant gastritis).*

The exact connection between *H. pylori* and peptic ulcer disease, both gastric and duodenal, and *H. pylori* and other conditions such as nonsteroidal anti-inflammatory drug (NSAID)-induced ulcer development, is not yet fully understood. One problem is that a substantial, age-dependent proportion of the adult population tests positive for *H. pylori* in the gastric mucosa.

Endoscopic findings in Helicobacter pylori gastritis

H. pylori is not thought to be responsible for a specific type of endoscopic gastritis. However, it may be responsible for what has been described as endoscopic erythematous exudative gastritis. The mucosa, especially in the antrum, is usually erythematous (Fig. 7.9), and the duodenum may also be involved. There may be an accentuation of the areae gastricae pattern in *H. pylori* gastritis (Fig. 7.10). Duodenitis manifests as erythema and erosion (endoscopic erythematous exudative duodenitis) (Figs. 7.11 and 7.12). Other associated conditions include varioliform gastritis (Fig. 7.13) and gastric ulcer surrounded by mucosa revealing *H. pylori*-positive gastritis (Fig. 7.14).

Endoscopic Atrophic Gastritis

If the normal stomach is fully distended with air (carefully avoiding overdistension), vessels typically become visible, especially in the fundic region. In atrophic gastritis, mucosal and submucosal capillaries and vessels are visible without excessive distension with air because of marked atrophy and thinning of the mucosa (Figs. 7.15 and 7.16). In addition to visible blood vessels, other abnormalities in atrophic gastritis include a decrease in the rugal fold prominence, which may progress to fold disappearance, and mucosal unevenness or slight nodularity (Fig. 7.17). In addition there may be larger hyperplastic or adenomatous polyps.

▼ **A**   ▼ **B**

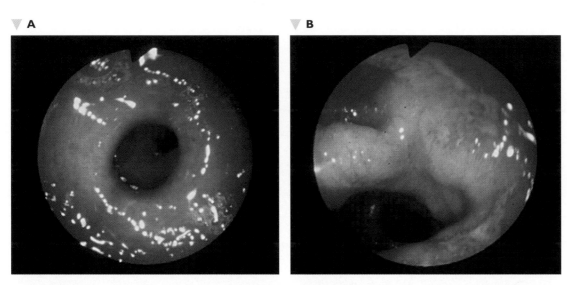

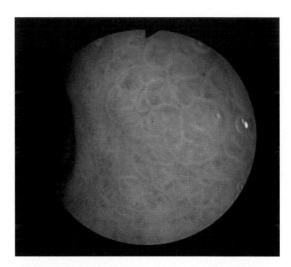

Figure 7.9 (**A** and **B**) Two examples of H. pylori endoscopic erythematous exudative gastritis. The antrum is primarily involved. The mucosa is erythematous, with small superficial erosions.

Figure 7.10 H. pylori gastritis with coarse areae gastricae mucosal pattern.

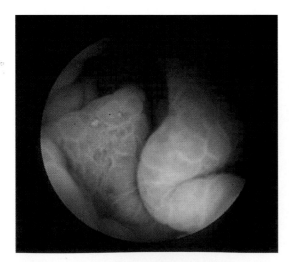

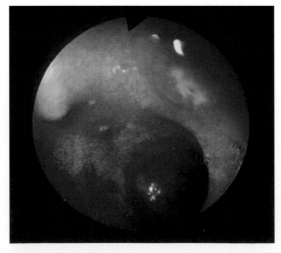

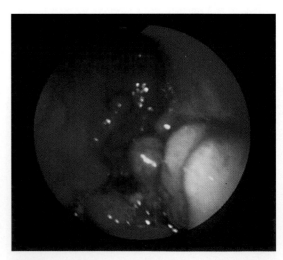

Figure 7.11 The duodenal bulb mucosa in this patient with H. pylori infection appears erythematous and reticulated (endoscopic erythematous exudative duodenitis).

Figure 7.12 Duodenitis in a H. pylori-positive patient. Erythema, nodularity and small erosions are noted (endoscopic flat erosive duodenitis).

Figure 7.13 Endoscopic raised erosive gastritis in a patient with H. pylori endoscopic erythematous exudative gastritis.

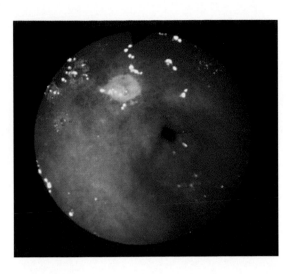

Figure 7.14 Antral ulcer and surrounding antral gastritis caused by H. pylori. The ulcer is small and benign appearing, the surrounding mucosa is diffusely erythematous.

There are two types of atrophic gastritis. Autoimmune atrophic gastritis is characterized by mucosal atrophy in the fundus and corpus region. The mucosa of the antrum is normal or shows only evidence of mild gastritis. In the second type, *H. pylori*-related gastritis, the inflammation occurs mainly in the antrum.

Intestinal metaplasia may occur in conjunction with atrophic gastritis. This may be seen endoscopically as gray–white patches with a villous and slightly opalescent appearance (Figs. 7.18 and 7.19). Such areas may be either slightly raised or depressed (Figs. 7.20 and 7.21), and may be more readily identified with dye-spraying techniques, such as with a 0.5% solution of methylene blue (Fig. 7.22). Not uncommonly, xanthelasma with a peculiar yellowish appearance may be seen in atrophic gastritis (Fig. 7.23), or hyperplastic polyps may be noted (Fig. 7.24). Intestinal metaplasia may be a

▼ **A** ▼ **B**

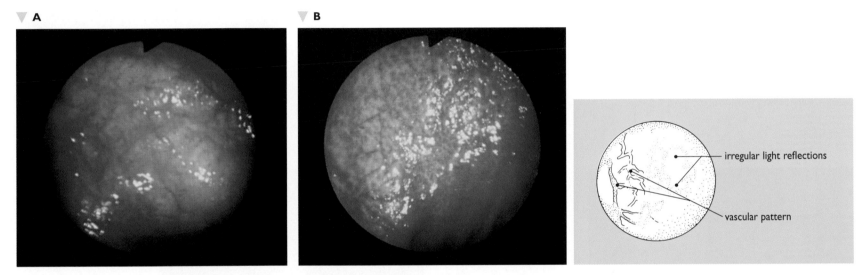

Figure 7.15 (A) Early atrophic changes in the corpus mucosa. Note the appearance of a delicate vascular pattern. (B) More pronounced atrophic gastritis with a conspicuous vascular pattern and irregularities of light reflections, indicative of mucosal unevenness.

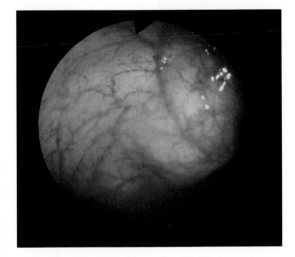

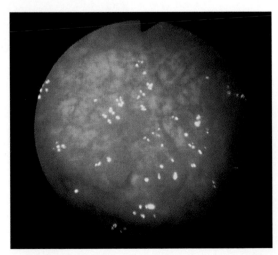

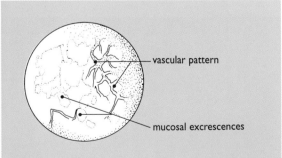

Figure 7.16 Severe atrophic gastritis with marked visibility of vascular pattern. Usually vessels are visible only with distension of the stomach by air.

Figure 7.17 Tiny mucosal excrescences contrast with slightly depressed areas of atrophy. Visible vascular ramifications are also evident.

precursor of gastric adenocarcinoma of the intestinal type. Moreover, gastric adenoma, which carries a risk of cancerous degeneration, is commonly found in intestinal metaplasia and may occur in patients with autoimmune atrophic gastritis and pernicious anemia (Fig. 7.25). There also seems to be an increased prevalence of hyperplasia of endocrine-like cells in the corpus and fundus mucosa and of gastric carcinoids.

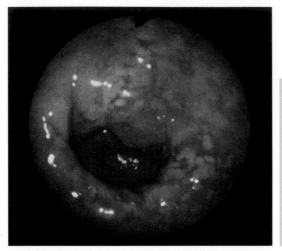

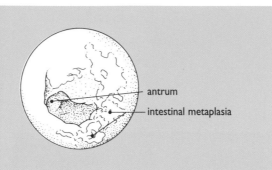

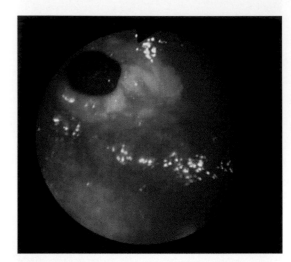

Figure 7.18 *View of distal stomach with gray–white areas of intestinal metaplasia. This condition, which may occur in conjunction with atrophic gastritis, may be a precursor of gastric adenocarcinoma.*

Figure 7.19 *Distal antral intestinal metaplasia. The white zones are slightly raised and extend into the pyloric channel, contrasting with reddened areas of surrounding mucosa.*

Figure 7.20 *Patchy white flat discolored mucosa with intestinal metaplasia.*

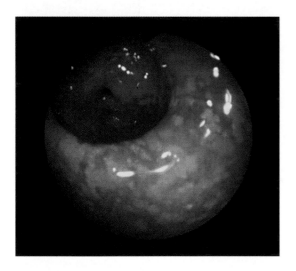

Figure 7.21 *Extensive elevated intestinal metaplasia.*

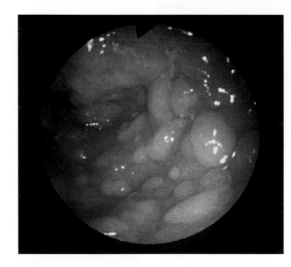

▼ **A**

▼ **B**

Figure 7.22 *Areas of pronounced, slightly raised intestinal metaplasia in the antrum (**A**) are accentuated after spraying with methylene blue dye (**B**).*

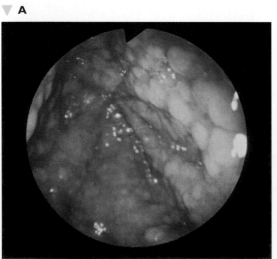

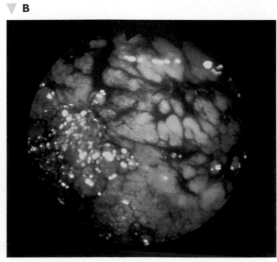

Because of the increased risk of cancer, some physicians recommend regular gastroscopic screening of patients with autoimmune atrophic gastritis and achlorhydria, with or without pernicious anemia. Others feel that the risk is too low to justify regular screening.

Benign gastric ulcers often occur in association with antral and corpus atrophic mucosa. Such patients are often hypochlorhydric and are thought to develop gastric ulcers because of a reduction in mucosal defenses rather than because of hypersecretion.

Endoscopic Flat Erosive Gastritis

Flat erosions are superficial necrotic lesions of the mucosal lining, limited to the muscularis mucosae (Fig. 7.26). Typically they have a white or yellowish base surrounded by a narrow zone of erythema. These erosions may be multiple and vary in size. They are fairly simple to detect endoscopically because of the sharp distinction between the exudate over the base and the surrounding erythematous mucosa. They frequently occur over the crests of gastric folds, especially just proximal to the pylorus (Fig. 7.27), and often heal within days although they may persist longer.

Endoscopic Raised Erosive Gastritis

Raised or varioliform erosions have an elevated, inflamed border surrounding a small depressed central necrotic patch (Fig. 7.28). The center may be initially hemorrhagic, but after 1–2 days it turns yellow–gray as a patch of fibrinous exudate forms. These nodular elevations usually measure between 5 and 10 mm. Raised erosions are usually multiple and may develop in the antrum, but they are also found in the corpus and fundus. Quite often, raised erosions are aligned along a fold directed towards the pylorus (Fig. 7.29).

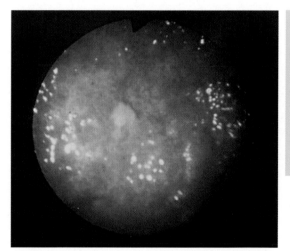

Figure 7.23 *Atrophic gastritis with xanthelasma. Note the yellowish appearance of this defect.*

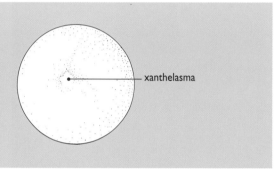

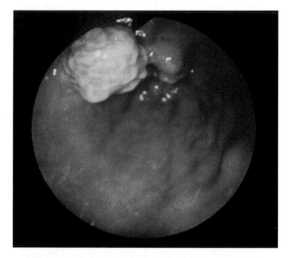

Figure 7.24 *Hyperplastic polyp in atrophic gastritis. Biopsy or removal is necessary to differentiate hyperplastic from adenomatous polyps.*

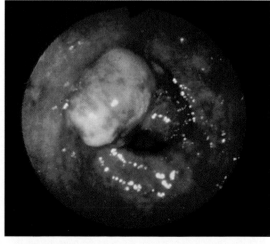

Figure 7.25 *Adenomatous polyp in the antrum was found in a patient with atrophic gastritis and pernicious anemia.*

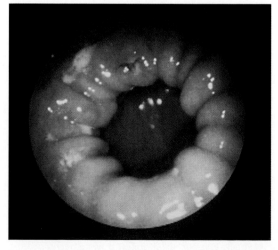

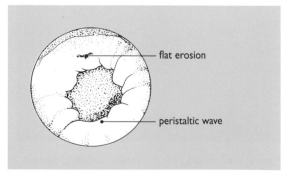

Figure 7.26 *Flat superficial erosion on top of a peristaltic wave. A minute amount of bleeding is observable. Surrounding patches of whitish mucoid material are easily distinguished from erosions. Advantage should be taken of peristaltic activity to visualize all of the mucosa in detail.*

Endoscopically, these erosive areas have a specific appearance. They often present as a series of nodules or bulges on the crests of the folds, characteristically in the antrum. The distinguishing characteristic, apparent on endoscopic and radiographic appearance, is a central depression or erosion. When not healed, they often are covered with a white or brown exudate. When they heal, the depression in the center is covered with mucosa that appears normal. Although these lesions may heal in a few days, they may persist for months or years.

Raised erosions may evolve into hyperplastic polyps, presumably as a result of foveolar hyperplasia in the borders surrounding the central crater (Fig. 7.30). Some investigators feel that this progression is substantiated by the appearance of the tip of the polyp, suggesting a healed erosion (Figs. 7.31–7.34). Others do not accept this hypothesis and feel that raised erosions and hyperplastic polyps are different types of response to injury.

Lymphomatous or metastatic lesions in the stomach occasionally mimic the appearance of raised erosions (Fig. 7.35). The endoscopist should always be alert to the fact that multiple biopsies are required whenever an atypical-appearing lesion is observed.

Drug-Induced Mucosal Damage

The gastric mucosa is vulnerable to injury by drugs, especially aspirin and other NSAIDs. Endoscopically identifiable lesions develop in virtually all patients at the start of aspirin therapy. However, this seems to be caused by an acute topical effect. The real problem lesion is the gastric or duodenal NSAID-induced ulcer. A gastric ulcer is noted in 15–20% of arthritis patients taking NSAIDs chronically; duodenal ulcer is much less common. Both gastric and duodenal NSAID ulcers can cause serious complications such as perforation and hemorrhage. The cause of these chronic lesions is thought to be prostaglandin depletion, a systemically mediated effect of the NSAID. The reduction in prostaglandin levels leads to a postulated decrease in mucosal defense and thus an increased chance of developing an ulcer.

We are only now becoming fully aware of the extent of NSAID-induced ulcer and ulcer complications. There are an estimated 37 million people in the USA with arthritis, approximately 17 million of whom take NSAIDs for the relief of symptoms, and there are an increasing number of NSAIDs available – many of which are extremely potent. The Food and Drug

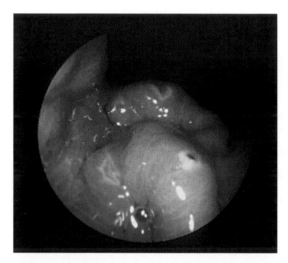

Figure 7.27 *Flat erosion on the crest of a fold surrounded by erythematous mucosa.*

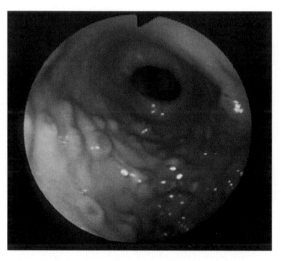

Figure 7.28 *Numerous raised erosions scattered over the corpus region of the stomach. Note the central depression revealing whitish or reddish discoloration.*

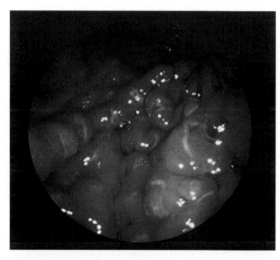

Figure 7.29 *Raised erosions. These discrete nodular bulges aligned along the fold show central erosive patches.*

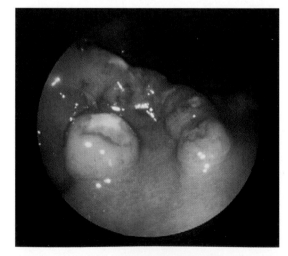

Figure 7.30 *Large, raised erosions with deep central defects covered by a white fibrinous exudate. Some endoscopists suspect that such nodules may lead after healing to formation of hyperplastic polyps.*

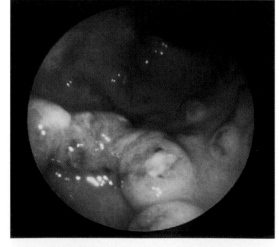

Figure 7.31 *Early partial healing of raised erosions. Proximally, erosions still manifest a white necrotic slough. Distally, the erosive defect has healed, as indicated by the appearance of an intensely red fleck in the center of the nodule.*

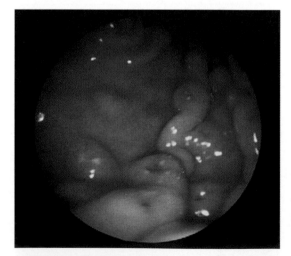

Figure 7.32 *Raised erosions during follow-up. Necrotic central depressions become smaller, to be exchanged with a reddish fleck, indicative of regenerating epithelium.*

Administration of the USA estimates that 2–4% of patients on NSAIDs for 1 year risk developing a symptomatic ulcer, or an ulcer bleed or perforation. It is estimated that as many as 200 000 people may be hospitalized each year in the USA for NSAID-induced ulcer complications, and that up to 20 000 deaths may occur each year as a result.

When aspirin injures the stomach, often the lower body of the stomach and antrum are involved; however, acute mucosal damage can also involve other gastric areas. The endoscopic appearance of drug-induced mucosal damage is variable. The lesions often radiate from the pylorus, and range from a red hemorrhagic dot to a confluence of dots, merging into a streak (Fig. 7.36).

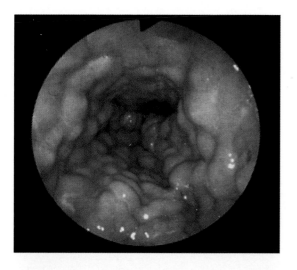

Figure 7.33 Final healing stage of raised erosions. Only the nodular elevations remain, giving the mucosa a coarsely nodular aspect. Epithelial defects have disappeared.

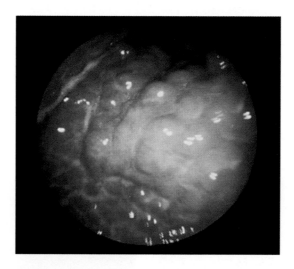

Figure 7.34 Detail of coarsely nodular cobblestone-like deformity that developed after healing of raised erosions.

A

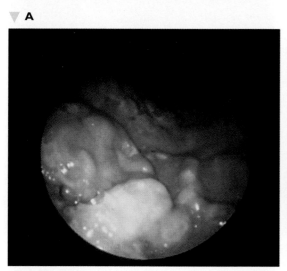

B

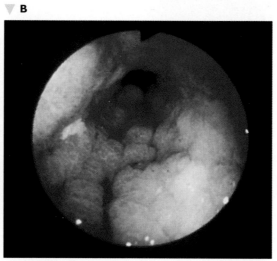

Figure 7.35 Certain malignant diseases in the stomach may mimic the nodularity of raised erosions. (**A**) Non-Hodgkin's lymphoma. (**B**) Metastatic breast cancer.

A

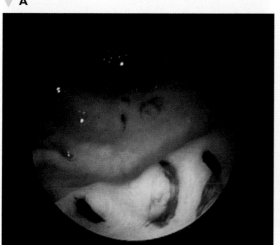

B

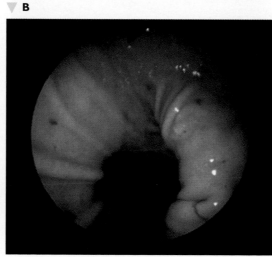

Figure 7.36 (**A** and **B**) Aspirin-induced acute mucosal bleeding. Small petechiae and small bleeding erosions are noted.

A small erosion with a white center and surrounding erythema is also typical of NSAID injury (Fig. 7.37). These lesions may progress to larger erosions. Eventually ulcers may form (Figs. 7.38–7.40). NSAIDs can also cause a jejunal ulcer in a patient with a gastroenterostomy (Billroth II) (Fig. 7.41).

Aspirin or other NSAIDs may also induce the formation of larger ulcers (over 1.5 cm in diameter). These ulcers often occur without endoscopic evidence of erythema or erosions in the surrounding mucosa. Usually no evidence of chronic gastritis is seen on biopsy of the mucosa surrounding a medication-induced ulcer. Chronic gastritis is found in biopsy of mucosa surrounding an *H. pylori* associated ulcer. In NSAID-induced gastric ulcer the incidence of *H. pylori*-associated gastritis is reported to be the same as for an age-controlled population.

Drug-induced erosive lesions may heal after several days, even with continued ingestion of anti-inflammatory drugs. Large ulcers associated with anti-inflammatory agents heal completely once the offending drug is stopped. These ulcers will heal if the patient is placed on acid suppressive therapy (Figs. 7.42 and 7.43). It is best if the aspirin or NSAID therapy is stopped.

Endoscopic Hemorrhagic Gastritis

Endoscopic hemorrhagic gastritis is often drug-induced, particularly by aspirin or related compounds. Mucosal or submucosal hemorrhagic spots are the predominant lesions in this type of gastritis. Endoscopically, these spots are reddish or brownish-black, of variable size, and usually sharply delineated (Figs. 7.44–7.46). Occasionally they may be indistinguishable from focally dilated vascular structures (Fig. 7.47). Necrotic erosive areas may also be present. Thrombocytopenia may present with gastric purpura, which must be differentiated from drug-induced mucosal damage or hemorrhagic gastritis (Fig. 7.48).

Three grades are used to describe hemorrhagic gastritis. In mild disease, one or two spots or areas of mucosal hemorrhage are visible. In moderate disease more numerous mucosal hemorrhages are seen, associated with edema. In severe disease, there is a large area of mucosal hemorrhage with active bleeding or widespread involvement of the stomach.

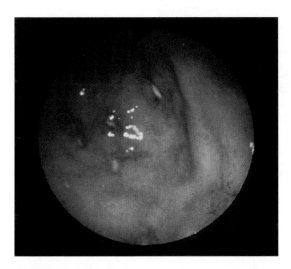

Figure 7.37 *NSAID-induced mucosal erosions in the antrum. The surrounding mucosa is red.*

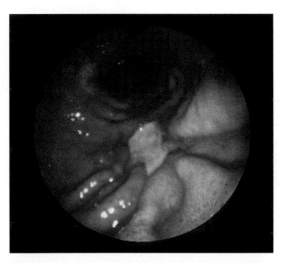

Figure 7.38 *NSAID-induced gastric ulcer with clearly visualized radiating folds.*

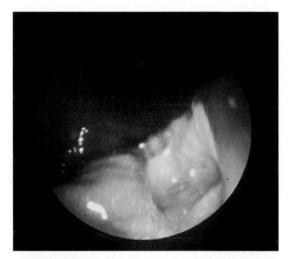

Figure 7.39 *NSAID-induced deep gastric ulcer. The exudate in the base is bile stained.*

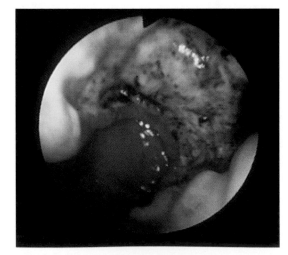

Figure 7.40 *Huge NSAID-induced gastric ulcer with evidence of bleeding.*

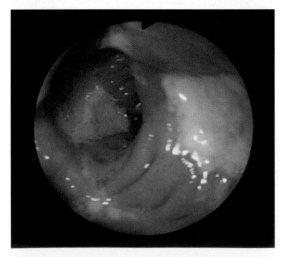

Figure 7.41 *NSAID-induced ulcer in a Billroth II stomach, which appears similar to a peptic jejunal ulcer but the surrounding mucosa does not show signs of inflammation.*

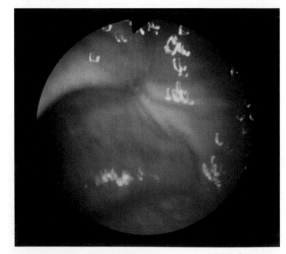

Figure 7.42 *NSAID-induced gastric ulcer has healed after 6 weeks of ulcer therapy and discontinuance of the NSAID. A depressed scar with radiating folds is noted, the ulcer is almost entirely healed. Large NSAID-induced ulcers may take months to heal, small ulcers heal more quickly.*

Stress-Induced Gastric Mucosal Damage

Stress-related gastric mucosal damage is usually associated with severe trauma, hypotension, sepsis, jaundice, renal failure, respiratory failure, surgical procedures, major burns (Curling's ulcer), and neurosurgery (Cushing's ulcer). Acute stress-related mucosal damage is often preceded by shock, which is thought to decrease gastric mucosal blood flow. Once the primary disease is

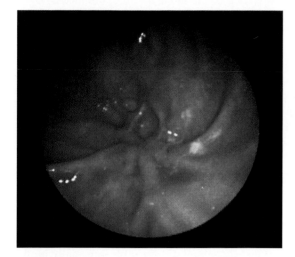

Figure 7.43 *Marked scarring and deformity on greater curve of stomach after NSAID ulcer healed.*

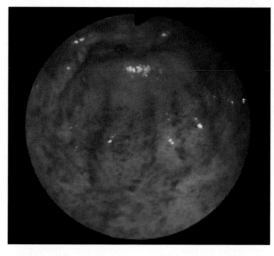

Figure 7.44 *View of aspirin-induced gastritis in the antrum. Hemorrhages appear as linear petechial streaks.*

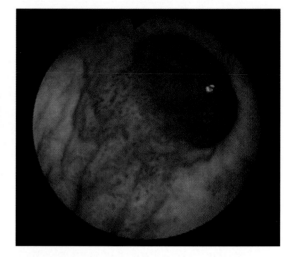

Figure 7.45 *In this view, hemorrhagic gastritis is characterized by brownish-black flecks in a sharply delineated area.*

▼ **A**

▼ **B**

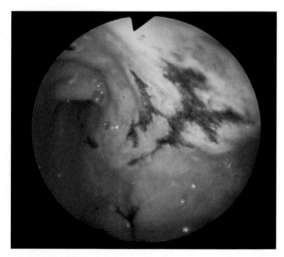

Figure 7.46 *Hemorrhagic gastritis with an area of active bleeding.*

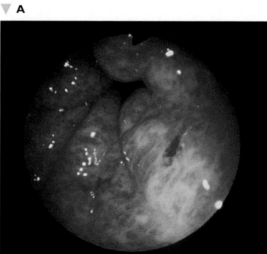

Figure 7.47 *(A and B) Two examples of antral telangiectasia in patients with liver cirrhosis may simulate hemorrhagic gastritis.*

▼ **A**

▼ **B**

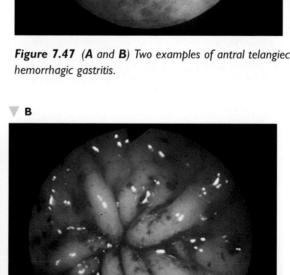

Figure 7.48 *(A and B) Gastric purpura caused by severe thrombocytopenia associated with leukemia.*

successfully treated, mucosal regeneration usually occurs, and the integrity of the gastric mucosa is restored. Lesions occurring after intracranial trauma are often deeper than those associated with other causes. Acute stress-related lesions begin minutes or hours after the trauma especially in areas of mucosal pallor. Shallow erosions occur in the fundic region of the stomach. In the next 24 hours, petechiae and multiple shallow red-based erosions may be observed in the fundus. After 48 hours, the erosions deepen and may look black-based with raised margins. The erosions may spread to involve the entire corpus and antrum. The necrotic process may extend to the submucosal layer and lead to ulceration. Because major blood vessels may be present in the submucosa, these deep lesions are more likely associated with severe hemorrhage.

These patients are examined because of upper gastrointestinal bleeding. Typically, they are hospitalized in intensive care units, often intubated and on assisted ventilation when examined. Some experience is necessary to insert even a small caliber endoscope past an endotracheal tube in the posterior pharynx. Inspection with a laryngoscope may assist the passage of the endoscope through the cricopharyngeus sphincter.

Endoscopic Rugal Hyperplastic Gastritis
Gastric rugae are considered enlarged when the folds are wider than 8–10 mm (Fig. 7.49). Enlarged or giant folds that do not flatten during maximum insufflation suggest an inflammatory or infiltrative process. Giant folds may occur over the entire stomach but usually are present only in the corpus–fundus area. Areas of fold enlargement may begin abruptly or gradually (Fig. 7.50).

Biopsy with a standard biopsy forceps is insufficiently deep to demonstrate the findings necessary to make a diagnosis such as foveolar and glandular hyperplasia; therefore, use of a large caliber biopsy forceps is recommended. Alternatively, macroparticle biopsy taken with a polypectomy diathermy snare yields specimens 1–3 mm in depth, extending into the submucosal layer and averaging about 10 mm in diameter. After ensnaring a portion of large fold, the electrosurgical snare is tightened and the gastric fold is lifted up and away from the gastric wall during the excision to limit depth of damage. The resected sample is then grasped with the snare and retrieved. This biopsy technique can result in an unexpectedly large and deep biopsy. It has a higher complication rate than the large caliber forceps biopsy technique.

The most common causes of enlarged gastric folds are Ménétrièr's disease, hypertrophic (hypersecretory) gastritis, Zollinger-Ellison syndrome, lymphoma, carcinoma, peptic ulcer disease, postoperative stomach, granulomatous disease, and gastric varices.

Ménétrièr's disease is characterized by hyperplasia of mucus-producing cells and foveolar elongation with cystic dilation of gastric glands and regression of glandular tubules. Parietal and chief cells are decreased in number, resulting in acid hyposecretion. There may or may not be an increased number of intraepithelial lymphocytes. The most characteristic appearance endoscopically is that of significantly enlarged giant folds, especially in the corpus area, which do not flatten upon maximum insufflation (Fig. 7.49). The folds may be convoluted and occasionally appear erythematous. Variations in caliber are common. There is a conspicuous increase in mucus secretion resulting in strands of mucus covering the folds (Fig. 7.51). Enlarged

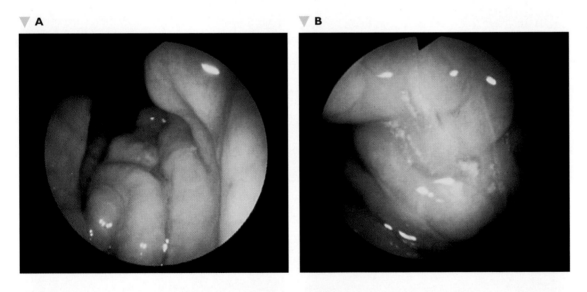

A **B**

Figure 7.49 Ménétrièr's disease. (**A**) There are true giant folds in the corpus area, as evidenced by their persistence despite maximum insufflation. (**B**) A detailed view of the giant folds with adherent mucus strands.

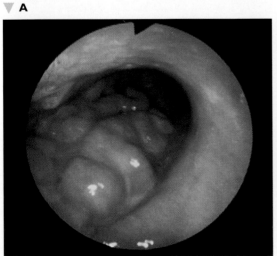
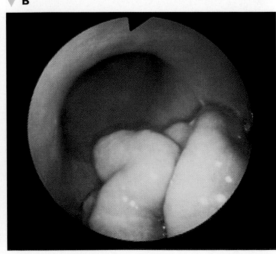

A **B**

Figure 7.50 Ménétrièr's disease. (**A**) A cluster of enlarged folds are seen along the greater curve and persist despite maximum air insufflation. Note the mucus strands. (**B**) The abrupt onset of enlarged folds in obvious in this view.

folds may also occur in the antrum, often with polypoid structures (Fig. 7.52). The question of eventual malignant degeneration has been raised. The appearance of the folds may simulate malignancy (Fig. 7.53).

Hypertrophic (hypersecretory) gastritis has a similar endoscopic appearance to Ménétrièr's disease but is characterized by hypertrophy of the glandular and foveolar layers (Figs. 7.54 and 7.55).

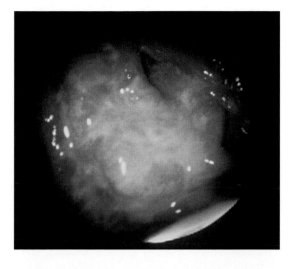

Figure 7.51 *Ménétrièr-like changes of the greater curve occurred after a pancreatic cystogastrostomy.*

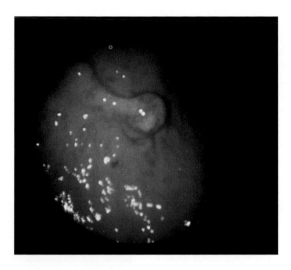

Figure 7.52 *Antral polypoid lesions in Ménétrièr's disease. Giant folds can occur in the antrum but are less often seen than polyps.*

▼ **A**

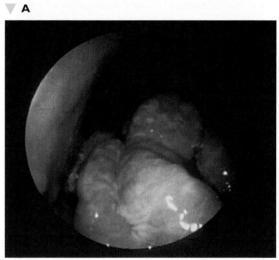

▼ **B**

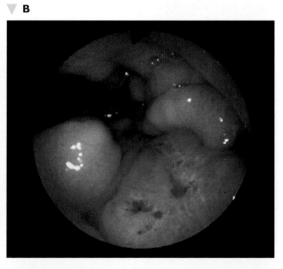

Figure 7.53 *(A and B) Two cases of Ménétrièr's disease. Giant folds here simulate malignancy.*

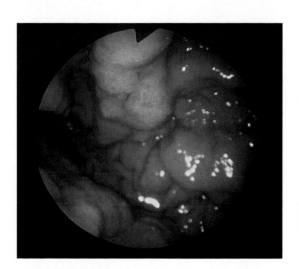

▼ **A**

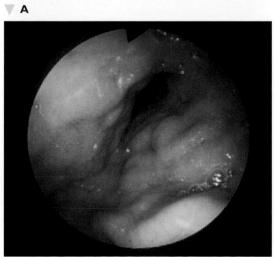

▼ **B**

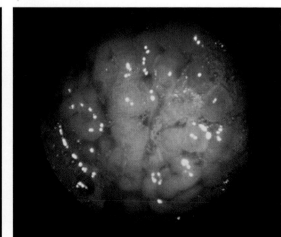

Figure 7.54 *Hypertrophic gastritis with coarsely enlarged fold pattern.*

Figure 7.55 *Hyperplastic gastritis. (A) Narrowing of the lumen with coarse nodular deformity and broadening of the fold pattern. (B) Detail of coarse nodular deformity shows mucus strands between the cobblestone-like appearance of the broadened folds.*

In Zollinger-Ellison syndrome, glandular hyperplasia is caused by the trophic action of gastrin produced in excess quantities by a gastrinoma. The mucosal thickness may be increased to 2–3 mm (Fig. 7.56). In most patients the folds are only slightly enlarged and covered with copious amounts of clear, very acidic fluid. Occasionally, the folds are slightly irregular or finely nodular. There may also be a conspicuous increase in the size of the areae gastricae (Figs. 7.57 and 7.58). Concomitant gastric ulceration is rare except when there is stasis associated with delayed gastric emptying because of peptic ulcer disease or scarring in the duodenal bulb or postbulbar duodenum. Diffuse inflammation with erosive defects may also be found in the bulb and descending duodenum (Fig. 7.59). Large deep ulcers may be present in the bulb and in the postbulbar duodenum down to the duodenal jejunal flexure (Fig. 7.60).

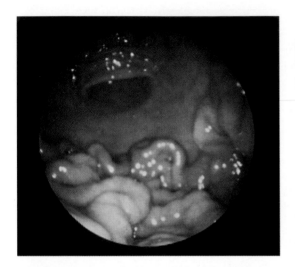

Figure 7.56 *Zollinger-Ellison syndrome, marked by an enlarged fold pattern.*

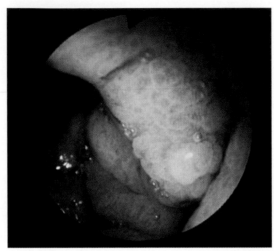

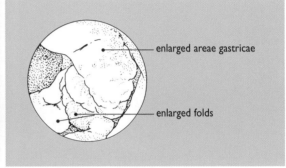

Figure 7.57 *Zollinger-Ellison syndrome. Massive enlargement of fold pattern and marked accentuation of areae gastricae pattern are evident.*

▼ **A**

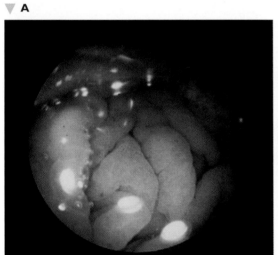

▼ **B**

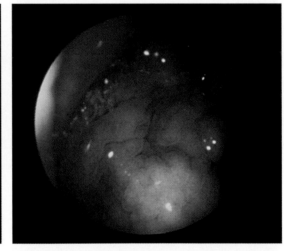

Figure 7.58 *(A) A patient presented with ulcus jejuni pepticum. After a partial resection (Billroth II), a Zollinger-Ellison-like pattern of accentuated folds developed. (B) Accentuation of areae gastricae can be seen.*

▼ **A**

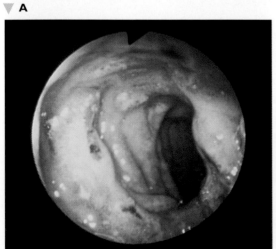

▼ **B**

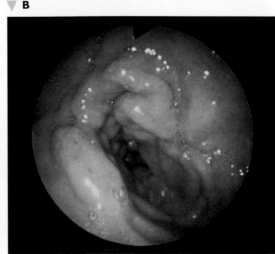

Figure 7.59 *(A) Zollinger-Ellison syndrome with extensive bulboduodenitis. (B) Healing of bulboduodenitis after 3 weeks of omeprazole therapy.*

Irregular gastric folds may also occur in lymphoreticular malignancies. They are usually seen in combination with atypically shaped ulcerative and erosive defects (Figs. 7.61 and 7.62).

Enlarged gastric folds may also occur in pseudolymphoma of the stomach, also called benign lymphatic hyperplasia. Occasionally, superficial or deep irregular epithelial defects may be present in addition to irregular enlargement of the fold pattern. Cobblestone-like deformity of the mucosal surface may be seen, especially in the antrum and corpus (Fig. 7.63). The characteristic histologic finding in this condition is the presence of mature lymph follicles with germinal centers; the inflammatory infiltrate is of polyclonal character.

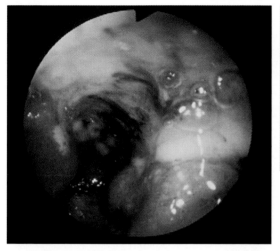
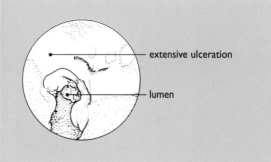

Figure 7.60 Zollinger-Ellison syndrome. Extensive ulceration of the second part of the duodenum is due to acid hypersecretion.

▼ A

▼ B

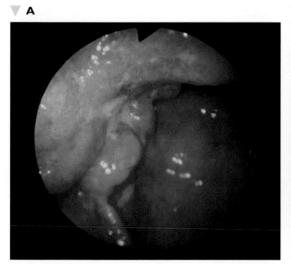
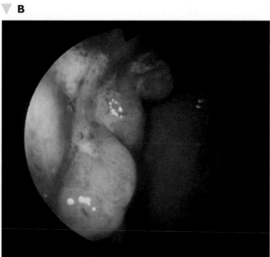
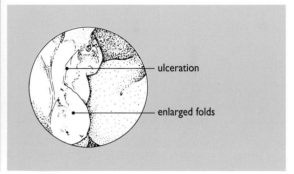

Figure 7.61 Irregular gastric folds due to lymphoma. (A) Coarse, enlarged, nodular deformity of fold pattern. (B) Detail of irregular ulceration in the center of enlarged folds.

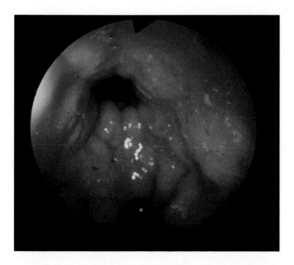

Figure 7.62 Abnormal folds in linitis plastica. This appearance is most often seen as a manifestation of adenocarcinoma, but can also appear in benign conditions such as gastric syphilis.

Radiation-Induced Mucosal Damage

Radiation therapy delivered to the upper abdomen may damage the gastric mucosa, producing varying degrees of erythema and friability. Prominent gastric folds with reduced pliability may be noted (Fig. 7.64). This injury varies in form. The initial injury is characteristically acute inflammation with erythema (Fig. 7.65). If the injury progresses, shallow or deep ulcers may occur and can perforate. As ulcers heal, scarring may occur with marked retraction of the lumen. Scar formation can obstruct the gastric outlet. A characteristic of radiation-induced gastric injury, also noted in colonic injury, is the formation of telangiectasia. Several of these characteristic findings may be noted in one patient (Figs. 7.66 and 7.67).

Differentiation between radiation damage and recurrent malignancy is sometimes difficult. Prominent ulcerative folds of a thickened nature are common to both radiation damage and tumors such as recurrent lymphoma. Multiple biopsies are necessary to make a diagnosis of lymphomatous invasion. Endosonography may also help in the diagnosis of diffuse tumor invasion.

Granulomatous Lesions

Several conditions affect the stomach, producing lesions characterized by granulomas. These include granulomatous gastritis, Crohn's disease, and sarcoidosis.

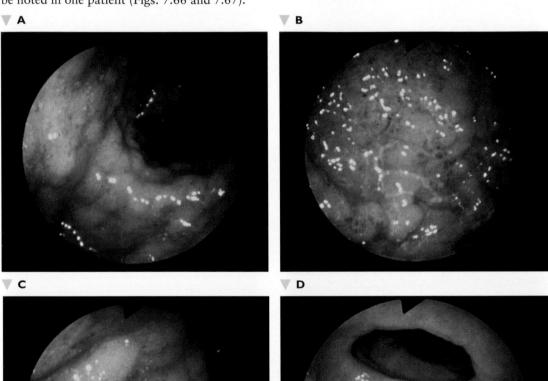

A   **B**

C   **D**

Figure 7.63 *Gastric pseudolymphoma.* (**A**) *Coarse cobblestone-like deformity of the fold pattern.* (**B**) *Coarsely nodular deformity of the rugal pattern.* (**C**) *Close-up of the nodular fold deformity and inflammatory changes.* (**D**) *A gaping, immobile pyloric sphincter area in this same patient.*

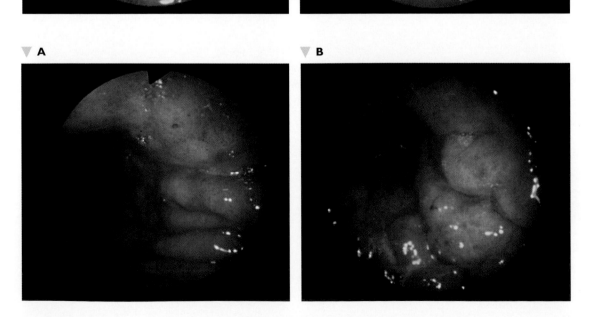

A   **B**

Figure 7.64 (**A** *and* **B**) *Postradiotherapy gastric changes show enlarged folds and erythematous flecks in two patients.*

Primary idiopathic granulomatous gastritis affects the elderly and usually involves the proximal stomach. Endoscopic findings are nonspecific, ranging between normal mucosa, scattered areas of erythema, fine or coarse granularity of the mucosa, and obvious irregular nodular deformity of the folds (Figs. 7.68 and 7.69).

In Crohn's disease, involvement of the upper gastrointestinal tract may occur in conjunction with involvement elsewhere in the bowel. The frequency of gastric involvement is variable. Crohn's lesions are indistinguishable from those due to other causes such as NSAIDs. The diagnosis is nearly impossible to make without involvement of other areas of the bowel. Overall, the

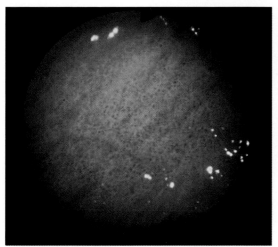

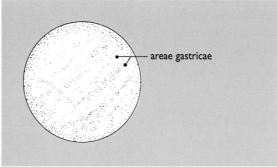

Figure 7.65 *Mild radiation damage. Numerous red islands of areae gastricae are separated by connecting, pale, linear areas of lineae gastricae.*

▽ **A**

▽ **B**

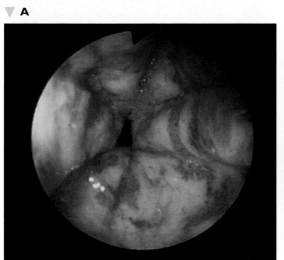

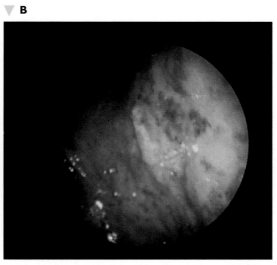

Figure 7.66 *Radiation-induced mucosal damage. (A) In the antrum, conspicuous telangiectasia and antral narrowing are apparent. (B) Corresponding radiation-induced telangiectatic changes in the corpus–fundus region.*

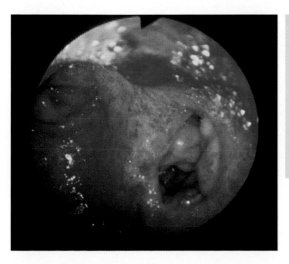

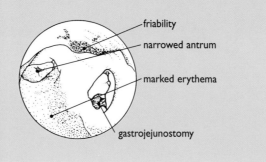

Figure 7.67 *Severe radiation damage with pronounced erythema and friability. A gastrojejunostomy was necessary because of gastric outlet obstruction, caused by marked antral narrowing.*

endoscopic findings include erythema, mucosal nodularity, aphthoid erosions, and linear or serpiginous ulcers. The prepyloric antrum is a commonly involved site. Typically, aphthoid erosions are seen focally in the prepyloric antrum with the intervening mucosa uninvolved (Fig. 7.70). The mucosa between the ulcerations may be nodular or polypoid, resulting in a cobblestone-like appearance. In addition, there may be considerable scarring and deformity of the antrum. If the pyloric channel is narrowed, the stomach may be dilated. Antral peristalsis is diminished. Stricturing may give rise to symptoms of gastric outlet obstruction (Fig. 7.71). Aphthoid erosions and small or large serpiginous ulcers may also occur in the body of the stomach or may develop around a gastrojejunostomy performed for gastric outlet obstruction (Fig. 7.72).

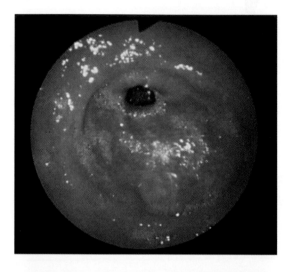

Figure 7.68
Granulomatous gastritis in the antrum. Patchy areas of erythema are apparent.

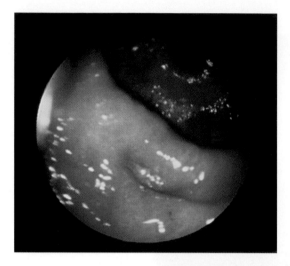

Figure 7.69
Granulomatous gastritis in the corpus with a small punched-out ulcer.

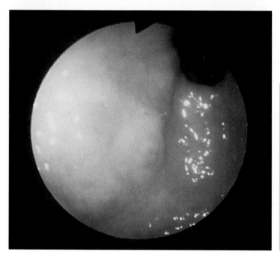

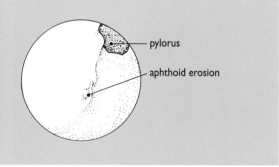
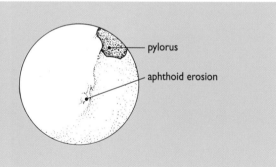

pylorus

aphthoid erosion

Figure 7.70 *Crohn's disease of the stomach. A tiny aphthoid erosion in the antrum is typical.*

Figure 7.71 *Crohn's disease of the stomach, with pinpoint gastric outlet obstruction. An ulcer is noted with adjacent nodularity.*

Figure 7.72 *Superficial ulcers have developed around a gastroenterostomy in a patient with Crohn's disease involving the stomach. The original outlet obstruction was caused by the Crohn's disease.*

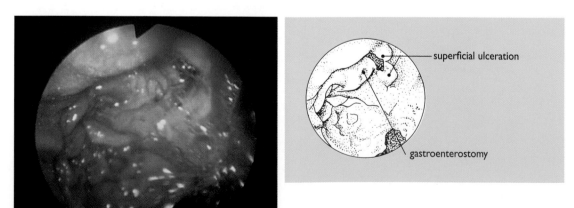

superficial ulceration

gastroenterostomy

Sarcoidosis may also affect the stomach and should be included in the differential diagnosis of granulomatous lesions. The antrum is often involved with prominent folds and deformity. Ulcers may occur. Nodules and the loss of pliability may make it difficult to distinguish sarcoid from an infiltrating neoplasm such as linitis plastica.

Enterogastric reflux gastritis

Gastritis caused by recurrent alkaline or biliary reflux may occur in patients because of an incompetent pylorus. Edema and marked hyperemia are the usual findings (Fig. 7.73). Such changes may also be seen after an episode of prolonged vomiting. Red mucosa is typical in a Billroth II stomach (Figs. 7.74 and 7.75).

OTHER MUCOSAL ABNORMALITIES

MASTOCYTOSIS

Gastric and duodenal involvement in mastocytosis can result in erosive or ulcerative defects that may bleed. The gastric folds may appear thickened with focal erythema, edema, and flat round urticaria-type lesions.

CAUSTIC GASTRIC DAMAGE

Common agents causing caustic gastric damage include sulfuric, acetic, and hydrochloric acids. Less common ones include nitric, formic, and chromic acids. Alkali and lye burns are usually due to caustic soda and bleach. Endoscopy provides information on the extent and severity of the injury. It is a reasonably safe procedure in the absence of evidence of perforation or transmural necrosis. The procedure is usually performed with a small caliber endoscope. Examination of the oropharynx and hypopharynx should always precede endoscopic examination. The presence of an oropharyngeal burn increases the possibility of an esophageal or gastric burn being present. However, as with esophageal injury, there is no correlation between oropharyngeal involvement and presence or severity of lesions in the stomach.

Areas of physiologic narrowing within the esophagus should be carefully examined; damage is often most severe at the lower end. The proximal esophagus may be relatively spared. Involvement of the stomach is usually most severe along the lesser curvature and in the region of the antrum Concentrated acids or bleach produce isolated gastric damage in a substantial percentage of patients.

Caustic damage or burn to the gastric mucosa may be graded in three stages: mild (grade 1), moderate (grade 2), and severe (grade 3). In grade 1

▼ A

▼ B

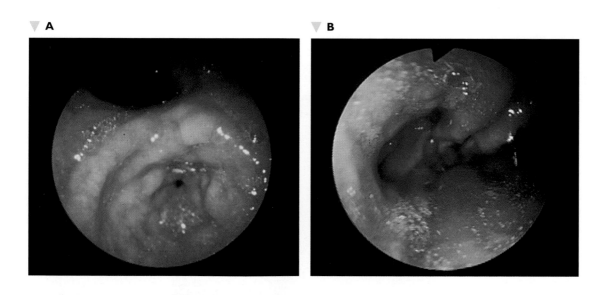

Figure 7.73 Enterogastric reflux in the intact stomach. (**A**) The antrum has patchy erythema. (**B**) Corresponding view of the corpus–fundus area shows erythema and an abundance of bile-stained liquid.

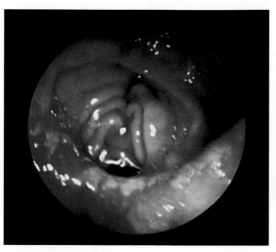

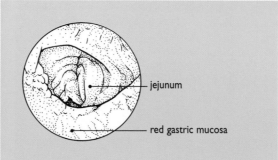

jejunum

red gastric mucosa

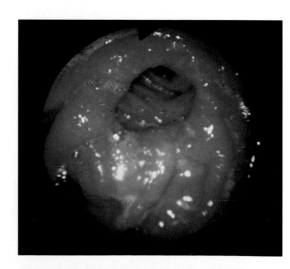

Figure 7.74 Enterogastric reflux gastritis in a Billroth II stomach. The gastric mucosa is red just proximal to the anastomosis.

Figure 7.75 Billroth II stomach with red gastric mucosa proximal to the anastomosis.

the only abnormalities are focal or linear streaks of erythema (Fig. 7.76). In grade 2 a few ulcerations are visible in addition to the hyperemia, and there may be slight hemorrhage. The ulcers are usually superficial and smaller than 5 mm in diameter. Areas of necrosis are limited to a portion of the esophagus or stomach. In grade 3 there are multiple erosions indicating extensive necrosis of the mucosal lining involving the entire esophagus or stomach, or both, or major parts of the upper digestive tract (Fig. 7.77). In addition to deep ulcerations, there may be massive hemorrhage. Esophageal and gastric complications after caustic damage include esophageal stricture, gastric perforation, scarring (Fig. 7.78), and gastric outlet obstruction.

UPPER GASTROINTESTINAL BLEEDING

Bleeding from the upper gastrointestinal tract is a commonly encountered problem in clinical medicine. The estimated incidence in the USA is about 100 cases per 100 000 per year. The mortality for upper gastrointestinal bleeding has remained at 10% for the past 40 years, although in view of the aging US population and consequent changes in underlying illnesses, this observation may not be meaningful.

Injection therapy and banding therapy of esophageal varices are presented in Chapter 4. Gastric varices are considered to be injectable if they are at the esophagogastric junction. Varices in the fundus of the stomach are more difficult to inject successfully. However, injection with the cyanoacrylate Histoacryl immediately adjacent to the bleeding point may effectively arrest the bleeding from fundal varices (Figs. 7.79 and 7.80).

ENDOSCOPIC DIAGNOSIS

Lesions that frequently occur with gastrointestinal bleeding include esophageal varices, gastric ulcers, and duodenal ulcers. When endoscopy is performed within 24 hours of the onset of bleeding, a definitive diagnosis is possible in 80–95% of patients. Figure 7.81 summarizes causes of bleeding in a series of 2225 cases collected and analyzed by the American Society for Gastrointestinal Endoscopy.

Routine endoscopic evaluation of all patients hospitalized with upper gastrointestinal bleeding has been criticized on the grounds that a precise diagnosis does not necessarily affect outcome. In a prospective randomized study of hospitalized patients who were not actively bleeding after the first 6 hours of admission, no difference was found in mortality or morbidity between those who underwent endoscopy and those who had an upper gastrointestinal x-ray.

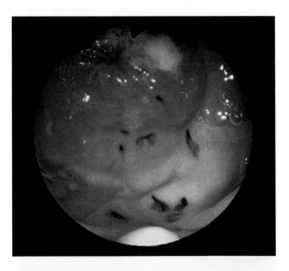

Figure 7.76 Linear streaking caused by mild chemical injury This is a grade 1 injury.

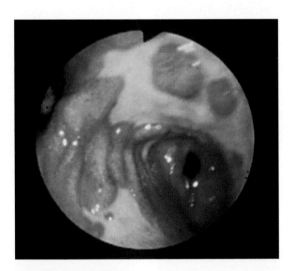

Figure 7.77 Extensive ulceration of the distal stomach after sloughing of necrosis. This damage was caused by ingestion of strong acid.

▼ **A**

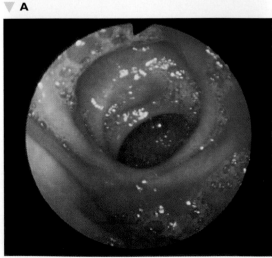

▼ **B**

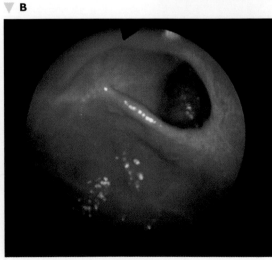

Figure 7.78 (**A** and **B**) Two examples of marked scarring, retraction, and deformity of the stomach as a result of previous extensive caustic damage.

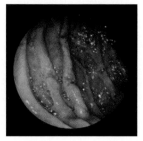

8

Small Bowel

In this chapter we review the endoscopic appearance of the normal pylorus, bulb, and duodenum. Abnormal findings related to extrinsic factors, peptic disease, and nonpeptic disease are presented, as well as vascular abnormalities and tumors of the small bowel.

THE PYLORUS

ENDOSCOPIC APPEARANCE OF THE PYLORUS

The pyloric channel is a tubular opening, 5 mm long, which expands to a diameter of 1.0–1.5 cm when relaxed. A larger channel is referred to as patulous. The antrum surrounding the pylorus may show folds radiating from the pylorus or relatively smooth mucosa (Fig. 8.1). Sometimes a prepyloric fold lies over the midpoint of the channel; although it may appear distorted, the channel itself is symmetrical (Fig. 8.2). The pyloric channel is usually in the center of the distal antrum, but sometimes lies eccentrically, adjacent to the greater or lesser curve (Fig. 8.3). A 13 mm diameter endoscope usually passes easily through the pyloric channel.

ENDOSCOPIC APPEARANCE OF THE DISEASED PYLORUS

Peptic ulcer disease is the most common abnormality of the pyloric channel (Fig. 8.4). If peptic ulcer disease is suspected, several careful passes of the endoscope are required to examine each quadrant for recessed or otherwise hidden ulcers, especially if the channel is deformed. Wide caliber instruments do not allow a detailed examination of the channel in one pass; a 9 mm instrument is preferable.

A smooth, perfectly symmetrical prepyloric antrum with intact mucosa in a patient with a narrowed, abnormal pylorus suggests benign ulcer stenosis, whereas an asymmetrical appearance or an ulcer with atypical features suggests malignancy. If pyloric folds are prominent, the margin of a benign pyloric channel ulcer may appear nodular or mass-like, especially if the ulcer is deep. A pyloric channel ulcer is indistinguishable from a malignancy if the margins are markedly irregular or heaped-up, and the base is not well seen and does not show a sharp differentiation from the surrounding mucosa. It may be difficult to distinguish heavy folds caused by a benign ulcer from those caused by a malignancy. Clues to a malignancy include indurated, irregular folds with an associated sessile or polypoid mass and either shallow or deep adjacent ulceration (Fig. 8.5). Ultimately, endosonography may be used to distinguish between a wall affected by ulcer scarring and that thickened by a tumor not apparent from the mucosal surface.

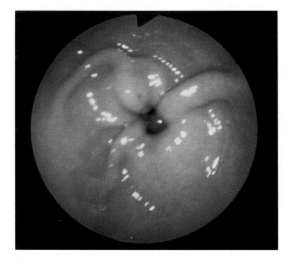

Figure 8.1 Pyloric channel. This view shows the opening with prominent radiating folds.

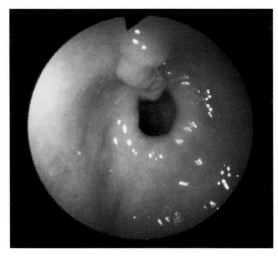

Figure 8.2 Pyloric channel. A prepyloric fold is located at its midpoint.

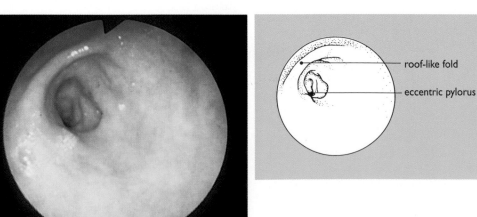

Figure 8.3 This eccentrically located pylorus has a roof-like fold.

Pyloric deformity may result from narrowing of the channel due to scarring from previous ulceration. A transverse, pyloroduodenal junction fold connecting the anterior wall of the channel with the posterior wall of the bulb may be related to scar deformity (Fig. 8.6). This fold may accentuate the anterior fornix. Scarring and retraction of bulbar ulceration may also cause pyloric changes, including an eccentric location or keyhole deformity (Fig. 8.7).

A double, or split, pylorus occurs when a fistula forms between the prepyloric antrum and the duodenal bulb as a consequence of a penetrating ulcer. This fistula is located adjacent to the original pyloric channel (Fig. 8.8). When this fistula heals, the new covering mucosa may appear normal, so that one may see a double pylorus with little evidence of the original ulcer and fistula.

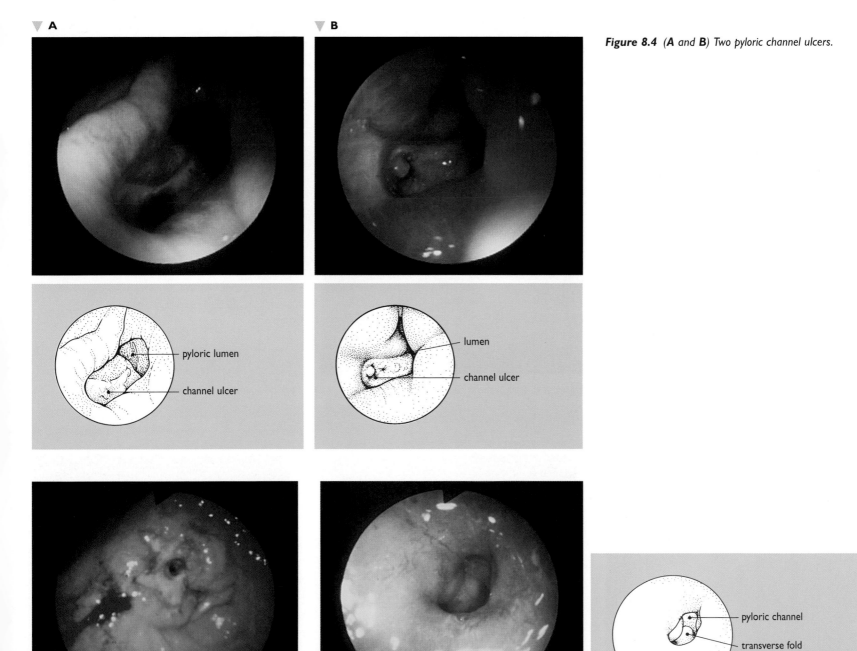

Figure 8.4 (**A** and **B**) Two pyloric channel ulcers.

Figure 8.5 Distal antral malignancy is infiltrating and narrowing the pyloric channel.

Figure 8.6 Deformity of the pyloric channel. A transverse pyloroduodenal junctional fold caused by ulcer scarring narrows the channel.

The channel is considered abnormally narrow when it measures less than 1 cm in diameter, has lost its compliance, and does not admit even a 9 mm endoscope. One must try to ensure that failure to pass the endoscope is not related to technique. It may be difficult in some cases to keep the pylorus centered in the endoscopic field as the tip is advanced. If the channel is less than 6 mm in diameter, pyloric stenosis is considered. Sometimes the pylorus is so small as to become difficult to identify. The pylorus is called stenotic when it is impossible to pass a small caliber endoscope (9 mm diameter or less) (Fig. 8.9).

Pyloric obstruction may lead to the formation of gastric bezoars. An ulcer in or adjacent to the already compromised pylorus may cause the channel to become obstructed as a result of inflammation and edema (Fig. 8.10).

In adult-type hypertrophic pyloric stenosis, the pyloric channel is elongated, extending over 2 cm. In addition, there are prominent circular prepyloric folds that extend into the lumen. The pylorus protrudes into the antrum with a mass-like deformity (Fig. 8.11). The hypertrophic pyloric musculature pushing the prepyloric and pyloric mucosa into the lumen causes the mass effect.

THE BULB AND DUODENUM

ENDOSCOPIC APPEARANCE OF THE BULB AND DUODENUM

The Duodenal Bulb

The duodenal bulb is a small, triangular structure 4–6 cm long and 2–3 cm wide that connects the anterior, intraperitoneal antrum with the posterior, retroperitoneal descending duodenum. The base of the bulbar triangle contains the angular fornices. The anterior and posterior walls extend distally to a third triangular terminal point called the apex.

In some patients, it may be possible to retroflex the endoscope tip inside the bulb and examine the fornices directly.

Because the bulb courses posteriorly, its most distal point (apex) is often seen in the 3 o'clock position of the visual field. The superior wall of the bulb is in the 12 o'clock position, and the inferior wall is in the 6 o'clock position.

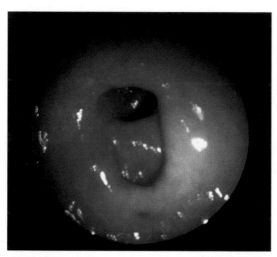

Figure 8.7 *Keyhole deformity of pyloric channel. Scarring and retraction due to bulbar ulcer disease have caused these changes.*

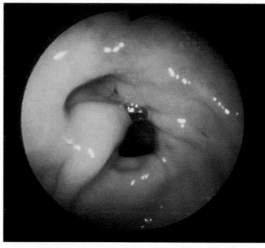

Figure 8.8 *Split pylorus. The fistula created above the original pyloric opening is the result of a penetrating ulcer.*

second opening
original pylorus

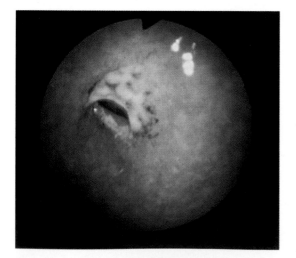

Figure 8.9 *Pyloric stenosis. In this patient, the narrowing occurred after pyloroplasty.*

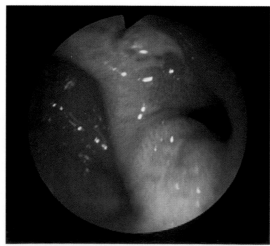

Figure 8.10 *Benign pyloric channel ulcer and deformity, thought on x-ray to be malignant.*

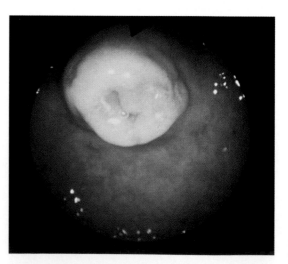

Figure 8.11 *Adult-type hypertrophic pyloric stenosis. Thickened pylorus muscle, which can easily be passed by a standard endoscope, bulges into the antrum.*

At the apex of the bulb there is often an abrupt angle at a fold leading into the descending duodenum. This is referred to as the superior duodenal angle. Heavy folds may appear at the apex, just proximal to entering the descending portion. The mucosa of the descending duodenum has circular Kerckring's folds that begin just beyond the apex of the duodenal bulb. This sign helps to determine when the tip of the endoscope leaves the smooth mucosa of the bulb and enters the circular folds of the descending portion.

The mucosa of the bulb is somewhat pale and yellow–gray compared with the orange–pink color of the stomach. When closely inspected, the fine villous texture of the mucosa can be appreciated as having a granular appearance with tiny dots of reflected light (Fig. 8.12). The vascular pattern, as seen with air insufflation, consists of tiny, short vascular structures.

Because the bulb is small, it can be difficult to examine unless approached in a careful and systematic fashion. A small caliber instrument is preferred, especially if bulbar pathology is suspected, because of its shorter turning length. Retroflexion may be necessary to examine the pylorobulbar junction and the fornices; this is accomplished by upward deflection with continued intubation in the midbulb using a small caliber endoscope with excellent tip bending characteristics.

Descending Duodenum

Several differences differentiate the descending duodenum from the stomach and the bulb. Bile may be noted as well as considerable luminal motility. When a hypotonic agent like glucagon has been administered, it is easier to inflate and examine the duodenum. Circular folds are seen (Fig. 8.13). Although the papillae are seen occasionally with an end-viewing endoscope, they are better examined with a side-viewing scope. The main papilla of Vater is located on the medial wall in the mid-descending duodenum. There may be a second or minor papilla of Santorini, which is characteristically proximal to the main papilla, smaller and fleshy in appearance.

The descending duodenum has a yellow–orange coloration compared with the yellowish-gray appearance of the bulb. Usually there is no mucosal vascular pattern seen. Especially in the presence of slow gastric emptying, some whitish discoloration may be present in the mucosa, due to lipid in the lamina propria lacteals (Fig. 8.14).

ABNORMALITIES OF THE BULB AND DUODENUM DUE TO EXTRINSIC FACTORS
Bulb Abnormalities

Enlargement of adjoining anatomic structures may impinge on the bulbar architecture and alter its shape. Examples include enlargement of the head of the pancreas, which can deform the bulb at its apex and along the inferior wall. Massive dilation of the common bile duct may compress the bulb at or just beyond the apex. Gall bladder enlargement may deform the anterior aspect of the bulb. Rarely, a gallstone can be seen penetrating into the bulb (Fig. 8.15). Apical stenotic deformity due to peptic ulcer disease may dilate the bulb giving the apex a contracted appearance with a pinpoint lumen. Bulbar dilatation may also be seen in association with scleroderma.

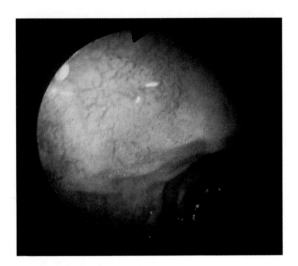

Figure 8.12 *Mucosa of the bulb has a villous appearance.*

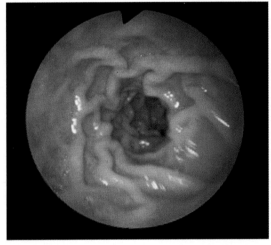

Figure 8.13 *View down second portion of duodenum. Beautiful normal folds are noted.*

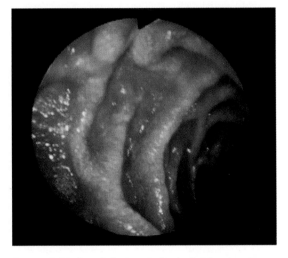

Figure 8.14 *Detailed view of whitish discoloration due to lipid accumulation in the mucosa covering Kerckring's folds.*

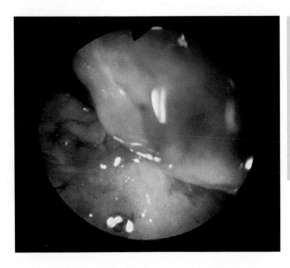

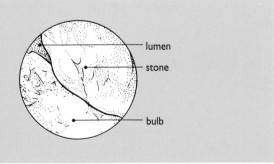

lumen
stone
bulb

Figure 8.15 *A gallstone is seen eroding and penetrating into the anterior wall of the duodenal bulb.*

Adjacent malignancy usually produces extrinsic compression from the anterior aspect of the duodenal bulb, a mass-like deformity can be seen obstructing the lumen at the apex. The bulb proximal to this appears dilated. Sometimes normal adjacent structures can cause a nonspecific compression of the posterior wall of the bulb, which must be distinguished from an adjacent malignancy (Fig. 8.16). Ultrasound endoscopy will be very useful for making this distinction.

Duodenal Abnormalities

Abnormalities of the descending duodenum include changes in the papilla or its immediate surrounding structures. Papillary changes include carcinoma of the papilla, adenoma of the papilla, and perivaterian diverticula. Adjacent structures may also cause an extrinsic impression on the descending duodenum. The descending duodenum is retroperitoneal and fixed in position. When compressed by an enlarged adjacent organ, such as a cyst of the pancreas (either a pseudocyst or a true cyst) or a carcinoma of the head of the pancreas, extrinsic pressure distorts the duodenal lumen. In these circumstances it may be difficult to identify the duodenal anatomy, and to locate and cannulate the papilla.

Endoscopically, extrinsic compression is commonly seen with carcinoma of the pancreas (Fig. 8.17). Swelling caused by a pancreatic abscess may be seen. The opening of a spontaneous fistula tract draining the abscess into the duodenal lumen is rare (Fig. 8.18). The bile duct runs in the duodenal wall, and if this structure is obstructed by a stone or cancer (of the pancreas, papilla or distal bile duct) the duct may bulge into the duodenal lumen. When this is noted, the opening of the papilla is usually seen at the distal end of the bulge (Fig. 8.19).

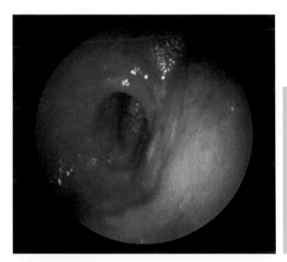 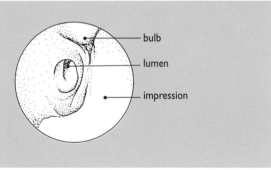

Figure 8.16 Nonspecific compression of the posterior wall of the bulb.

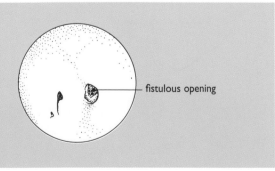

Figure 8.17 Duodenal wall deformity due to infiltrating suprapapillary pancreatic malignancy.

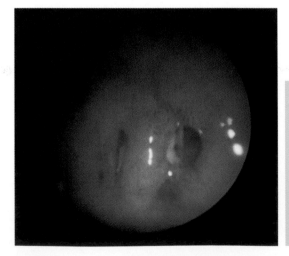 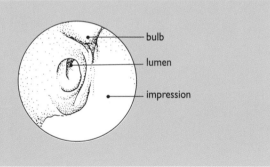

Figure 8.18 Fistulous opening in the duodenal wall, seen after spontaneous breakthrough of a pancreatic abscess.

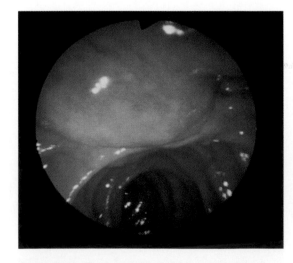

Figure 8.19 The impression of the duodenal wall is associated with a dilated common duct.

Penetration of the bile duct through the wall creates a weak spot that may form a diverticulum. For this reason the diverticula of the descending duodenum are usually next to the papilla (Fig. 8.20). An unusual type of diverticulum is an inverted diverticulum in which the opening appears next to the lumen of the descending duodenum. This is called a windsock diverticulum (Fig. 8.21). Such diverticula may be inflamed or contain food or secretions (Figs. 8.22 and 8.23), or may appear empty (Fig. 8.24).

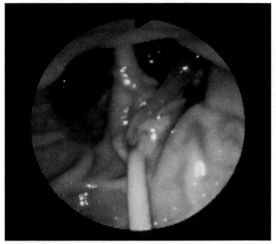

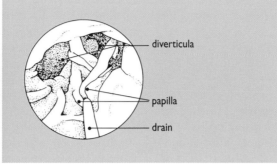

Figure 8.20 *Two diverticula adjacent to the papilla. Note the endoscopically placed drain projecting from the papillary orifice.*

▼ **A**

▼ **B**

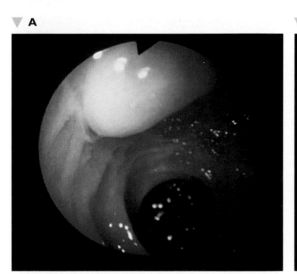

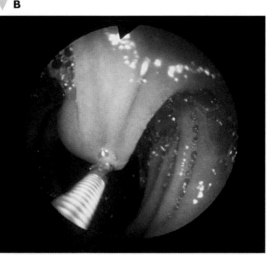

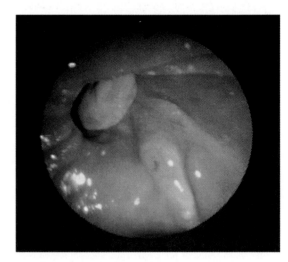

Figure 8.21 *(A) Windsock diverticulum extending into descending duodenal lumen. (B) The pliable nature of the diverticulum is noted. The orifice is not seen in these slides.*

Figure 8.22 *Peripapillary diverticulum. A concrement is evident in the papillary orifice.*

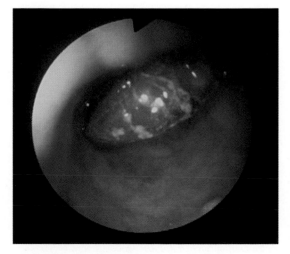

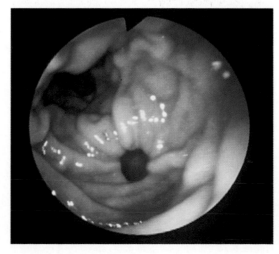

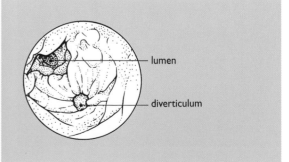

Figure 8.23 *Duodenal diverticulum. Bile-stained concrement fills the diverticulum.*

Figure 8.24 *Diverticulum of descending duodenum in a patient with multiple duodenal and jejunal diverticula.*

Occasionally, a congenital band or ring of pancreatic tissue surrounds the second portion of the duodenum and constricts it; this anomaly is termed annular pancreas. At endoscopy, a stenotic area may be seen, or there may be complete obstruction, generally beginning within 3 cm of the apex (Fig. 8.25). Just above the stenotic area, extrinsic compression from the lateral wall can be observed. The constriction is usually above the major papilla. If endoscopic retrograde cholangiopancreatography (ERCP) is technically feasible, it can confirm the presence of an annular pancreas with the pancreatic duct circling the duodenum. No other relevant endoscopic abnormalities are seen in most cases.

A congenital duodenal diaphragm or septum is a ring-like narrowing 5–10 mm wide, which may first become symptomatic in adult life (Fig. 8.26). At endoscopy, a characteristic, often slit-like, narrowing is seen in the midportion of the descending duodenum.

Dilation of the descending duodenum may occur because of mechanical obstruction of the third and fourth portion, due to stricturing malignancy, Crohn's disease, or vascular mesenteric root obstruction. In cases of duodenal involvement, the duodenum may dilate up to a diameter of 7 cm or more, which may decrease the size of or entirely flatten Kerckring's folds.

Postsurgical Abnormalities

Postsurgical deformity of the bulb and duodenum is usually due to a choledochoduodenal anastomosis. In the case of a proximal choledochoduodenostomy, the anastomosis is located at the posterior wall of the bulb (Fig. 8.27). At endoscopy, converging folds are seen on the posterior wall aspect of the apex; bile often drains from this area. In the case of a distal choledochoduodenostomy, a surgically created stomal orifice is seen just proximal and posterior to the normal-looking papilla (Fig. 8.28). Another postsurgical abnormality is a peripapillary fistula (Fig. 8.29). This is often seen just cephalad to the papilla and may result from an injury to the distal common bile duct by a stone or during biliary surgery.

Catheterization of a choledochoduodenostomy is usually possible. Occasionally, food residue may be seen through the stoma opening. Enlargement of a strictured anastomosis is possible over a distance of not more than 3–4 mm using a papillotomy wire or knife. This must always be done with utmost care because of the risk of bleeding or perforation. An alternative method is to dilate the opening with a balloon catheter.

When examining a patient with a Billroth II gastrojejunostomy, the endoscope enters the afferent loop and moves towards the papilla. It is important to identify the papilla or the surgically closed inverted duodenal stump to determine when the entire length of the afferent loop has been traversed (Fig. 8.30).

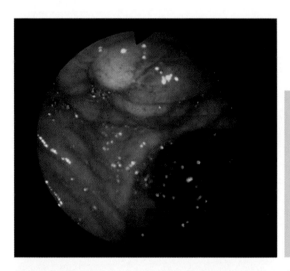
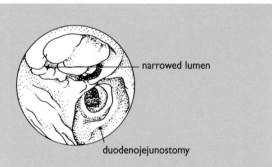

Figure 8.25 Annular pancreas. The duodenal lumen is markedly narrowed by pancreatic tissue. A duodenojejunostomy was surgically created to bypass the obstruction.

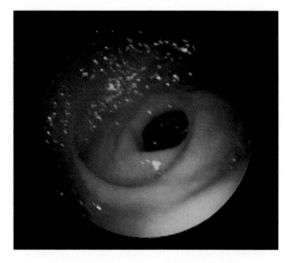

Figure 8.26 Congenital duodenal diaphragm. The abnormality becomes manifest in adulthood.

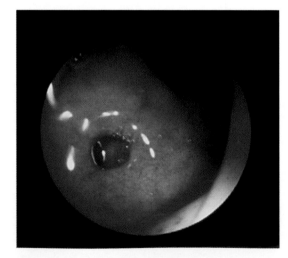

Figure 8.27 Normal-appearing choledochoduodenostomy on the posterior wall of the duodenal bulb.

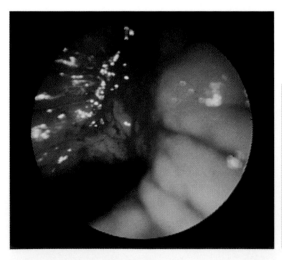
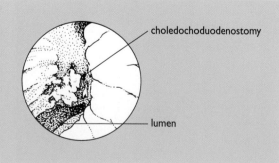

Figure 8.28 Postsurgical deformity caused by a recently performed suprapapillary choledochoduodenostomy. Minor inflammatory changes are also present.

Duodenitis

Duodenitis may be part of the spectrum of duodenal ulcer disease. Whether duodenitis is the precursor to or the healing state of duodenal ulcer is unclear. The relationship is variable between symptoms and presence or severity of duodenitis as assessed endoscopically or histologically. This has contributed to the confusion about the significance of this entity. On the basis of the available evidence, duodenitis seems to be a stage in the formation of an ulcer.

Endoscopic Erythematous Exudative Duodenitis

Patchy or diffuse reddening of the entire bulb is the most common finding in endoscopic erythematous exudative duodenitis. Focal erythematous areas usually measure 0.3–1.5 cm. Hypermotility usually accompanies erythema, and puckering folds prolapse back and forth within the bulb (Fig. 8.31).

Endoscopic Flat Erosive Duodenitis

Epithelial destruction with discrete focal erosions is the predominant feature in more severe inflammation with endoscopic flat erosive duodenitis, and may be the source of upper gastrointestinal bleeding (Fig. 8.32). However, this is not brisk bleeding like that which occurs with a duodenal ulcer with an artery in its base. Because of the adherent exudate, erosions usually appear as whitish areas, 1–3 mm in diameter or larger, often surrounded by a rim of striking erythema (Fig. 8.33). Patients with pronounced endoscopic erosive

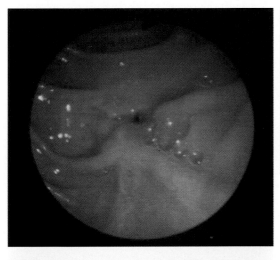

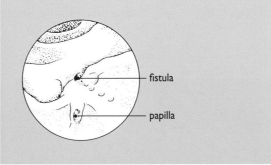

Figure 8.29 Iatrogenic peripapillary fistula. A fistulous opening is seen just above the papilla.

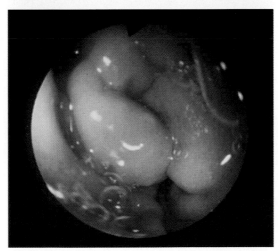

Figure 8.30 Closed inverted duodenal stump in a patient with a Billroth II anastomosis. The covering mucosa appears normal.

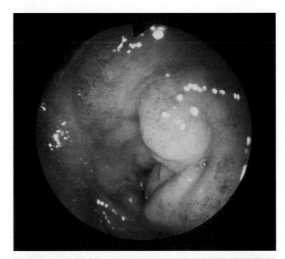

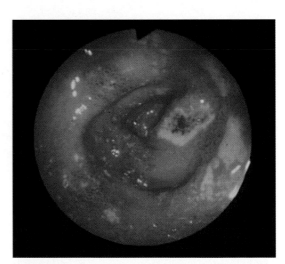

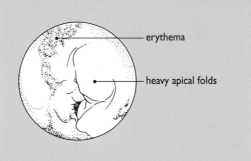

Figure 8.31 Mild endoscopic erythematous exudative bulboduodenitis. Swollen apical folds prolapse back and forth in this patient, who was previously treated for a duodenal ulcer. Patchy erythema is also discernible.

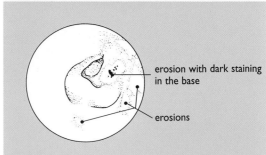

Figure 8.32 Endoscopic flat erosive bulboduodenitis. Multiple flat erosions are seen; one shows signs of recent bleeding.

duodenitis often have gastric hypersecretion. Endoscopic signs are copious amounts of acid fluid in the stomach and an accentuated pattern of areae gastricae in the corpus–fundus area (Fig. 8.34). In hypersecretion, the erosive defects may expand into the descending duodenum and may be the source of upper gastrointestinal bleeding (Fig. 8.35). This lesion may be pronounced in Zollinger-Ellison syndrome, in which lesions typically extend beyond the bulb.

Endoscopic Raised Erosive Duodenitis

Mucosal nodular deformity or excrescences are found in a minority of patients with duodenitis. Such nodules are usually concentrated in the bulb, and may be discrete and small (2–4 mm) or in the 5–10 mm range. If they continue into the descending duodenum, they may be accompanied by thickened Kerckring's folds. Such nodules may show apical erythema with or without tip erosions, although in some patients mucosal coloration is normal. Histologically, a variable degree of acute and chronic inflammation is usually present. Endoscopic raised erosive duodenitis is especially common in end-stage renal disease or in patients on chronic dialysis (Fig. 8.36).

NSAID-Associated Duodenitis

Duodenitis appearing as diffuse mucosal erythema and petechiae (endoscopic erythematous exudative duodenitis) (Fig. 8.37) or aphthous erosions (endoscopic flat erosive duodenitis) (Fig. 8.38) may be associated with nonsteroidal anti-inflammatory drug (NSAID) use.

PEPTIC ULCERATION OF THE BULB AND DUODENUM

Incidence and Etiology

Peptic bulboduodenal ulceration is a necrotic process in which the lesion extends into the submucosa or into the deeper muscle layers. It is common in the USA; about 10% of the population will experience duodenal ulcers sometime in their lives, men more often than women. For unknown reasons, however, the incidence has been decreasing over the last 30 years.

Of all factors that are pathogenetically significant in duodenal ulcer disease, *Helicobacter pylori* infection is the most important because cure of the infection cures the ulcer diathesis. The infection and the severe inflammation

▼ **A**

▼ **B**

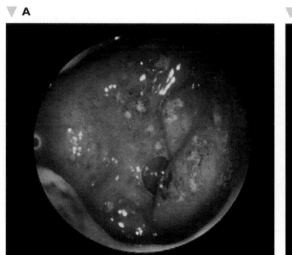
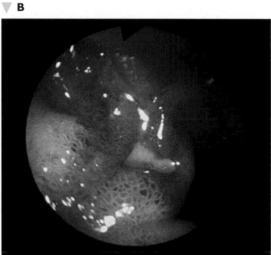
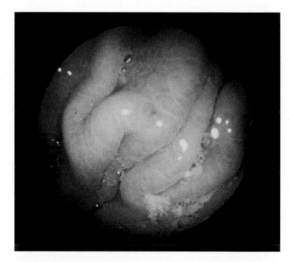

Figure 8.33 (**A**) Endoscopic flat erosive bulboduodenitis. Note the erythematous ring surrounding the defects. (**B**) A small ulcer is seen with severe bulbitis and erythema.

Figure 8.34 In patients with endoscopic erosive bulboduodenitis, there is often evidence of gastric hypersecretion. Pronounced areae gastricae and copious amounts of acid fluid are apparent in this view of the stomach.

▼ **A**

▼ **B**

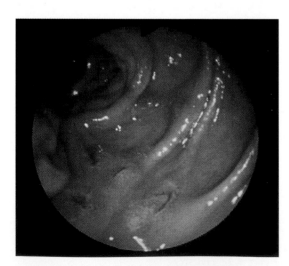
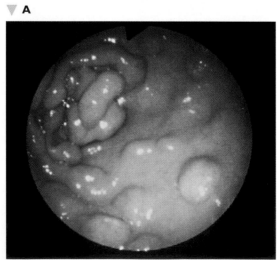
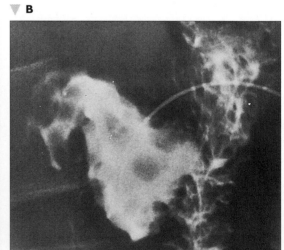

Figure 8.35 Endoscopic erosive defects in the descending duodenum, with evidence of mild bleeding.

Figure 8.36 (**A**) Nodular deformity of bulb in a patient on renal dialysis. This is the characteristic appearance of endoscopic raised erosive duodenitis. No alteration of the mucosal appearance can be seen. (**B**) Corresponding x-ray of bulb shows obvious nodularity.

in the stomach is largely restricted to the antrum leaving the corpus mucosa and the parietal and chief cell mass intact. Several findings support the notion of enhanced bacterial virulence in duodenal ulcer patients (more attachment, more phospholipase destroying the phospholipid barrier, more vacuolating, etc.).

As a consequence of antral inflammation, gastrin homeostasis is severely disturbed. Especially after meals there is excessive gastric release as a consequence of failing counter-regulation by the somatostatin-producing D cells. The resulting hypergastrinemia drives the faveolar cells to high acid production and, in the long run, to expansion of the parietal cell mass because of the trophic effect of the latter. As a consequence of the enhanced acid production and accelerated gastric emptying, acid flux in the bulb is enhanced. This bulbar hyperacidity is responsible for more extensive gastric mucosal-type metaplasia, creating the optimal niche for *H. pylori* spread from the stomach. Once infected, the metaplastic patches become inflamed, which leads to epithelial degeneration and exfoliation. The ensuing erosions coalesce and ultimately an ulcer crater forms. Drugs such as acetylsalicylic acid and other NSAIDs or potassium chloride medications can also cause

ulcers in the absence of *H. pylori* infection (Figs. 8.39 and 8.40), which usually heal rapidly after withdrawal of the offending medication.

Symptoms

The symptoms of a duodenal ulcer vary. The classic pattern in many patients is burning epigastric pain 2–3 hours after eating. The pain is often severe enough to awaken the patient at night, but is rarely present in the morning, and is usually relieved by antacids or food. Occasionally, ulcers may occur without pain; in these cases, patients may present initially with a complication such as bleeding. Sudden onset of an ulcer complication is reported to be more common in people using NSAIDs than in others. Fewer than 50% of patients on NSAIDs experience symptoms before a complication, compared with 75% of patients not using an NSAID.

Recurrence rates of over 80% in 1 year have been reported after healing of a duodenal ulcer with acid-reducing therapy if all patients are re-examined after healing regardless of the presence of symptoms.

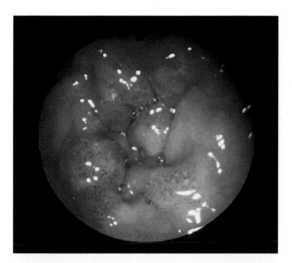

Figure 8.37 *Aspirin-induced endoscopic erythematous exudative duodenitis. The mucosa is red and the folds are edematous.*

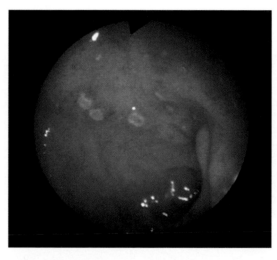

Figure 8.38 *NSAID-induced endoscopic flat erosive bulboduodenitis with aphthoid lesions in the bulb.*

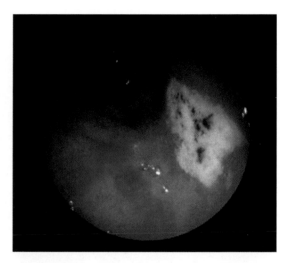

Figure 8.39 *Combined drug-induced duodenal and gastric ulcer. The duodenal ulcer shows signs of recent bleeding.*

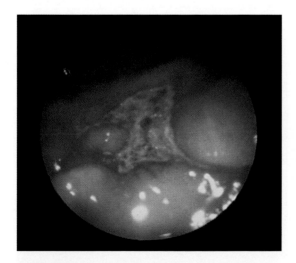

Figure 8.40 *Potassium chloride-induced ulcer in the bulb. Note the irregular shape and absence of inflammatory changes in the surrounding mucosa.*

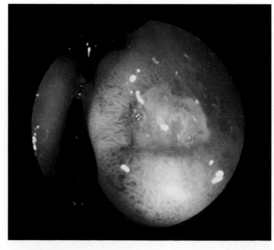
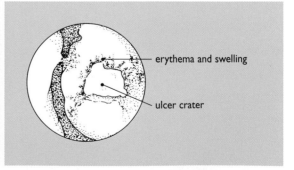

Figure 8.41 *Duodenal ulcer of the posterior wall. Conspicuous erythema and swelling are apparent.*

erythema and swelling

ulcer crater

Location

About 50% of all duodenal ulcers are located on the anterior wall. Ulcers on the posterior wall are less common (Fig. 8.41). The surfaces of the superior and inferior walls account for roughly 20% of all duodenal ulcers. Apical ulcers are relatively uncommon and are usually associated with prominent folds and scar deformity

About 15% of patients with a duodenal ulcer have a second ulcer, often within a short distance of the main ulcer. Common sites of multiple ulcers are the pylorobulbar junction, the anterior and posterior wall of the midbulb, and the apex. Ulcers on opposite walls of the same site are called 'kissing ulcers' (Fig. 8.42).

Size and Shape

The size of an ulcer may be estimated with reasonable accuracy by direct vision. Generally, error is on the side of underestimation. A more accurate estimation of ulcer size can be achieved using either the open biopsy forceps method or a calibrated probe (Fig. 8.43).

Most duodenal ulcers are under 10 mm in greatest dimension, with roughly 50% having a diameter of between 5 and 9 mm. Twenty-five per cent are large and have a diameter between 10 and 20 mm (Fig. 8.44). Giant duodenal ulcers can have a diameter exceeding 20–25 mm. Most duodenal ulcers are 1–2 mm deep. Superficial ulcers may be difficult to distinguish from erosive defects, whereas deep ulcers have a depth of greater than 3 mm.

The single most striking feature of an ulcer of the bulboduodenum is the shape of the crater, which also has some bearing on its response to medical therapy. The round or oval-shaped ulcer is the most common and responds most predictably to therapy (Fig. 8.45). The crater appears yellowish-gray; the margin is usually hyperemic and erythematous. Occasionally the ulcer crater may merge with an erosive patch. Histologically, the base shows a fibrinoid necrosis, whereas the erythematous rim shows features of acute duodenitis.

Irregularly shaped ulcers account for about 10% of all ulcers, and are usually associated with scar deformity (Fig. 8.46). Presumably because of such scarring, these ulcers do not heal as readily in response to therapy.

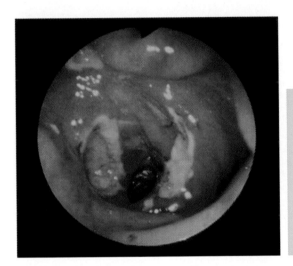
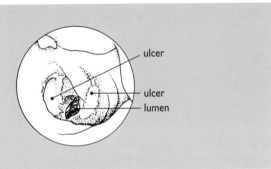
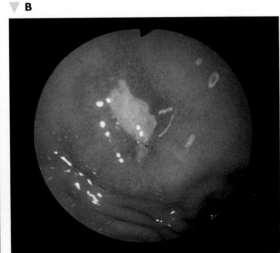

Figure 8.42 Kissing ulcers in the bulb are found on opposite walls at the same site.

Figure 8.43 Open biopsy forceps as a measuring device. This ulcer recurred within 10 days after a 6-month course of maintenance therapy with ranitidine.

▽ **A**   ▽ **B**

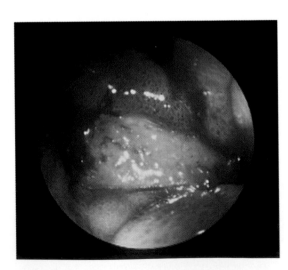
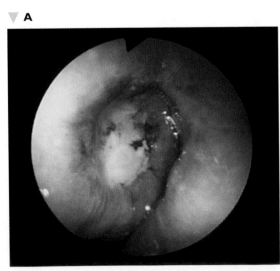

Figure 8.44 Large duodenal ulcer of the posterior wall with marked erythema and friability of the border.

Figure 8.45 (**A** and **B**) Typical duodenal ulcers with round appearance.

About 10–20% of all ulcers are linear. These are also commonly associated with scar deformity and may be found along the ridges of one or more of the deforming folds (Fig. 8.47). Linear ulcers are the least predictable in response to treatment.

The multifocal, patchy ulcer is distinctly less common. A discrete area of multiple, tiny ulcerations is seen on a background of intense erythema (Fig. 8.48). Such ulcers are generally less than 1 cm in diameter, are relatively slow to heal, and have a high recurrence rate.

In the rare mixed type, the ulcer pattern combines two or more of the above variations. Most often, the round or irregular shape is seen in combination with the linear appearance. This mixed type is commonly associated with scar deformity.

Healing and Scar Formation

Duodenal ulcers re-epithelialize from the periphery. During the healing phase, the crater becomes progressively smaller and shallower at the average rate of 1–4 mm per week. Usually the healing phase is characterized endoscopically by marked erythema of the surrounding edges (Fig. 8.49). After healing, prominent folding in a hypercontractile bulb may persist (Fig. 8.50).

Delayed healing may be seen in association with scar deformity, suggesting recurrent ulcer disease. As duodenal ulcers tend to recur, there is often evidence of previous ulceration and scarring together with fresh crater formation (Fig. 8.51). Thus, ulcer scarring should always alert the endoscopist to search for the presence of an ulcer crater. Scarring is presumably the result of repeated injury at the same location, causing mucosal and submucosal

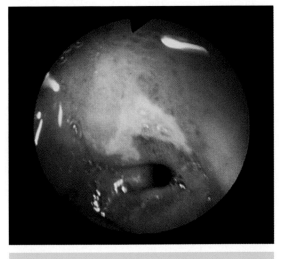

Figure 8.46 *Irregular-type duodenal ulcer in a scarred bulb.*

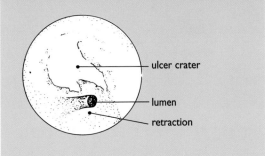

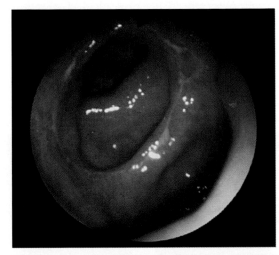

Figure 8.47 *Healing stage of linear ulceration located along the ridge of the fold. Note the characteristic pseudodiverticular malformation.*

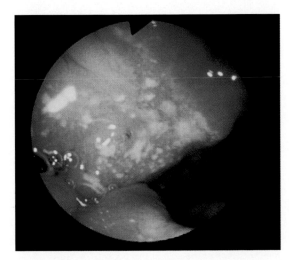

Figure 8.48 *Multifocal, patchy duodenal ulceration. Background mucosa shows erythema.*

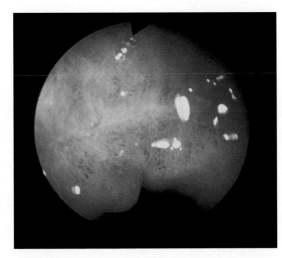

Figure 8.49 *Complete healing stage. Edges surrounding the scar are erythematous.*

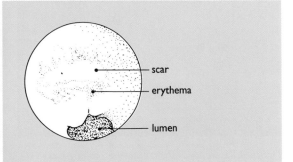

fibrosis with some muscle hypertrophy around the site of ulceration. The combination of fibrosis and muscle hypertrophy tends to pull the adjacent layers towards the point of recurrent ulceration, producing the characteristic converging folds radiating from the ulcer towards the periphery.

Between these folds, one may appreciate pseudodiverticula. These are single or multiple outpouchings in the bulb within zones of scar deformity, possibly formed as a result of a pulsion effect on the lesser or uninvolved portion of the duodenal wall (Fig. 8.52). A pseudodiverticulum may simply be the result of a stretching effect of the uninvolved wall by material entering the bulb between fixed points of scarring. Pseudodiverticula usually occur at the fornices and midportion of the bulb (Fig. 8.53).

Midbulb or apical deformity alone or together may be sufficient to contract the bulb, shortening it to less than 3 cm (Fig. 8.54). In advanced stages of foreshortening, the bulbous structure may virtually disappear. In a healed duodenal ulcer a circumferential fold may remain at the apex of the bulb (Fig. 8.55).

Breakthrough bulbar ulcers, observed during prolonged H₂-receptor blockade therapy, have a peculiar appearance. Most often such ulcers are small and superficial without intense erythema and swelling of the surrounding mucosa (Figs. 8.56 and 8.57). Occasionally, they may be difficult to distinguish from a large erosion. Patients with marked scarring and deformity are especially prone to breakthrough ulceration (Fig. 8.58).

Gastric Ulcers With Duodenal Ulcer

Peptic ulcers of the bulb may be associated with gastric ulcers. Characteristically, such ulcers are in the prepyloric antrum, adjacent to or within 2 cm of the pyloric channel (Fig. 8.4). Another common location for a secondary gastric ulcer is the angle along the lesser curve. The presence of prepyloric ulcers indicates the need for a detailed examination of the bulb. Such ulcers are notoriously difficult to heal and have a high recurrence rate.

In patients with ordinary duodenal ulceration, the gastric mucosa usually looks normal. Occasionally, upon careful inspection one sees lush gastric mucosa with somewhat thickened folds and a prominent areae gastricae pattern, especially in the corpus and fundic area (Fig. 8.59).

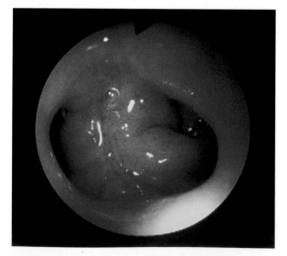

Figure 8.50 Heavy folds in a hypercontractile bulb after duodenal ulcer healing.

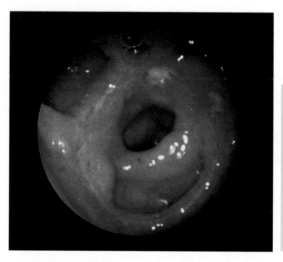
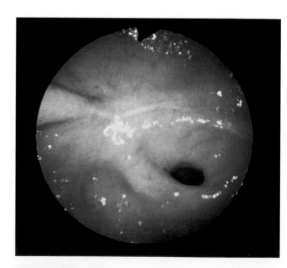

Figure 8.51 Recurrent duodenal ulcer. Fresh ulceration is seen together with scarring and deformity from previous ulcers.

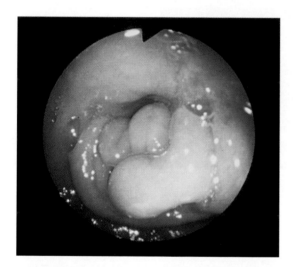
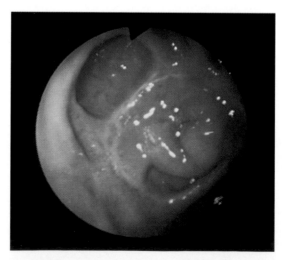

Figure 8.52 In this patient, excessive scarring and retraction caused pseudodiverticular formation, giving the appearance of a split pylorus.

Figure 8.53 Scar deformity with pseudodiverticula.

Figure 8.54 Extensive scarring and refraction caused foreshortening of the bulb in this patient.

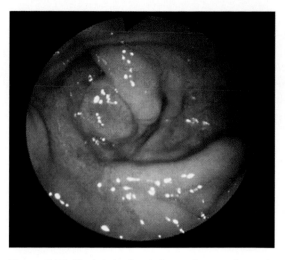

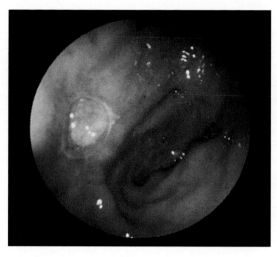

Figure 8.55 Healed duodenal ulcer with circumferential apical fold, caused by scar and contraction, remaining.

Figure 8.56 Breakthrough ulcer observed during H_2-receptor blockade maintenance therapy. This ulcer is small and superficial without prominent inflammatory changes in the surrounding mucosa.

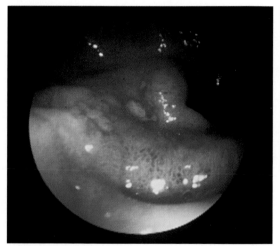

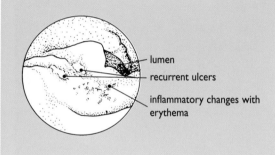

Figure 8.57 Breakthrough ulcers with more conspicuous inflammatory changes.

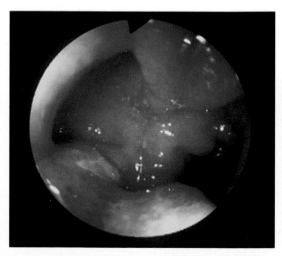

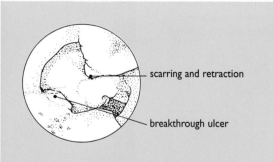

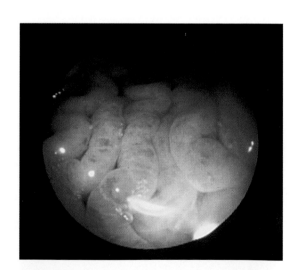

Figure 8.58 Breakthrough ulcer. In this patient, the bulb shows evidence of scarring and retraction, indicating a tendency for breakthrough ulcers.

Figure 8.59 Lush gastric mucosa with a prominent areae gastricae pattern is occasionally seen in patients with ordinary duodenal ulcer disease. This appearance is compatible with acid hypersecretion.

Gastrinoma-Related Ulcers

Multiple extensive ulcers of the bulb and descending duodenum may be associated with gastrinoma and acid hypersecretion (Fig. 8.35, Figs. 8.60 and 8.61). Superficial, erosive or ulcerative destruction of the duodenum usually appears on the uppermost portion of the prominent, somewhat enlarged Kerckring's folds. The presence of postbulbar, superficial or large, and extensive ulceration of the descending and horizontal parts of the duodenum should always suggest the possibility of gastrinoma or Zollinger-Ellison syndrome. In such cases, inspection of the stomach usually reveals enlargement of the fold pattern with accentuation of the areae gastricae. A careful evaluation to exclude a gastrin-producing tumor is essential in this situation.

Endoscopic Guidelines

A small caliber endoscope or a side-viewing instrument should be used when there is strong suspicion of an ulcer, especially along the proximal portion of the superior wall of the duodenum. In general, most ulcers are located within 1–2 cm of the pylorobulbar junction. Occasionally, an ulcer may be hidden between swollen folds (Fig. 8.62). Careful, gentle inspection and, if necessary, intravenous injection of antispasmodics such as glucagon usually allows identification of the ulcer.

Because of the risk of rupturing a deep, penetrating ulcer, it may be wise to forego entirely, or limit the number of attempts at, passing the endoscope

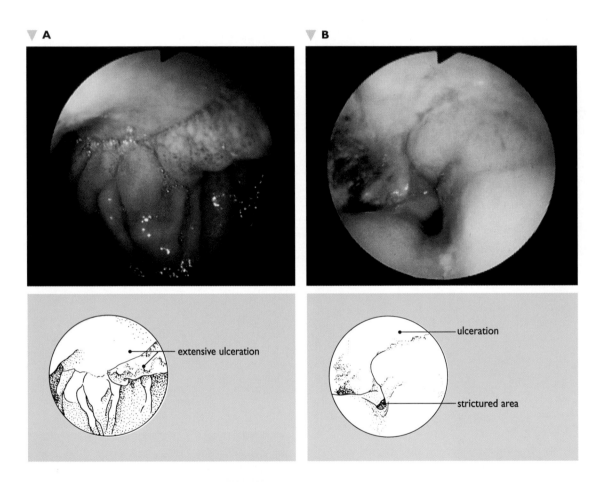

A **B**

Figure 8.60 (**A**) Giant postbulbar ulceration in the horizontal part of the duodenum is due to gastrinoma. (**B**) The same patient shows stricturing at the duodenojejunal angle.

extensive ulceration

ulceration

strictured area

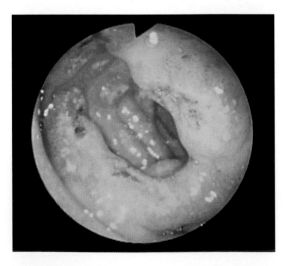

Figure 8.61 Extensive erosive duodenitis in a patient with gastrinoma.

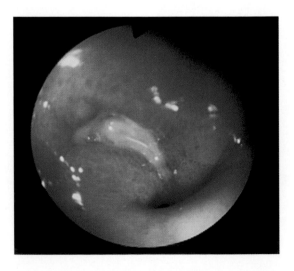

Figure 8.62 This oval duodenal ulcer was initially hidden between swollen folds and not immediately identified. Upon close inspection, however, it is readily seen.

for examination of the bulb in patients with severe symptomatic disease. This is especially true if antispasmodic medication does not sufficiently relax the bulb to allow easy passage of a small caliber endoscope. Excessive air insufflation is certainly to be avoided.

Complications

Major complications of severe ulcer disease include intractable pain (less common now because of antisecretory therapy), scarring causing gastric outlet obstruction, penetration, perforation, and bleeding. The presence of a complication may be preceded by a change in symptoms. For example, obstruction must be suspected when pain is no longer relieved by food ingestion, and is accompanied by nausea and vomiting.

Bleeding from a posterior wall ulcer is dangerous because of the proximity of major arteries involving the stem or side branches of the gastroduodenal artery. Occasionally a vessel may be visible in the base of such an ulcer (Fig. 8.63). Especially in severe bleeding, the overlying blood, or clot, or both, may obscure the crater itself. Jet irrigation may clear the blood sufficiently to allow visualization of the crater and of the bleeding spot. However, it can be difficult if not impossible in a contracted bulb to obtain a full view of the bleeding site, which is a prerequisite for treatment with laser photocoagulation, bipolar electrocoagulation, heater probe application, or local injection therapy, although targeting with the latter therapy is somewhat less critical.

NONPEPTIC DISORDERS OF THE DUODENUM

The duodenum may undergo degenerative or inflammatory changes as a result of infection by viruses, bacteria, fungi, or parasites. In addition, the bulboduodenal mucosa may be involved in various diseases such as Crohn's disease and diseases that cause malabsorption, such as gluten-sensitive enteropathy. Several other disorders can cause characteristic changes in the bulb or duodenum.

Parasitic Infections

Parasitic duodenitis caused by hookworm, *Strongyloides, Giardia,* or *Ascaris* appears as a pronounced focal erythema with edema and partial or complete disappearance of the Kerckring's folds (Fig. 8.64). Occasionally there is some nodular deformity. The lesions usually start in the postbulbar area and are diffusely spread. Duodenal aspiration and biopsy should be performed for diagnosis in patients with unexplained duodenal inflammatory changes that spare the bulb, especially if the patient has recently traveled in tropical areas.

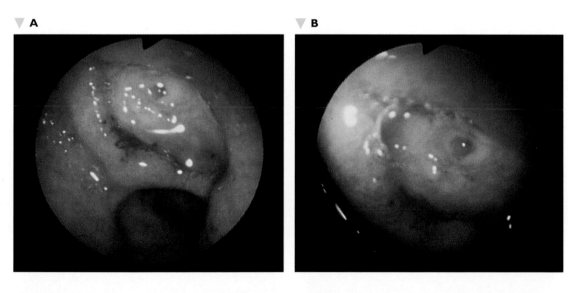

▽ **A** ▽ **B**

Figure 8.63 (**A**) A side branch of the gastroduodenal artery is visible in this posterior wall duodenal ulcer. (**B**) Bleeding is evident at the margin of the ulcer.

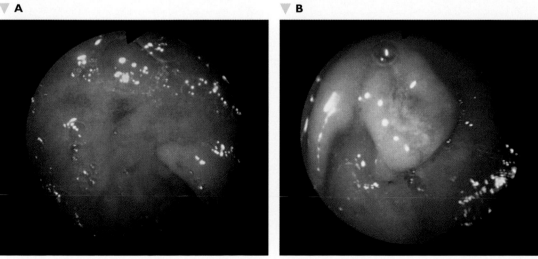

▽ **A** ▽ **B**

Figure 8.64 Parasitic duodenitis due to Strongyloides. (**A**) Small focal erythematous areas are clearly visible. (**B**) Strongyloides worms visible as tiny whitish threads.

Crohn's Disease

Of all patients with gastrointestinal Crohn's disease, 0.5–4.0% will have manifestations in the duodenum. Whether isolated duodenal involvement in Crohn's disease exists is uncertain. Generally the bulb is involved in conjunction with the descending duodenum or prepyloric antrum. Discrete aphthoid erosions and shallow ulcerations are seen in the prepyloric antrum, bulb, and proximal or entire duodenum (Fig. 8.65). Surrounding the aphthoid erosions is a rim of erythema; between the lesions the mucosa may appear normal. Occasionally nodular deformity may develop, creating a cobblestone-like appearance. There may be long or deep serpiginous ulceration within areas displaying a cobblestone pattern. In rare cases, discrete ulcers are present around a fistulous tract (Fig. 8.66). Other patients show only a nonspecific duodenal inflammation with erythema, exudate, and minor nodular deformity of the contour.

Stricturing with some obstruction of the proximal small intestine is not uncommon in Crohn's duodenitis (Figs. 8.66 and 8.67). The apex itself may be ulcerated and stenotic. In addition, the lesions usually extend into the proximal midportion of the descending duodenum, giving the mucosa a nodular and ulcerated appearance. In approximately 50% of the biopsies, epithelioid cell granulomas may be identified.

Gluten-Sensitive Enteropathy

In most patients with gluten-sensitive enteropathy, the mucosa appears normal; there are no petechiae and the mucosa does not traumatize easily. However, on closer examination, villous atrophy can be seen (Figs. 8.68 and 8.69). In some patients, the duodenal mucosa may appear pale and atrophic with a pronounced vascular pattern. In other cases, the mucosa is conspicuously erythematous. Sometimes a mottled appearance of pallor and erythema may be noted.

The most common mucosal feature is the loss of the normal velvet-like fine granular appearance. Instead, the mucosa appears smooth and shiny due to loss of villous excrescences, especially in the duodenal bulb. Sometimes a mosaic pattern or a finely convoluted appearance may be appreciated. Occasionally the openings of the crypts may be visible; such areas should be biopsied. Within the descending duodenum, the Kerckring's folds may be either normal, slightly prominent and erythematous, or – rarely – flattened.

A more detailed study of the mucosal surface morphology may be obtained using either indigo carmine or methylene blue dye-scattering techniques. Most characteristic is a flat mosaic appearance as the insufflated air forces the dye into the clefts between the islands of slightly elevated mucosa

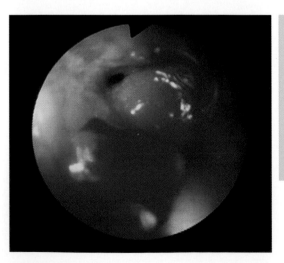
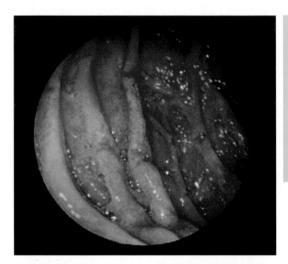
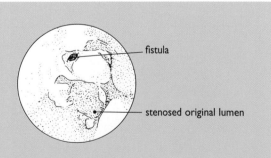
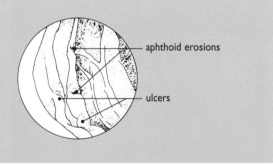

Figure 8.65 Duodenal Crohn's disease. Note the discrete aphthoid erosions and small ulcers at the crests of Kerckring's folds.

Figure 8.66 Crohn's disease of the postbulbar area can cause stricturing. In this case, stenosis of the lumen is seen along with a fistula leading to an intramural sinus.

devoid of villi (Fig. 8.68). Occasionally the dye enters the mouth of the slightly dilated crypts of Lieberkühn. The mucosa of the terminal ileum may appear atrophic in gluten-sensitive enteropathy. Often the disease in gluten-sensitive enteropathy is limited to the proximal small bowel (Fig. 8.69).

Other Nonpeptic Disorders

Patients with hypogammaglobulinemia or common variable immunoglobulin deficiency syndrome may have a flat, avillous mucosa, or nodular lymphoid hyperplasia, or both (Figs. 8.70 and 8.71). Raised 2–5 mm nodules

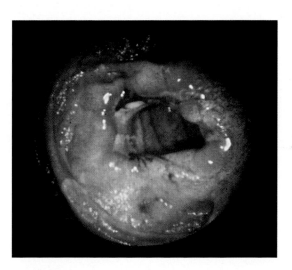

Figure 8.67 *Stricture of small bowel caused by Crohn's disease. The strictured area is ulcerated and the surrounding mucosa is red and nodular.*

A **B**

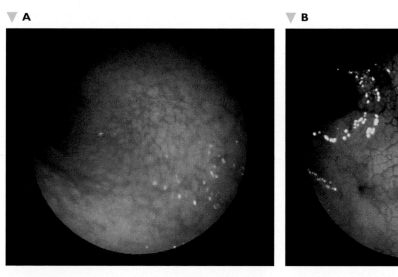

Figure 8.68 *Gluten-sensitive enteropathy. (A) Close examination of the mucosa shows complete villous atrophy. (B) Corresponding picture after methylene blue dye-spraying shows the characteristic mosaic pattern of the flat mucosa.*

A **B**

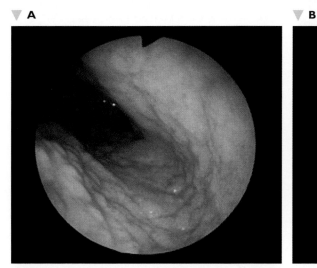
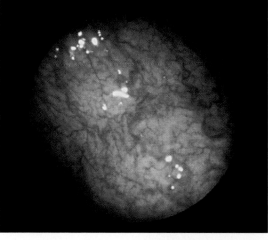

Figure 8.69 *(A) Flat mucosa in gluten-sensitive enteropathy. No villi are seen. (B) Atrophic mucosa of terminal ileum in severe sprue. The vascular pattern is abnormally prominent.*

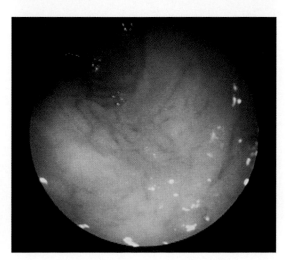

Figure 8.70 *Hypogammaglobulinemia. Total villous atrophy is seen. Giardiasis was present.*

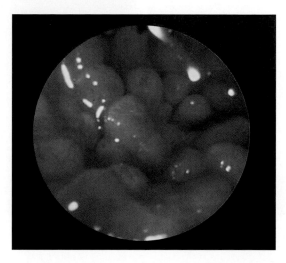

Figure 8.71 *Hypogammaglobulinemia is associated with nodular lymphoid hyperplasia in this presentation.*

may cover a portion of the mucosa. Usually they are a somewhat brighter color than the surrounding mucosa. The Kerckring's folds may be normal, or they may appear pink because of the abundance of superimposed nodules. In Bruton's agammaglobulinemia there is usually complete villous atrophy without nodular lymphoid hyperplasia (Fig. 8.72).

Whipple's disease has a characteristic endoscopic appearance with patchy, whitish discoloration, alteration of the villous pattern, and occasionally a markedly irregular mosaic pattern (Fig. 8.73). A related condition called

pseudo-Whipple's disease, caused by *Mycobacterium avium-intracellulare*, is regularly observed in patients with AIDS. Endoscopic abnormalities similar to Whipple's disease are seen with irregular coarsening of the villous pattern and conspicuous whitish discoloration due to stagnant lipid in the lamina propria (Fig. 8.74).

Lymphangiectasia or chylangiectasia is usually characterized endoscopically by shiny, whitish spots in an otherwise normal-looking mucosa. These white spots are due to light reflection from the ectatic lymph vessels filled

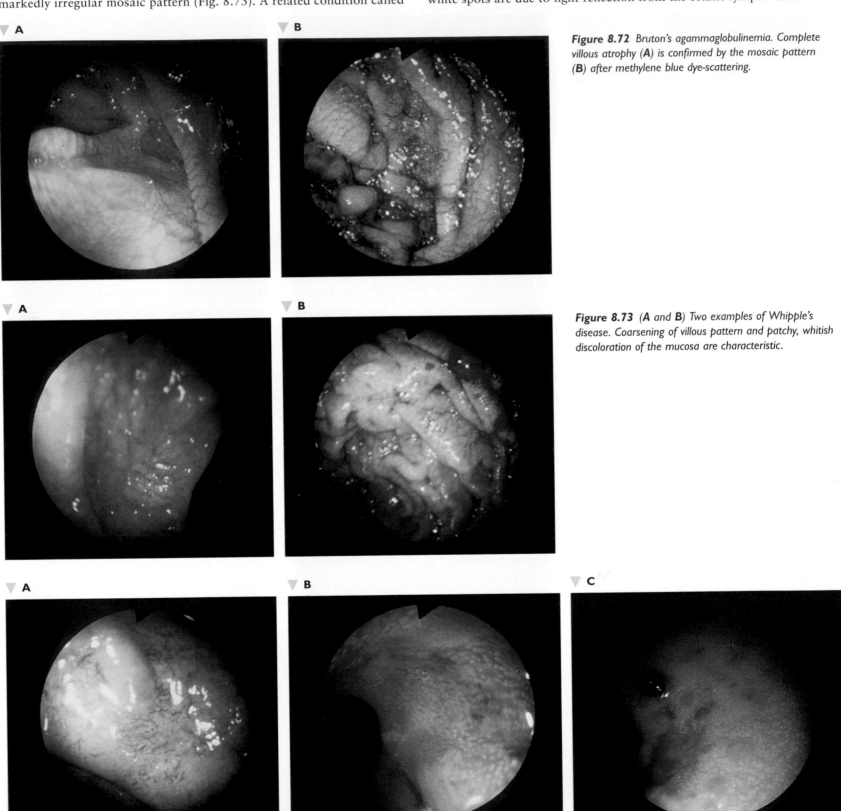

Figure 8.72 *Bruton's agammaglobulinemia. Complete villous atrophy (**A**) is confirmed by the mosaic pattern (**B**) after methylene blue dye-scattering.*

Figure 8.73 *(**A** and **B**) Two examples of Whipple's disease. Coarsening of villous pattern and patchy, whitish discoloration of the mucosa are characteristic.*

Figure 8.74 *(**A–C**) Three examples of pseudo-Whipple's disease in AIDS patients, caused by Mycobacterium avium-intracellulare.*

with chylomicrons (Fig. 8.75). In other patients, somewhat larger lymph or chyle cysts may be readily apparent. Yellow–white milky fluid may escape upon puncture of the cysts.

Duodenal melanosis is an unusual condition in which pigment is deposited in the mucosa (Fig. 8.76). Biopsies may show focal deposits of brownish-black pigment in the stroma of the villi.

VASCULAR ABNORMALITIES OF THE DUODENUM

Telangiectasis may be seen in Rendu-Osler-Weber syndrome. These irregular cherry red spots range in size between 2 and 4 mm (Fig. 8.77). Other types of vascular anomaly may also be seen in the duodenum, as well as elsewhere in the intestinal tract (Figs. 8.78 and 8.79).

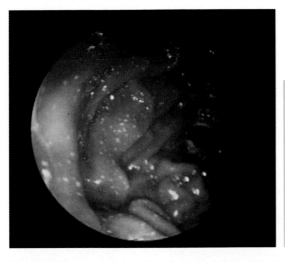
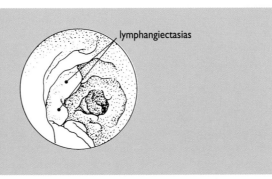

Figure 8.75 *Idiopathic small intestinal lymphangiectasia. Shiny white spots are characteristic of the ectatic lymph vessels.*

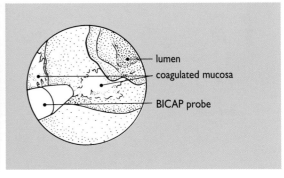

Figure 8.76 *Brown discoloration of the mucosa is due to duodenal melanosis.*

▼ **A**　　　　　　▼ **B**

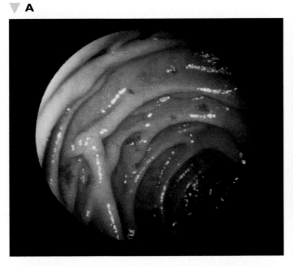
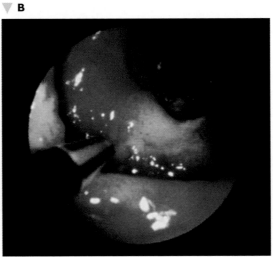

Figure 8.77 *Rendu-Osler-Weber syndrome.* **(A)** *Hemorrhagic telangiectasia of the duodenum may be seen in this hereditary disorder.* **(B)** *Coagulation can be accomplished with bipolar electrodes.*

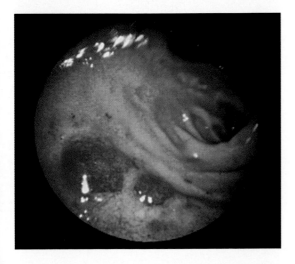

Figure 8.78 *Congenital vascular anomaly in duodenal bulb. This cavernous hemangioma is an example of blue rubber nevus syndrome.*

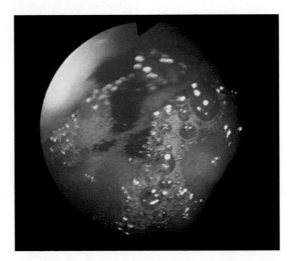

Figure 8.79 *Hemangiomas of duodenal bulb.*

The duodenum is occasionally the site of varices caused by extrahepatic portal hypertension or extensive malignancy of the pancreatic bed. Large, serpiginous, undulating, tortuous protuberances are seen running between Kerckring's folds, particularly on the posterior wall of the apex (Fig. 8.80). Sometimes they show a gray–blue or faint bluish discoloration; in other cases the color is that of the surrounding mucosa. These protruding nodular folds are soft and easily compressed when touched with a closed biopsy forceps, which is a useful clue to their identity. In portal hypertension, one may see hypertensive duodenopathy with swollen folds and vascular congestion (Fig. 8.81).

Rarely, ischemic damage occurs in the duodenum. The overall endoscopic appearance is nonspecific, with loss of the fold pattern, patchy focal erythema, and mild friability. In more severe cases, a diffuse erosive or ulcerative defect may be seen, covered with a dirty exudate. The cause is usually unknown.

TUMORS OF THE BULB AND DUODENUM

Tumors of the proximal small bowel are uncommon. The etiology varies from benign conditions to invading malignancies.

Benign Polypoid Lesions

Polypoid lesions of the bulb and duodenum usually occur as multiple small mucosal nodules. When there is no flat mucosa between the elevated surfaces, the terms nodularity or mamillation may be preferred; otherwise, the term polypoid excrescence is appropriate. There is virtually no effective visual feature for distinguishing polypoid lesions of epithelial origin from those of submucosal origin.

Multiple Polypoid Lesions

Multiple small polypoid excrescences can be hyperplastic, adenomatous, inflammatory, or they may be due to heterotopic gastric mucosa, Brunner's gland hyperplasia, or lymphoid hyperplasia.

Hyperplastic inflammatory polyps presumably correspond to the healing stage of nodular bulbitis. The mucosa can be histologically normal or it can show nonspecific duodenitis. At endoscopy the polyps appear as discrete, 2–4 mm elevations covered with normal-appearing mucosa. They may be found in the bulb alone or in descending duodenum also. Larger polyps of this type may become erythematous and even superficially eroded.

Polypoid lesions may also be composed entirely of heterotopic gastric mucosa. Heterotopic gastric epithelium is a common finding in bulboduodenal biopsies. Usually, several small 1–3 mm sessile excrescences are tightly grouped to form a granular, slightly elevated plaque. These excrescences are usually conical or round, and have a translucent appearance with a pale pink or slightly reddened coloration (Figs. 8.82–8.84). In other cases a slightly raised, irregular, illdefined patch of mucosa is seen, which has a fine cobblestone-like appearance (Fig. 8.85). Heterotopic gastric mucosa is located preferentially in the proximal part of the bulb. Sometimes a single whitish polyp about 5 mm in size is seen in the second portion of the duodenum. Histologically, the lesion consists of full thickness corpus-type gastric mucosa with parietal and chief cells. Heterotopic or ectopic gastric mucosa should not be confused with gastric or antrum-type metaplasia, which is presumably an acquired reaction in relation to acid reflux in the bulb.

In Brunner's gland hyperplasia, multiple nodular elevations about 5 mm in size are spread throughout the descending duodenum. In most cases the bulb is not involved. The nodular elevation is mainly due to accumulation of somewhat enlarged Brunner's glands (Fig. 8.86). Nodular lymphoid hyperplasia is seen endoscopically as multiple small sessile nodules covered with shiny mucosa that is otherwise unremarkable.

Single Polypoid Lesions

Many conditions in the bulboduodenum typically cause a single polypoid lesion. Single hyperplastic inflammatory polyps amidst normal mucosa are common. Their size (3–6 mm) and eroded appearance may cause the endoscopist to suspect an adenoma. Single, submucosal polyps are either leiomyoma, lipoma, carcinoid, Brunner's gland adenoma, hamartoma, or adenoma. Other benign small bowel tumors such as fibromas, angiomas, lymphangiomas, and myomas are rarely encountered.

▼ **A**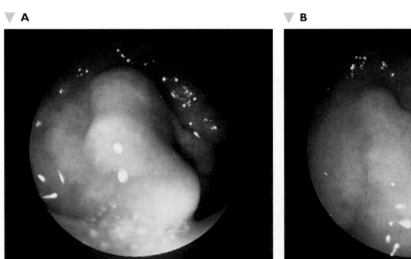

▼ **B**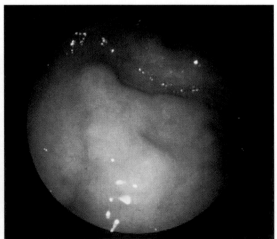

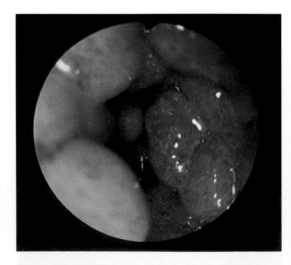

Figure 8.80 (*A and B*) *Varices of the duodenum are discernible here as large, tortuous, slightly bluish protuberances.*

Figure 8.81 *Portal hypertensive duodenopathy. Folds are swollen and congested with red lesions caused by vascular congestion.*

Leiomyomas are usually larger than 1 cm and are located at the junction of the apex of the bulb and the proximal descending duodenum (Fig. 8.87). Occasionally they may have a central ulceration or umbilication. Lipomas also occur preferentially at the bulboduodenal junction. They are yellowish and have a smooth surface. Unlike leiomyomas, they are usually not umbilicated or ulcerated. Most submucosal lipomas are 1–6 cm and form intramucosal sessile growths that eventually become pedunculated. Once pedunculated, the polyp is soft, freely movable on a stalk, and covered with normal shiny-looking duodenal mucosa.

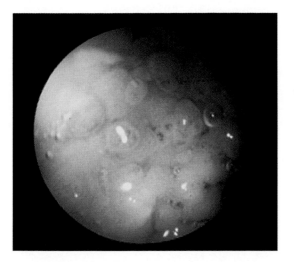

Figure 8.82 Heterotopic gastric mucosa in the bulb. A cluster of slightly elevated, pinkish, opalescent polyps, 5 mm in size, is readily apparent. Note the central red spot in several of the polyps.

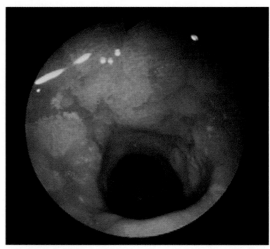

Figure 8.83 Heterotopic gastric mucosa, giving a flat appearance.

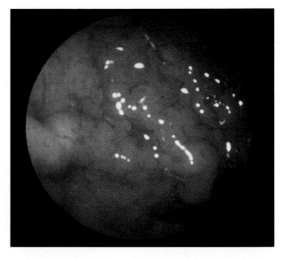

Figure 8.84 In this case, heterotopic gastric mucosa in the bulb presents a diffusely nodular appearance.

▼ **A**

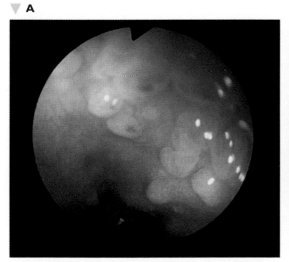

▼ **B**

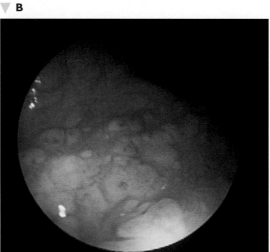

Figure 8.85 (*A* and *B*) Heterotopic gastric mucosa in the duodenal bulb with raised appearance in two patients.

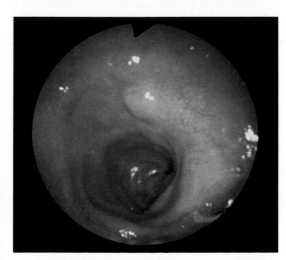

Figure 8.86 Brunner's gland hyperplasia with a single nodular elevation occurring in the apex of the bulb.

Figure 8.87 This submucosal polypoid lesion, consistent with a leiomyoma, is found at the apex of the bulb.

A Brunner's gland adenoma may appear as a sessile or pedunculated polypoid mass, 2–4 cm wide. These rare lesions are usually confined to the proximal part of the duodenum and are covered with normal-looking mucosa (Fig. 8.88) or slightly erythematous mucosa (Fig. 8.89).

Hamartomatous polyps in Peutz-Jeghers syndrome vary in size, are usually irregularly shaped, and have a somewhat dark-brownish color compared with surrounding mucosa (Fig. 8.90).

Adenomatous polyps in the duodenum are rare. Most are 1 cm or larger and may be single or multiple, sessile or pedunculated. The surface mucosa is usually finely mamillated. Such polyps are seldom large enough to cause obstruction. Intussusception is also not a problem because of the anatomical fixation of the duodenum. If a pedunculated polyp is endoscopically accessible, polypectomy should be considered. Regularly, small adenomatous lesions are seen in the duodenum in patients with familial polyposis coli (FPC) (Fig. 8.91). There may be multiple small bowel adenomatous polyps in both FPC and Gardner's syndrome (Figs. 8.92 and 8.93).

▼ **A** ▼ **B**

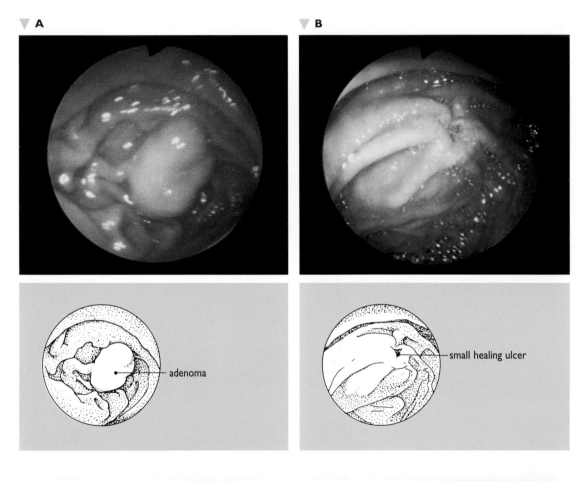

Figure 8.88 (**A**) Brunner's gland adenoma located in the proximal duodenum. (**B**) A small healing ulcer with converging folds remains after endoscopic removal with snare polypectomy.

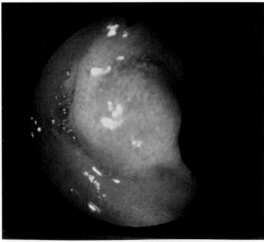

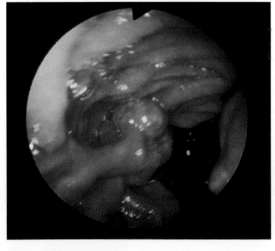

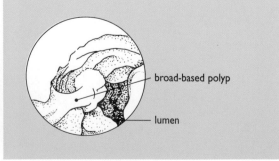

Figure 8.89 Brunner's adenoma of duodenum with slightly erythematous surface mucosa.

Figure 8.90 Hamartomatous polyp in the duodenum caused by Peutz-Jeghers syndrome.

An association between FPC or Gardner's syndrome and adenoma of the papilla is regularly observed. These lesions may be the precursor of adenocarcinoma of the papilla. When the association is clarified, patients may have to be screened with side-viewing duodenoscopy to rule out adenoma or carcinoma of the papilla. If there is a question concerning the papilla during endoscopy, biopsy and cytology are indicated.

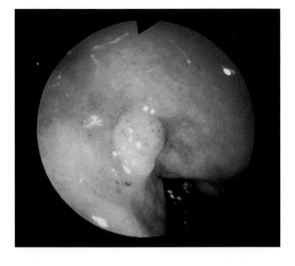

Figure 8.91 A small adenomatous polyp at the bulboduodenal junction is seen in this patient with familial polyposis coli and polyposis of the stomach.

An association between FPC and neoplasia of the upper gastrointestinal tract is also apparent. In patients with FPC, polyps are commonly found both in the stomach and in the duodenum. In the stomach, the polyps are rarely adenomas; typically they are nonadenomatous gastric fundal polyps. In the duodenum, however, polyps are frequently adenomatous.

A communication from St. Mark's Hospital in London reports on a study of 102 patients with FPC. Of these, 88 had duodenal polyps. The areas of maximal involvement were the second and third portions of the duodenum. Multiple duodenal polyps were very common, with 39 patients having 5–20 polyps and 37 patients having more than 20. The duodenal polyps were larger than gastric polyps, with a mean size of 9.4 mm and a range of 1–50 mm. In 86 of the 88 patients, polyps were adenomatous. The periampullary region was reported as histologically abnormal in 87 of 97 patients in whom a biopsy was taken and 72 of these 87 patients had adenoma. Biopsies of the papilla were more likely to show adenoma (81%) than the periampullary region (41%). These impressive data add to the growing body of knowledge regarding the increased risk of duodenal adenomas and adenocarcinoma in these patients, especially involving the periampullary region of the duodenum. St Mark's reports that they are screening most of their patients who have mild or moderate duodenal polyposis every 3 years and in those with severe polyposis, endoscopy is repeated yearly.

Optimal therapy for duodenal gastrointestinal adenomas has not yet been established. The adenomas are multiple and may recur, therefore treatment is complex. As data collect from careful screening programs of the type

▼ **A**

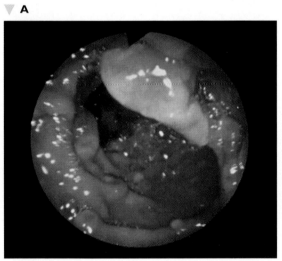

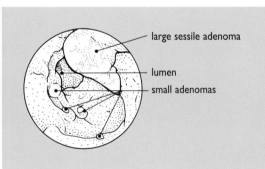

large sessile adenoma

lumen
small adenomas

▼ **B**

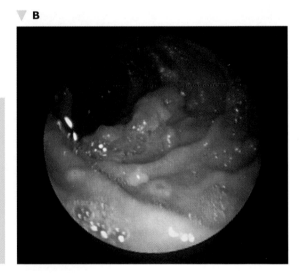

Figure 8.92 (**A** and **B**) Diffuse adenomatosis in small bowel in a patient with familial polyposis coli. The polyps vary from small to large in size.

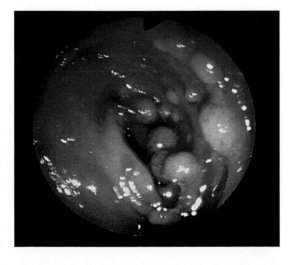

Figure 8.93 Small intestinal polyposis in Gardner's syndrome. Adenomas of various sizes are seen.

described at St. Mark's, we will gain a better understanding of the association between FPC, adenomatous polyps and duodenal cancer. Eventually we hope to be able to recommend firm guidelines for screening intervals, and procedures for identifying those FPC patients at high risk of developing duodenal cancer. Continued study should also help to clarify the best therapy for these adenomatous conditions.

Villous adenoma, a rare lesion of the duodenum, appears similar to villous lesions found in the colon. They are often sessile, irregular on the surface, and moderately large, often wider than 1–2 cm. Classically, a large, multilobed soft sessile polyp with a shaggy surface is seen at endoscopy (Fig. 8.94). Occasionally the villous adenoma appears limited to involving one portion of a Kerckring's fold (Fig. 8.95). In exceptional cases there is diffuse

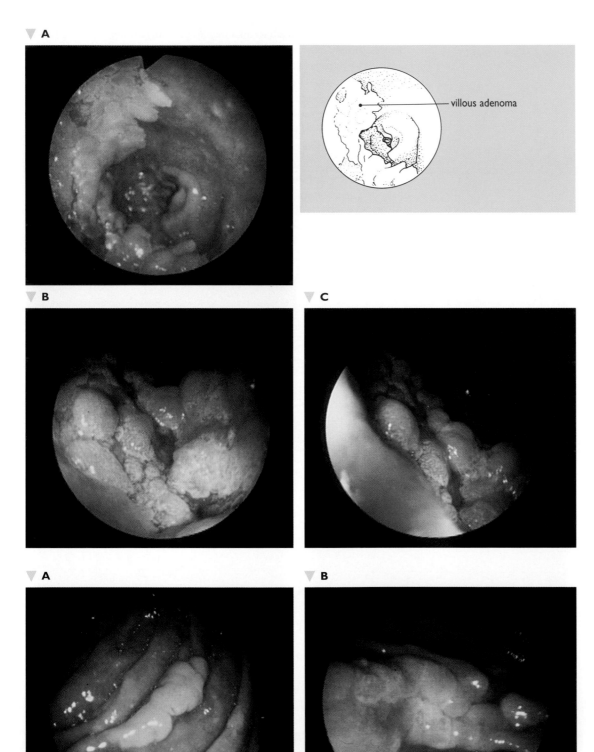

Figure 8.94 *Villous adenoma of the bulb.* (**A**) *Soft multilobular polyps are shown in this view.* (**B** *and* **C**) *Details of the adenomatous tissue show the cauliflower-like appearance of this tumor.*

Figure 8.95 (**A**) *A single, small adenomatous fold with severe dysplasia.* (**B**) *Villous adenoma involving a single fold in the descending duodenum. Note the shaggy, irregular surface and the difference in mucosal color.*

adenomatosis of the whole proximal small intestine in conjunction with FPC Fig. 8.96). Endoscopic resection should not be attempted unless the tumor is small and pedunculated because of the danger of transmural damage. Biopsies may miss a deep-seated carcinoma.

Duodenal Malignancies

Primary duodenal cancer is rare. The tumor usually appears as a nodular, ulcerated, exophytic, polypoid mass confined to the medial wall in the second portion of the duodenum (Fig. 8.97). This cancer may be limited or involve an entire segment of the duodenal wall.

Carcinoma more commonly arises directly from the duodenal papilla (Fig. 8.98). The papilla is enlarged to two or three times its normal size, appearing as a mass. Usually a bulky raised tumor mass projects out from the hooded fold. In the typical case, the cancer infiltrates circumferentially, lifting the peripheral portion of the orifice in relation to a central depressed area, and causing an excavated appearance. Tumor nodules and ulcerations may be seen within the excavated area.

Biopsies are obtained preferentially from the nodular periphery and from the excavated portion. Where the papillary malignancy is covered largely with normal-looking mucosa, the diagnostic yield of direct biopsy may be enhanced by performing a limited papillotomy with a standard papillotome, a precut papillotome, or a papillotomy knife to expose the deep layers.

Direct extension of pancreatic cancer is the most common cancer of the duodenum. A widespread, ill-defined nodular mass of the medial wall is seen, usually involving the papilla and in some cases replacing the entire medial wall (Fig. 8.99). The mass often consists of 2–3 cm nodules.

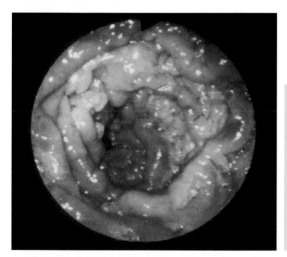
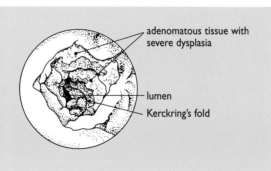

Figure 8.96 *Diffuse adenomatosis and dysplasia of the whole proximal small intestine. Note the color difference between adenomatous tissue and uninvolved Kerckring's folds. This rare presentation may be found in patients with FPC.*

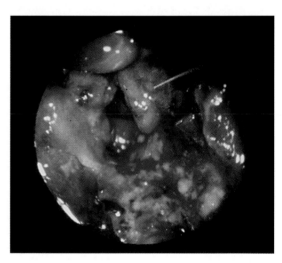

Figure 8.97 *Primary cancer of the apical region of the bulb. An exophytic ulcerating mass is clearly discernible.*

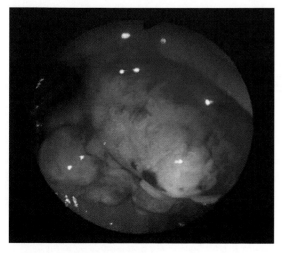

Figure 8.98 *Cancer of the ampulla of Vater. A large, multilobulated, friable mass is seen.*

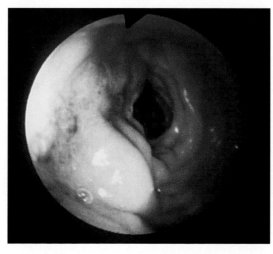
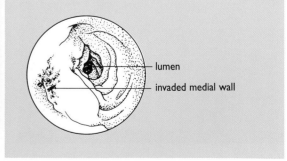

Figure 8.99 *Invasion of the medial wall of the duodenum by pancreatic cancer. Note asymmetry of the duodenal lumen.*

Metastasis to the duodenum from a distant primary cancer is rare. When it does occur it is usually from a malignant melanoma; in this case, lesions may be small and pigmented or large with an ulcerated central portion and pigmented periphery. Other tumors that can metastasize to the duodenum include bronchus, breast, kidney, and uterine cervix. The typical metastatic implant appears as a 1–2 cm ulcerated mass set apart from the papilla (Fig. 8.100).

Malignant lymphoma of the duodenum occurs most often in association with gastric lymphoma, which may extend through the pylorus. Multiple polypoid masses (Fig. 8.101) or large ulcerations may replace extensive portions of the bulb or duodenum, or the mucosa may have a diffusely infiltrated appearance with nodularity (Fig. 8.102). Primary duodenal lymphoma may appear as nodular, sessile, ulcerated masses (Fig. 8.103). In generalized lymphosarcoma, the characteristic multiple tiny whitish, slightly elevated lesions

in the duodenum can be easily overlooked (Fig. 8.104). Usually the stomach is also involved (Fig. 8.105).

Several other malignancies may occur in the bulb or duodenum. Duodenal infiltration caused by leukemia may appear as plaque-like thickening of folds or as diffuse elevated nodular lesions and polypoid masses.

Kaposi's sarcoma appears as variably sized, reddish-brown lesions, often associated with gastric lesions (Fig. 8.106). These may occur in the duodenal bulb (Fig. 8.107) and descending duodenum (Fig. 8.108). The surface of the lesion characteristically is bright red or reticulated and it has a similar appearance elsewhere in the bowel. Duodenal involvement by leiomyosarcoma usually occurs as a nodular, centrally ulcerated lesion and is associated with massive destruction of the duodenal wall. Concomitant lesions may be observed in surrounding structures such as the stomach (Fig. 8.109).

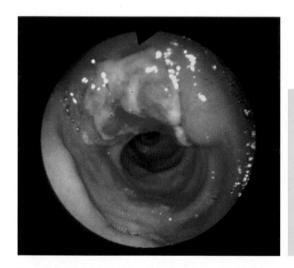

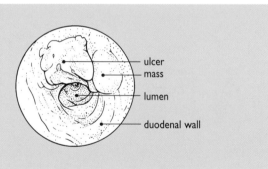

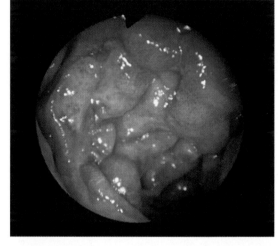

Figure 8.100 *Duodenal wall invasion by a renal cell adenocarcinoma occurring as an ulcerating mass. The patient presented with an upper gastrointestinal bleed.*

Figure 8.101 *Duodenal lymphoma with multiple polypoid masses.*

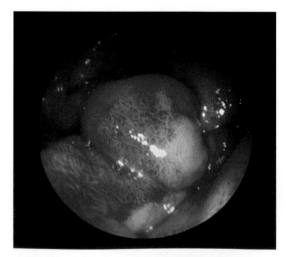

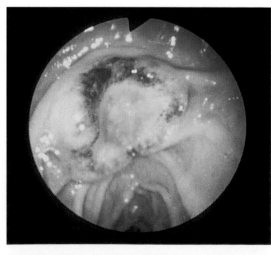

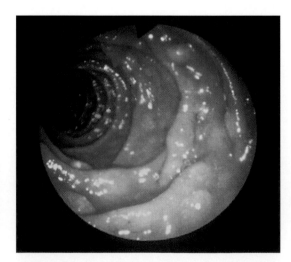

Figure 8.102 *Lymphoma involving duodenum with infiltrated, enlarged, erythematous folds appearing as nodules.*

Figure 8.103 *Centrally ulcerated mass caused by primary lymphoma of the duodenum.*

Figure 8.104 *Generalized lymphosarcoma of the duodenum is seen as patchy, discrete, white lesions.*

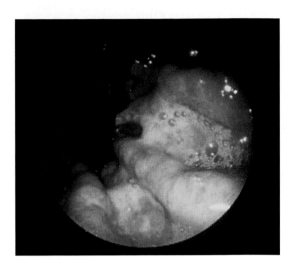

Figure 8.105 *Generalized lymphosarcomatous involvement of the stomach in the patient in Figure 8.104. Note irregularity and broadening of folds.*

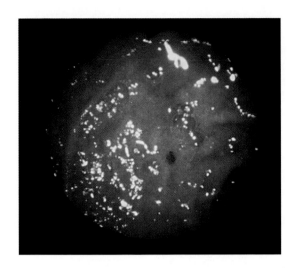

Figure 8.106 *A minute reddish-brown lesion, characteristic of Kaposi's sarcoma of the duodenum.*

▼ **A** ▼ **B**

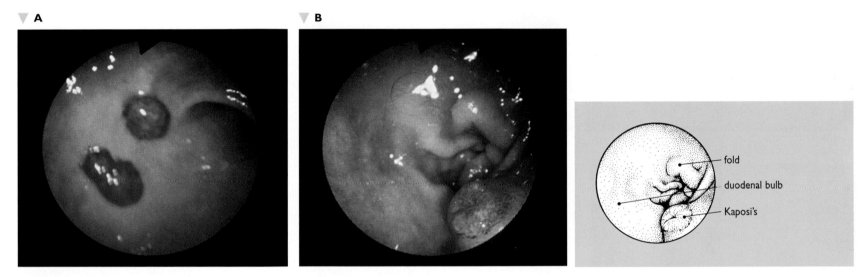

Figure 8.107 *(A and B) Kaposi's sarcoma of the duodenal bulb in a patient with AIDS. Elevated, red or reticulated surface covers these lesions (5 o'clock).*

▼ **A** ▼ **B** ▼ **C**

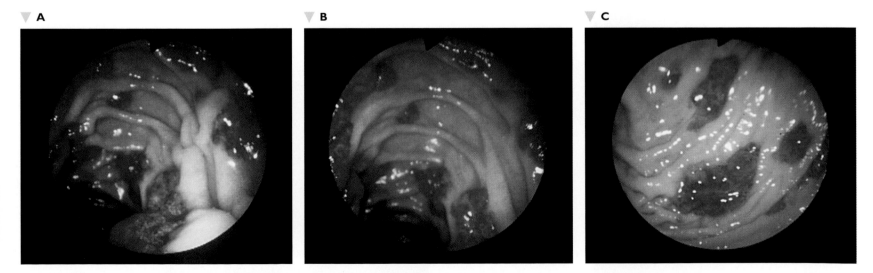

Figure 8.108 *(A–C) Kaposi's sarcoma involving the descending duodenum in three AIDS patients. Multiple red, elevated lesions are noted.*

Endosonography of Duodenal Masses

Endoscopic ultrasound can greatly facilitate evaluation of the duodenal wall and papilla of Vater. Endosonography can also be used to evaluate the head of the pancreas, the bile ducts, blood vessels surrounding the duodenum, the liver and other structures through the duodenal wall. Some examples of this are shown in Chapter 9. Here we show one example, a leiomyoma of the duodenal wall as evaluated with endosonography (Fig. 8.110).

POLYPOID LESIONS OF THE TERMINAL ILEUM

The terminal ileum has a relatively small caliber lumen. In some cases villi may be seen (Fig. 8.111). In teenagers and young adults, the mucosa may appear somewhat uneven because of irregularly distributed, small nodular elevations corresponding to the presence of prominent lymphoid follicles (Fig. 8.112). Sometimes the mucosa is carpeted with tiny 1–2 mm lymphoid nodules, giving it a granular appearance. This abundance of visible lymphoid

▼ **A**

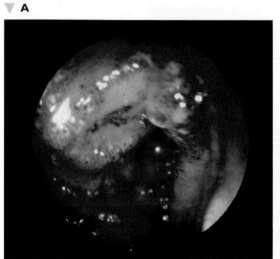

▼ **B**

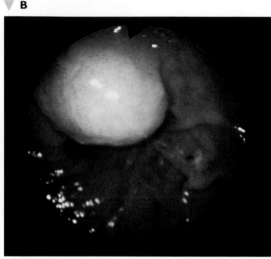

Figure 8.109 (A) Destruction of the duodenal wall caused by leiomyosarcoma. *(B)* Leiomyosarcomatous mass causing impression in the antrum. Endosonography is very helpful in examining this type of lesion.

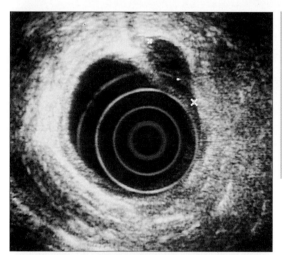

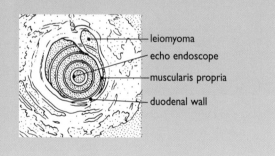

Figure 8.110 Duodenal leiomyoma. The hypoechoic homogeneous lesion is limited to the wall, does not extend into the periduodenal tissues and seems contiguous with the muscularis propria layer of the duodenal wall. *(Courtesy of Dr T.L. Tio)*

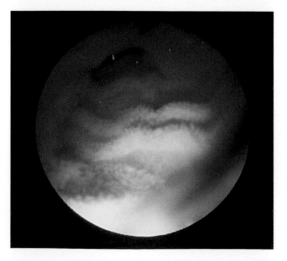

Figure 8.111 Normal terminal ileum; villi are seen.

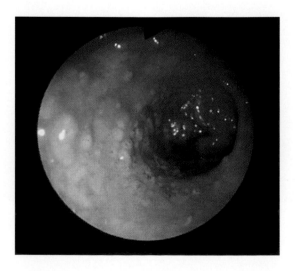

Figure 8.112 Lymphoid follicles in the terminal ileum.

tissue may produce mucosal surfaces ranging from flat through granular to a cobblestone-like appearance (Fig. 8.113). Some endoscopists grade the appearance of the terminal ileum in four classes, 0–3.

Grade 0 – absence of lymph follicles or only a few minute follicles distributed sporadically.

Grade 1 – diffusely but sparsely distributed tiny follicles.

Grade 2 – diffusely and densely distributed follicles, usually without conglomerations between follicles.

Grade 3 – diffuse and densely distributed follicles; individual follicles gen-erally large; interfollicular conglomerations or fusions evident; covering epithelium sometimes hyperemic or pale; large conglomerations referred to as Peyer's patches (Fig. 8.114).

OTHER LESIONS OF THE TERMINAL ILEUM

Other lesions may be visible in the terminal ileum. These include vascular anomalies that may cause recurrent gastrointestinal bleeding (Fig. 8.115); Crohn's disease (Fig. 8.116); and Peyer's patches, which may be mistaken for Crohn's disease (Fig. 8.117).

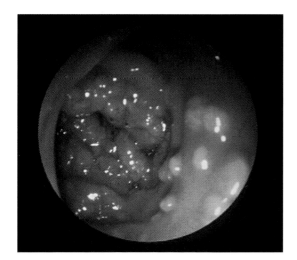

Figure 8.113 *Cobblestone-like appearance of coalescing lymphoid follicles in the terminal ileum.*

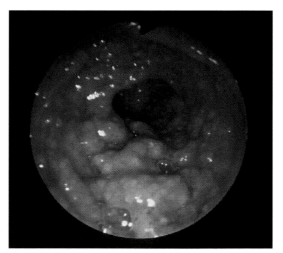

Figure 8.114 *Peyer's patches in the terminal ileum, with a slightly erythematous surface.*

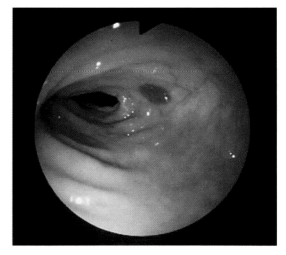

Figure 8.115 *Small vascular anomaly in the terminal ileum.*

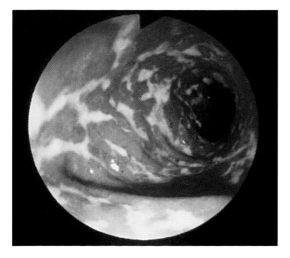

Figure 8.116 *Crohn's disease involving the new terminal ileum after a resection and anastomosis. Multiple linear ulcerations are noted.*

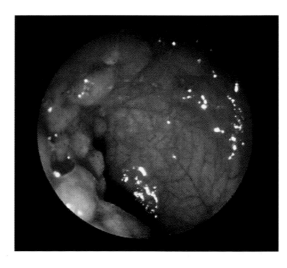

Figure 8.117 *Normal Peyer's patches of the terminal ileum. This case was misinterpreted initially as Crohn's disease.*

The pancreatic duct is usually in the center, or slightly to the right, of the papilla, although this may vary. The common bile duct is often in the left upper segment of the papilla, as viewed endoscopically (Fig. 9.5). The direction of approach to the pancreatic duct is towards the right and horizontally (Fig. 9.6); the direction of approach to the common bile duct is cephalad and towards the left upper margin of the papilla (Fig. 9.7). The papilla may undergo minor trauma during ERCP and cannulation; edema and a small amount of bleeding might be observed (Fig. 9.8).

▼ **A**　　　　　　　　　　　　　　　▼ **B**

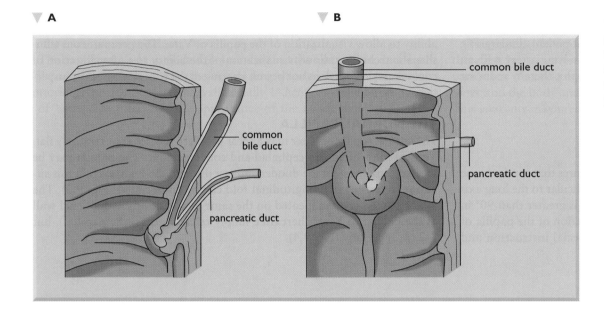

Figure 9.5 Longitudinal section (**A**) and endoscopic front view (**B**) of papilla of Vater. The orifice of the common bile duct on the papilla is located to the left and cephalad. The pancreatic duct is in the center of the papilla.

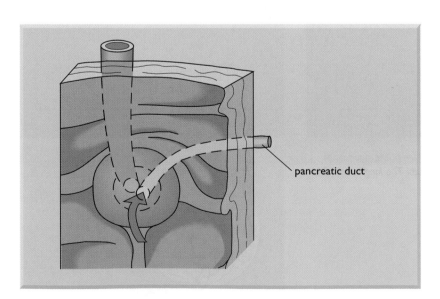

Figure 9.6 *Front view of papilla of Vater. The most successful direction of approach to the pancreatic duct is to the right and horizontal.*

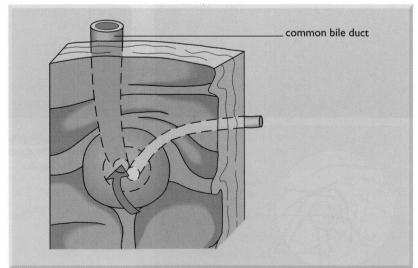

Figure 9.7 *Front view of papilla of Vater. The direction for cannulation of the common bile duct is up and to the left of the papilla. Bowing of the cannula may permit a cephalad orientation.*

THE ABNORMAL PAPILLA

After one has become familiar with the characteristics of the normal papilla, it is possible to appreciate abnormalities. If findings are ambiguous, biopsy and cytology may be helpful to exclude a neoplasm (carcinoma or adenoma). If the biopsy and cytology results are normal, it is prudent to re-examine the patient, and in some instances an ERS incision of the papilla is performed to permit biopsy of deeper tissues. Endoscopy can be repeated after a few weeks or months. If the papilla appears definitely abnormal, further evaluation for a periampullary carcinoma should proceed, even if biopsy and cytology results are negative. Endoscopic ultrasonography may prove useful in the examination of the ampullary region for detection of a tumor, a stone, dilated ducts or an adjacent mass.

Papilla with impacted stone

A bile duct stone impacted in the papilla may cause inflammation, with erythema of the overlying mucosa. A necrotic area may subsequently develop in the mucosa (Fig. 9.9). The papilla may bulge prominently and protrude into the lumen of the duodenum (Fig. 9.10). This bulge represents the intramural common bile duct, greatly distended as a result of obstruction. The opening of the papilla is found at the caudad margin of this bulge. Often, a small amount of exudate is present on, or exudes from, the papillary opening.

Acute infection of the biliary system (cholangitis) is an indication for immediate ERCP and treatment with ERS. In most patients, stones pass spontaneously after incisions of the papilla, resulting in immediate relief of obstruction and infection. In severe cholangitis, pus may drip from the papilla (Fig. 9.11).

Adenoma of the Papilla

Genetic predisposition to intestinal neoplasia is an increasingly important issue in gastroenterology. The clinical implications of the inherited polyposis syndromes are just now becoming apparent. An example is the association of duodenal and periampullary adenoma and carcinoma with familial polyposis coli. A characteristic 'lava flow' appearance has been described for the abnormal papilla in familial polyposis coli; often this appearance suggests an adenomatous change of the papilla, a possible forerunner of carcinoma (Fig. 9.12). The association of papillary problems and familial polyposis coli may be sufficiently strong to warrant periodic screening of the duodenum and papilla with a side-viewing endoscope.

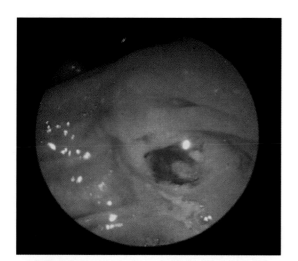

Figure 9.8 Normal papilla showing minor trauma caused by ERCP.

▼ A
▼ B

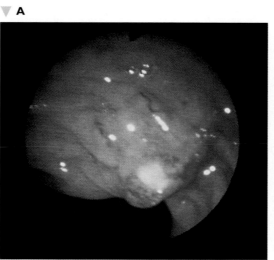

Figure 9.9 (*A and B*) The white necrotic area on the tip of the papilla resulted from an impacted stone in the common bile duct.

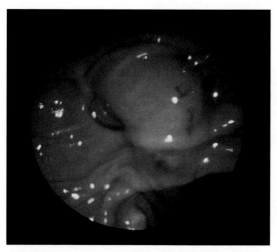

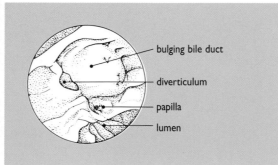

bulging bile duct
diverticulum
papilla
lumen

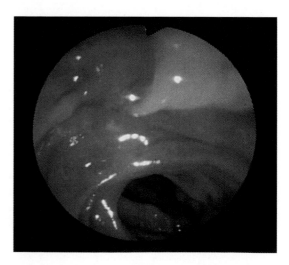

Figure 9.10 An impacted stone in the common bile duct causes the intramural portion of the duct to bulge. The papillary opening is at the tip of the bulge. A small perivaterian diverticulum is also seen.

Figure 9.11 In this case of severe cholangitis caused by an obstructing stone, pus can be seen exuding from the papilla.

Papilla affected by mucus-secreting pancreatic tumor

In patients with mucus-secreting pancreatic tumor, the papilla may be covered with mucus originating from a mucus-secreting pancreatic tumor (Fig. 9.13).

Suprapapillary Fistula

A fistulous opening may be noted between the common bile duct and the duodenum. This may result from complications of common bile duct stones or from injuries that occurred during biliary surgery (Fig. 9.14).

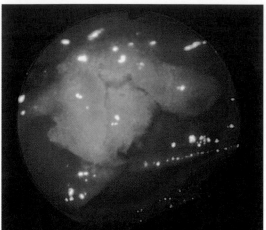
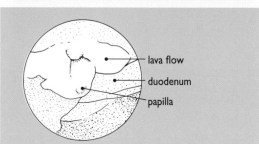

Figure 9.12 *This abnormal papilla shows the characteristic 'lava flow' appearance of an adenoma associated with FPC. The mucosa over the papilla appears pale and seems to spill over the papilla and adjacent tissue.*

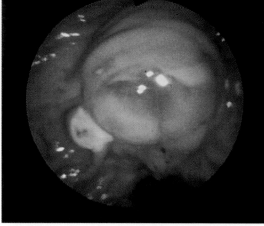
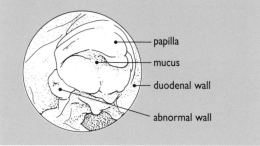

Figure 9.13 *Mucus is seen covering an enlarged papilla in this patient with mucus-secreting pancreatic carcinoma. As mucus is not normally seen over the surface of the papilla, this should always suggest disease. The abnormal white area immediately adjacent to the papilla should be biopsied and brushed for cytology.*

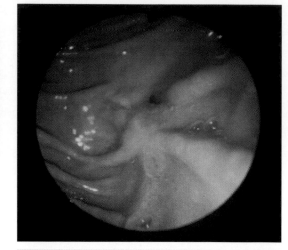
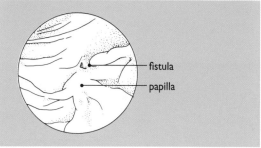

Figure 9.14 *A suprapapillary choledoduodenal fistula is seen just cephalad to the papilla. Bile exits from the fistula.*

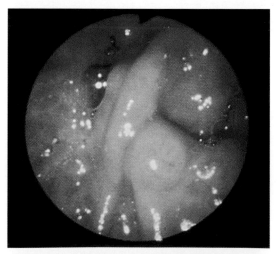
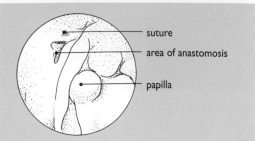

Figure 9.15 *A silk suture from a previous choledochoduodenostomy is seen. The orifice of the anastomosis is not well seen.*

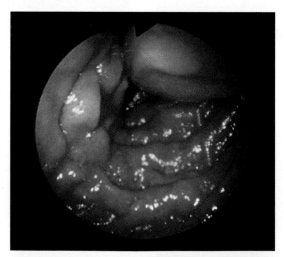
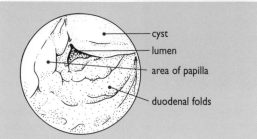

Figure 9.16 *Large duodenal cyst located in the periampullary area. The papilla itself is not well seen.*

Papilla after surgery

Postoperative changes occasionally may be seen. In Figure 9.15, a suture is apparent cephalad to the papilla, in the area of the remnant of a surgical choledochoduodenostomy performed several years earlier.

Periampullary duodenal cyst

A cyst involving the duodenal wall may distort the duodenal anatomy (Fig. 9.16).

Balloon dilation of the papilla

A saucer-shaped balloon catheter can be passed into a strictured papilla to dilate the orifice. This technique may be used in patients with stenosis after having undergone biliary surgical sphincterectomy (Fig. 9.17).

ERS

Precise, specific diagnoses of diseases of the hepatobiliary or pancreatic ducts are possible using ERCP. Another important aspect of this new technology is the ability to treat the patient endoscopically at the time of ERCP. This procedure is referred to as endoscopic retrograde sphincterotomy (ERS).

ERS has made endoscopic biliary surgery possible. Impacted bile duct stones can be pulled out using a balloon catheter or grasped with a basket. Ultrasound probes and lasers of varying frequency can be used in the duct to shatter the stones. Wire baskets can be used to crush stones mechanically. Currently, mechanical lithotripsy is used more often to fragment large stones, and then to grasp and extract the fragments. A temporary nasobiliary drain can be passed to relieve benign or malignant strictures, or permanent biliary stents can be placed.

TECHNIQUE OF ERS

ERS relies on both endoscopic and radiographic techniques. Fluoroscopy is essential to evaluate the state of the ducts, to ascertain the extent of disease, to monitor the position of the catheters during ERS and for placement of drains and stents. Endoscopy is essential to locate and cannulate the papilla, to perform ERS, and to direct the insertion of the various catheters and drains.

The first step in ERS is to locate the papilla. The endoscope must be positioned to visualize the papilla *en face*. Next, the papilla is cannulated as in a routine ERCP. Contrast is injected and the diagnosis established. A guidewire can be placed through this catheter to assist in placement of a papillotome if needed.

After ERS has been selected as the appropriate therapeutic procedure, the diagnostic catheter is replaced with a papillotome. A papillotome is a catheter with an exposed wire at the tip. Under fluoroscopic control, the papillotome must be deeply inserted into the papilla and up the common bile duct. If this is not possible, an initial small incision of the papilla may be necessary to allow passage of the papillotome. This is called a precut procedure (Fig. 9.18). The precut is just long enough to permit the papillotome to be passed

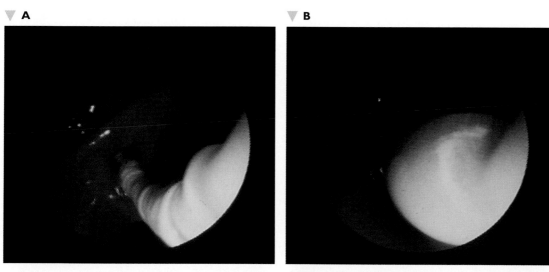

Figure 9.17 Stricture of the papilla after surgical sphincterotomy. (**A**) A saucer-shaped balloon catheter is introduced into the papilla. (**B**) On direct vision, the balloon is inflated to dilate the stricture.

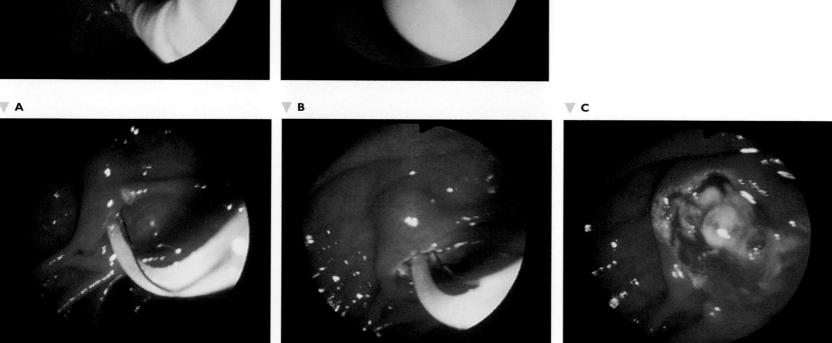

Figure 9.18 Precut procedure. (**A**) A modified papillotome is inserted into the papillary orifice to make a small incision. (**B**) The small incision allows deep insertion of the regular papillotome. (**C**) ERS has been completed.

into position for the full ERS. Some endoscopists separate the precut from the definitive ERS by days, whereas others perform the ERS immediately after the precut.

An alternative to a precut is to use a papillotomy knife. The instrument may be used in a manner similar to the precut papillotome to incise the papilla so that a regular papillotome can be passed (Fig. 9.19).

The technique of ERS is demonstrated sequentially in Figure 9.20. After locating the papilla and cannulating it, a papillotome is passed into the common duct. When the position of the papillotome in the bile duct has been confirmed using fluoroscopy, the wire is pulled taut and the tip bowed. The location of the wire relative to the papilla is critical. Endoscopically, the wire appears in the upper left quadrant between the positions of 9 o'clock and 12 o'clock, corresponding to the location of the intramural portion of the common bile duct. In any other position the wire may cut laterally, away from the roof of the papilla, causing a perforation or injuring the pancreas. Only the intramural portion of the distal common bile duct can be safely incised during ERS. A diathermic current is then passed down the papillotome. A ground plate in broad contact with the patient completes the electrical circuit. A cutting current, occasionally mixed with coagulation current, is used to make the incision of the sphincteric fibers surrounding the distal bile duct.

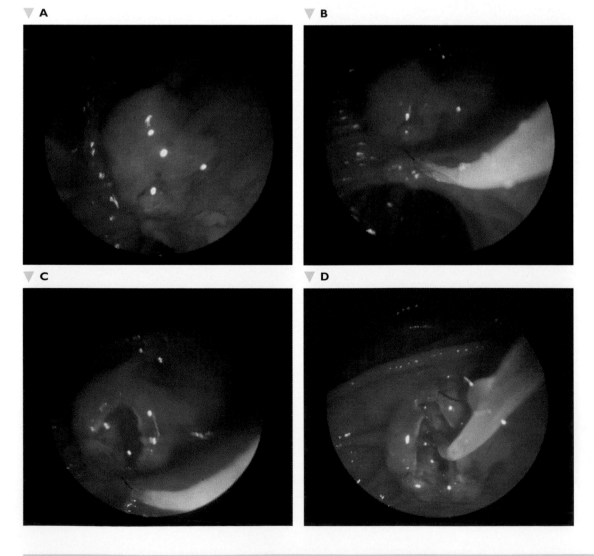

Figure 9.19 *Papillotomy knife sequence.* **(A)** *It was not possible to insert the papillotome into the papilla of Vater.* **(B)** *A papillotomy knife is used to incise the papilla.* **(C)** *A small incision is made.* **(D)** *The regular papillotome was then inserted and full papillotomy incision completed. The wire can be seen at the cephalad border of the incision.*

Under endoscopic guidance, a partial cut is made, followed in a stepwise fashion by a complete cut, 1.0–1.5 cm long. A balloon catheter can now be passed up the duct, inflated, and withdrawn to calibrate the size of the papillotomy. If a common bile duct stone does not pass spontaneously into the duodenum, a balloon catheter can be passed above the stone, the balloon inflated, and the catheter withdrawn, pulling the stone out of the papilla.

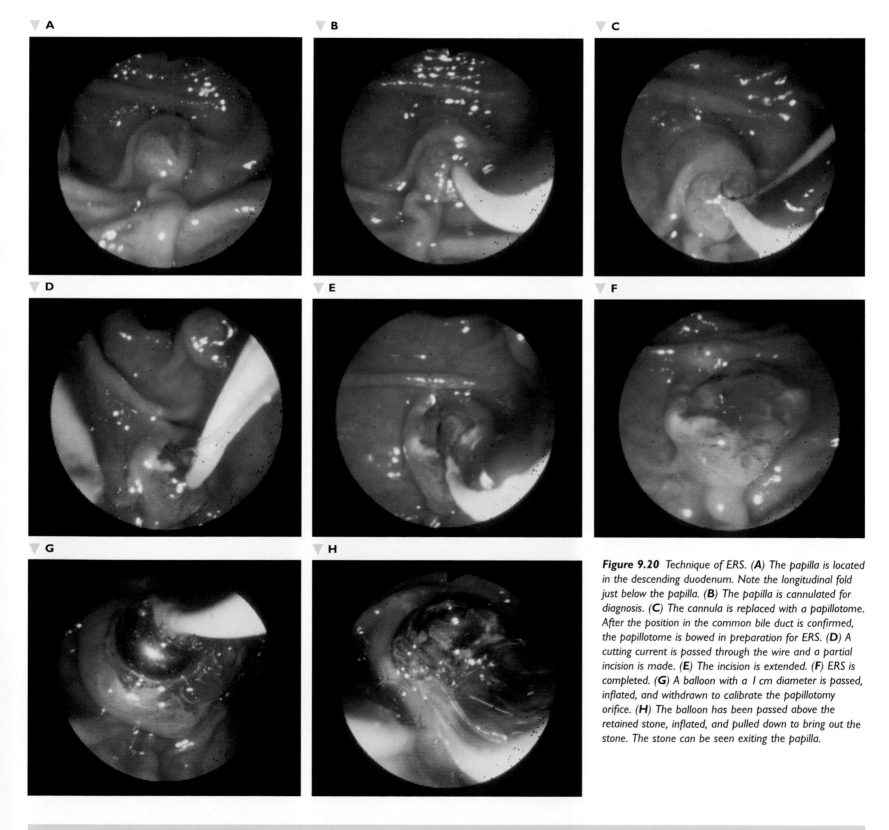

Figure 9.20 Technique of ERS. (**A**) The papilla is located in the descending duodenum. Note the longitudinal fold just below the papilla. (**B**) The papilla is cannulated for diagnosis. (**C**) The cannula is replaced with a papillotome. After the position in the common bile duct is confirmed, the papillotome is bowed in preparation for ERS. (**D**) A cutting current is passed through the wire and a partial incision is made. (**E**) The incision is extended. (**F**) ERS is completed. (**G**) A balloon with a 1 cm diameter is passed, inflated, and withdrawn to calibrate the papillotomy orifice. (**H**) The balloon has been passed above the retained stone, inflated, and pulled down to bring out the stone. The stone can be seen exiting the papilla.

The endoscopic appearance of the papilla after ERS varies with time. Acutely, there is whitening of the mucosa surrounding the incision, edema (Fig. 9.21), and occasionally a small amount of bleeding. After 1 week, the periampullary tissue is less edematous, and the white coagulated appearance is replaced by a lacy, erythematous-appearing mucosa (Fig. 9.22). The opening of the common bile duct may be seen, which is unusual in the normal, nonincised

▼ **A**

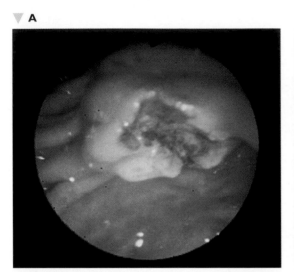

▼ **B**

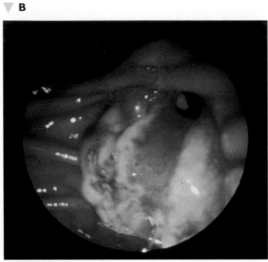

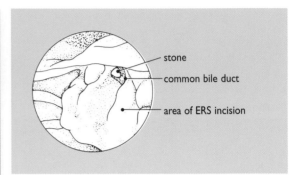

Figure 9.21 (**A**) Immediately after ERS, the incised tissue is edematous. (**B**) With a slightly different position of endoscope it is possible to see into the distal common duct and observe a retained stone.

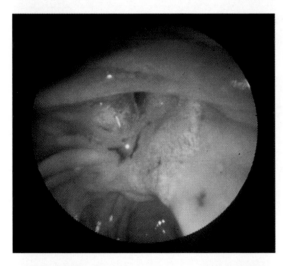

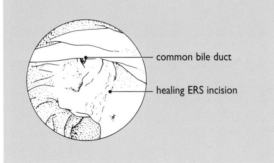

Figure 9.22 The papilla 1 week after ERS, with less edema and whitening of the mucosa. Instead, a lacy erythematous appearance is noted. The common bile duct opening is also visible.

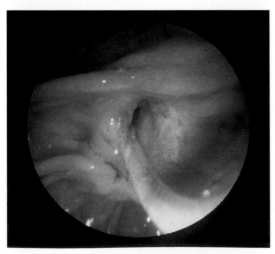

Figure 9.23 Papilla 1 week after ERS. Cannula is easily placed into the papilla.

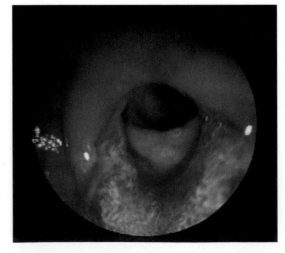

Figure 9.24 Six months after ERS, the papilla is still open and one can see into the common bile duct. There is no evidence of stenosis and no residual evidence of inflammation.

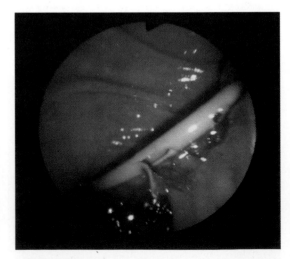

Figure 9.25 A biliary prosthesis from the common bile duct into the duodenum. The side flaps reduce the chance of migration.

papilla (Fig. 9.23). At 6 months, the papilla is usually less inflamed and is permanently open. It may be possible to look directly into the distal common bile duct (Fig. 9.24).

APPLICATION OF STENTS AND DRAINS

An exciting aspect of ERS is the ability to drain obstructions of the biliary ducts. In the past, patients with unresectable tumors had surgery simply for palliation. With ERS, a palliative bypass can be accomplished without invasive surgery.

First, a diagnostic ERCP is performed to determine the radiographic diagnosis, the location of the blockage, and the degree of stenosis. The extent of duodenal wall invasion must be noted. Obvious tumor masses are biopsied or brushed for cytology.

If a stent is to be passed, this can be accomplished with or without ERS. The latter eases the passage of stents and drains but is not necessary in all cases. ERCP and ERS may be performed with a standard side-viewing endoscope. After papillotomy, the smaller endoscope is removed and a side-viewing scope with a large channel is passed into the duodenum. A Teflon catheter, usually containing a guidewire, is then passed into the papilla and up the bile duct. If the catheter will not pass the obstruction, the spring-tipped guidewire is advanced from the catheter to see whether it will

pass. If the guidewire passes, the catheter is then advanced over the wire above the narrowed area. The advancement of the catheter and wire is monitored fluoroscopically.

A pusher tube then pushes the stent down the endoscope channel over the catheter. The stent is advanced into the bile duct and positioned with fluoroscopic guidance until the proximal tip is above the stricture. The catheter and wire are then removed, followed by the pusher tube, leaving the distal end of the stent free in the duodenum, protruding 1–2 cm from the papillary orifice. If the catheter and wire cannot be passed through the stricture, dilating catheters or balloon-tipped catheters may be used to enlarge it so that the catheter and wire can be passed above the stricture to guide the stent.

If a nasobiliary drain is selected to drain the duct temporarily, the tip of the drain is placed above the narrowed area. The proximal end of the drain is brought out through the mouth and then repositioned to exit from the nose.

Drains and stents are kept in place by having either a pigtail curvature on the end or a series of small spur-like protuberances on either end. These features help to anchor the stent and reduce the chance of migration (Fig. 9.25). Figure 9.26 demonstrates ERS for a malignant obstruction, with the passage of a prosthesis or stent for drainage. In complicated cases, which often involve malignant duct obstruction, multiple stents and drains may be necessary (Fig. 9.27).

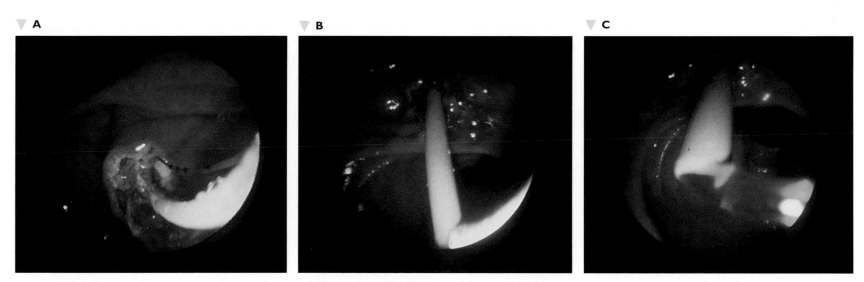

Figure 9.26 (A) ERS in a patient with malignant jaundice caused by an unresectable lesion in the bile duct. (B) A biliary prosthesis and pusher tube are inserted over a guidewire, which cannot be seen here. (C) After removal of the guidewire and pusher tube, bile exits from the drain.

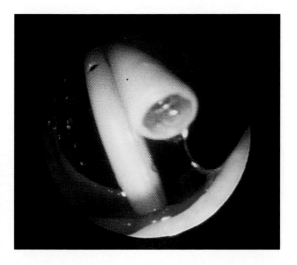

Figure 9.27 In this case two drains are seen exiting from the papilla. Multiple drains are used if the obstruction cannot be bypassed with a single drain, for example, if a tumor obstructs both the left and right main intrahepatic ducts.

Occasionally, drains become plugged with debris (Fig. 9.28). Figure 9.29 shows a clogged biliary stent, its endoscopic removal, and the endoscopic passage of a new stent. The limiting factor in the diameter of the stent or drain placed endoscopically is the diameter of the biopsy channel of the endoscope. Endoscopes with large 3.8 mm and 4.2 mm channels are available.

Recently, to delay clogging of the plastic stents, self-expanding metal stents have also been used in the common bile duct to bypass an area of obstruction. Several types of self-expanding stents are available; because the diameter of the stent in the constraining membrane is small, such stents are often correctly positioned in the bile duct without much difficulty.

ERCP AND ERS IN PERIVATERIAN DIVERTICULA

Of those patients undergoing ERCP, 10–15% have diverticula of the duodenum in the periampullary region. The diverticulum is most often seen as an opening adjacent to the papilla, although sometimes there may be a diverticulum on both sides of the papilla (Fig. 9.30). The papilla is located, characteristically, on the rim of diverticulum, often in the 4 o'clock position. Normally, the papilla in this position cannulates easily (Fig. 9.31). If the papilla is located inside the diverticulum (Fig. 9.32), it may be impossible

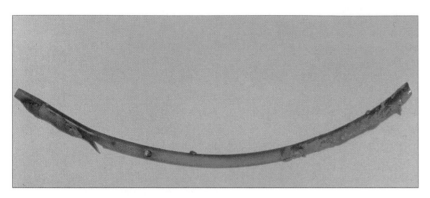

Figure 9.28 Clogged biliary endoprosthesis.

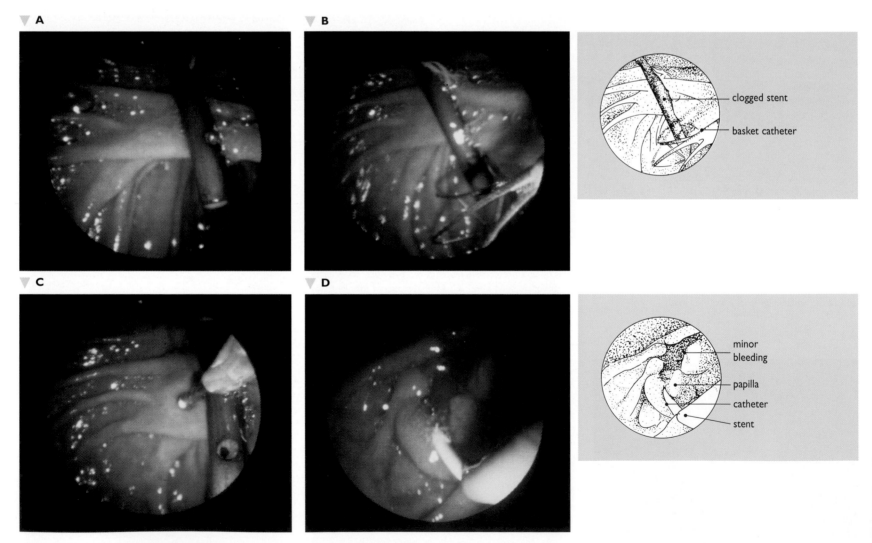

Figure 9.29 Clearing a clogged stent. (**A**) A biliary stent exiting from the papilla. The stent is clogged and has ceased to function. (**B**) A basket catheter has been passed and opened to grasp the end of the stent. (**C**) The basket has been tightened on the stent. The drainage hole in the stent is clogged with debris. (**D**) After removing the clogged stent, a guidewire and catheter are placed into the common bile duct and a new stent is about to be inserted into the duct.

Figure 9.30 *A papilla with a diverticulum on either side.*

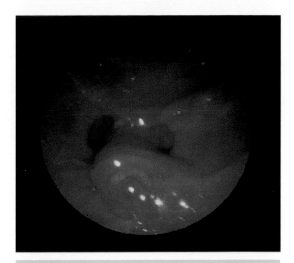

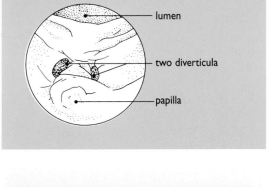

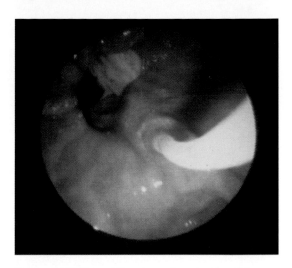

Figure 9.31 *The papilla is located on the rim of the perivaterian diverticulum. Note the debris in the diverticulum. The papilla is easily cannulated.*

Figure 9.32 *The papilla located inside a duodenal diverticulum.*

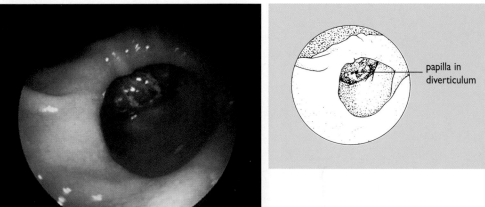

▼ **A**

▼ **B**

Figure 9.33 *(A) Here, the papilla is located inside a diverticulum. (B) With manipulation and suction via the endoscope channel, the papilla is everted out of the diverticulum.*

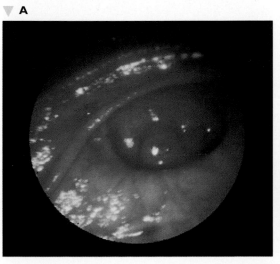

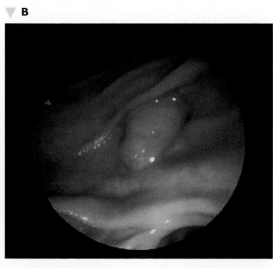

to cannulate; however, in some instances the papilla can be everted out of the diverticulum with gentle suction (Fig. 9.33) or gentle manipulation with a catheter, and then cannulated. In most instances the papilla can be cannulated directly in the diverticulum (Fig. 9.34).

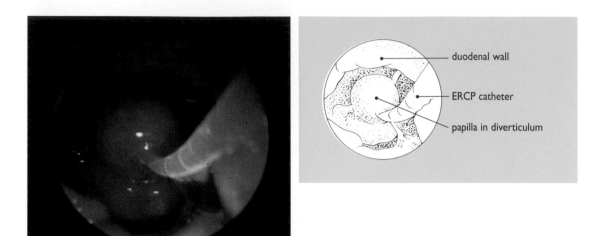

Figure 9.34 *The papilla is being cannulated inside a duodenal diverticulum.*

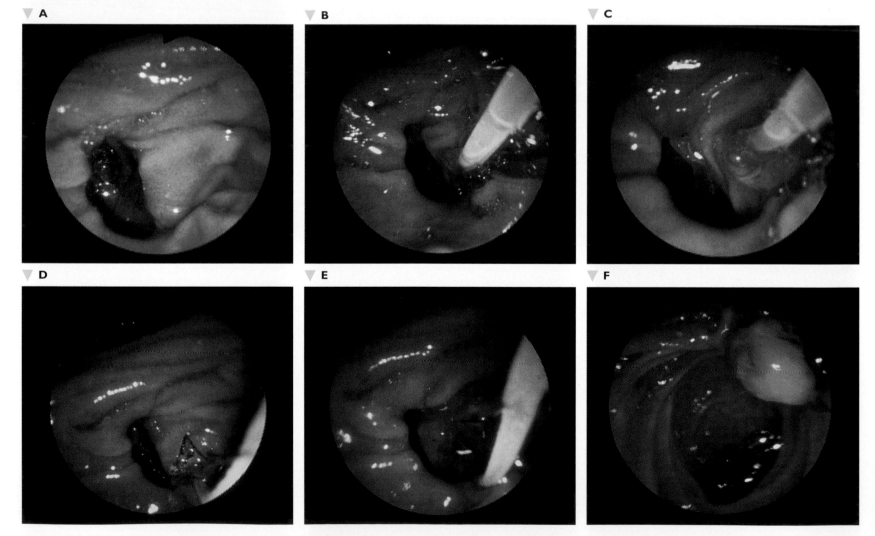

Figure 9.35 *ERS in perivaterian diverticula. (A) A perivaterian diverticulum in the descending duodenum. The papilla is inside the diverticulum and cannot be seen. (B) With gentle manipulation using an ERCP catheter, the papilla is everted out of the diverticulum. (C) The papilla is then cannulated. (D) and (E) ERS is performed. (F) The stone freed by ERS is seen in the duodenum.*

Initially, endoscopists were reluctant to perform ERS on patients with perivaterian diverticula because of the risk of perforating the diverticulum or the duodenal wall. However, it is now well accepted that ERS can be performed safely in these cases (Fig. 9.35). It is also possible to place drainage tubes to bypass bile duct obstruction in patients with diverticula (Fig. 9.36).

Anatomically, the common bile duct and pancreatic ducts pass through the duodenal wall at the level of the papilla of Vater, a site referred to as the duodenal window. This window may create a weak spot through which the duodenal mucosa can bulge and form a diverticulum. The same explanation may account for the association of colonic diverticula and penetrating blood vessels.

ERCP AND ERS IN PERIAMPULLARY CARCINOMA

Periampullary carcinoma usually has an appearance distinct from that of the normal papilla. The papilla may appear enlarged, irregular, multilobed, discolored (that is, not a fine, erythematous, lacy color, but rather white or yellowish), friable, and in some cases necrotic (Figs. 9.37–9.39). Periampullary carcinoid tumors may be seen as masses, occasionally with an ulcer at the tip (Fig. 9.40). A pancreatic carcinoma may be seen invading the duodenal mucosa and the papilla (Figs. 9.41 and 9.42).

If a periampullary carcinoma is encountered, the endoscopist should obtain a sheathed brush cytology specimen and several directed biopsies. A

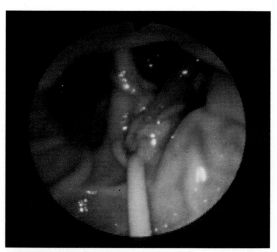

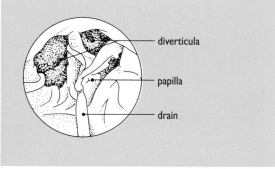

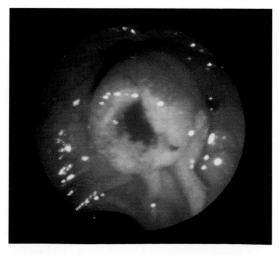

Figure 9.36 A nasobiliary drain has been placed into the papilla for drainage above a biliary obstruction. Diverticula are seen on either side of the papilla.

diverticula

papilla

drain

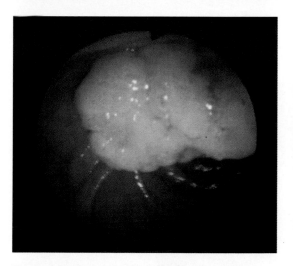

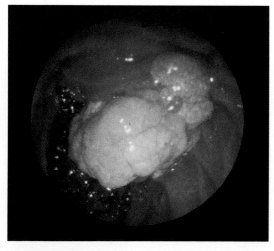

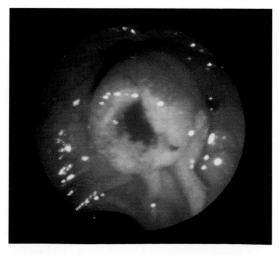

Figure 9.37 Periampullary carcinoma, seen as a large, pale mass in the area of the papilla. The surface is multilobed, slightly yellow, and irregular.

Figure 9.38 Multilobed periampullary carcinoma. Tumor appears to extend above and to the right of the papilla.

Figure 9.39 Periampullary cancer involving the papilla. The center is hemorrhagic and friable.

▼ **A**

▼ **B**

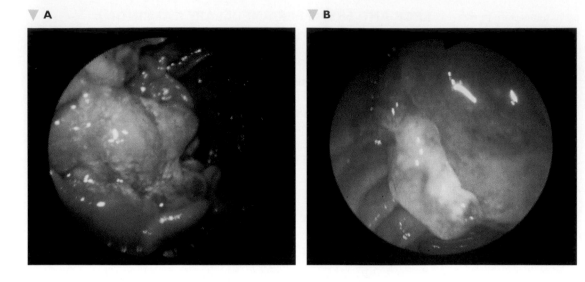

Figure 9.40 (**A**) and (**B**) Periampullary carcinoid tumors present as masses, sometimes with ulcerations (**B**).

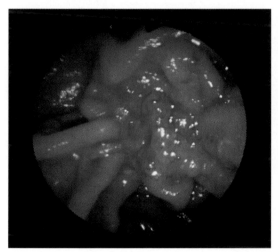

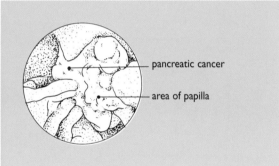

Figure 9.41 A pancreatic carcinoma has invaded the duodenal wall just above the papilla. The folds are irregular and nodular.

Figure 9.42 Infiltration of papilla by acinar-cell cancer of the pancreas.

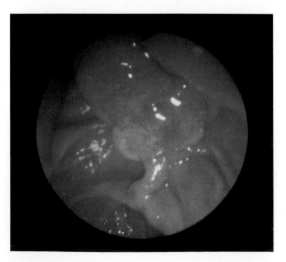

Figure 9.43 Periampullary carcinoma with an area of minimal bleeding in the center, cannulated for ERCP.

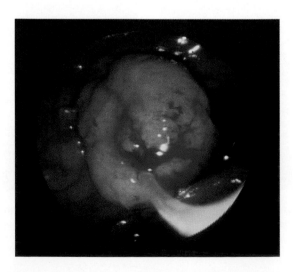

decision must be made concerning further diagnostic procedures to be performed during that session. In many instances, it is appropriate to cannulate the carcinomatous papilla to make a diagnosis and determine the extent of the obstruction by the tumor (Fig. 9.43). Endoscopic ultrasound may be useful to delineate the depth of infiltration and the presence of enlarged lymph nodes.

ERS may be performed in periampullary carcinoma for two reasons: first, to obtain a specimen of the deeper tissue of the papilla for histologic diagnosis; and second, to pass drainage tubes and stents for temporary (if surgery is planned) or permanent (if the problem is considered inoperable) relief of obstruction (Figs. 9.44 and 9.45).

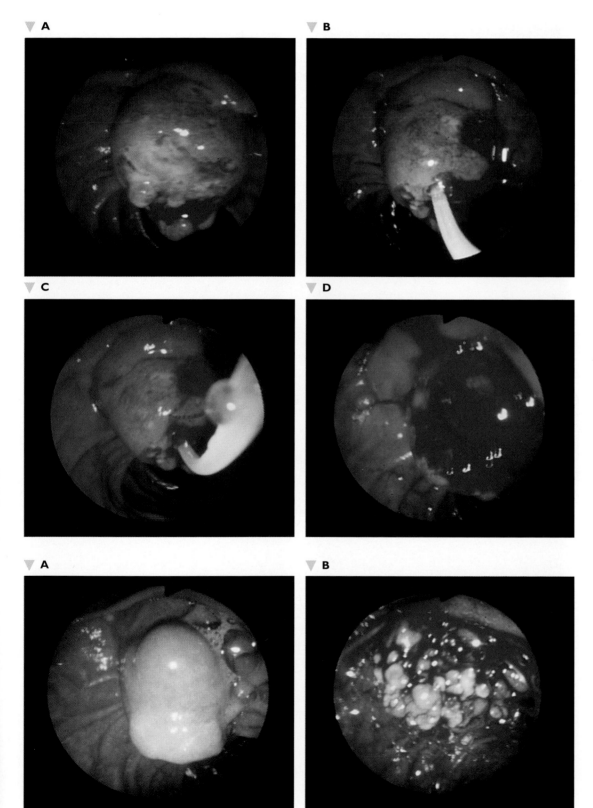

Figure 9.44 *ERS in periampullary carcinoma. (**A**) The carcinoma appears as a friable, bleeding mass. (**B**) A cannula is inserted. (**C**) After ERCP, a papillotome is passed for ERS. The taut wire can be seen making an incision. (**D**) After ERS, a small amount of bleeding occurs. The open papilla allows for biopsy of the mass and/or placement of stents or drains to relieve obstruction.*

Figure 9.45 *(**A**) Carcinoma of the papilla with a mass projecting into the duodenal lumen. (**B**) After papillotomy there is a small amount of bleeding and the deeper tissue of the mass is exposed, facilitating biopsy and drainage.*

CHOLEDOCHOSCOPY

In rare circumstances, a small-caliber end-viewing endoscope may be passed into the common bile duct, either through the papilla or through a chole-dochoduodenal anastomosis. One may then visualize the common bile duct, common hepatic duct, and even the bifurcation of the major right and left intrahepatic ducts (Fig. 9.46). This technique may occasionally allow visualization of ductal stones and other pathology such as villous adenoma or carcinoma.

HEMOBILIA
Bleeding Phase

ERCP is also of importance in the detection of hemobilia. During the acute bleeding phase, blood may be seen exuding from the papillary orifice. After bleeding has stopped, clots may occasionally be seen escaping from the papilla. Upon retrograde choledochography, clots that have a characteristic radiologic appearance may be noted in the biliary system.

RADIOLOGIC INTERPRETATION

ERCP requires expert interpretation of x-rays. This is often accomplished best by having the endoscopist work closely with a gastrointestinal radiologist. In this section, we present a series of x-rays showing neoplastic and non-neoplastic diseases of the biliary tree and pancreatic ducts. Images taken during endoscopic biliary therapeutic procedures are also included (Figs. 9.47–9.66). (All x-rays courtesy of Dr Charles Rohrmann.)

ENDOSONOGRAPHY OF THE PANCREAS AND BILIARY DUCTS

One of the original goals of endosonography was to obtain images of the pancreas, but it is now often used to study normal and abnormal pancreatic structures (Figs. 9.67–9.71). Endosonography is also used to examine the

▼ **A**

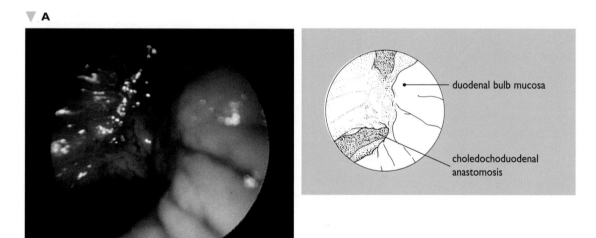

▼ **B**   ▼ **C**

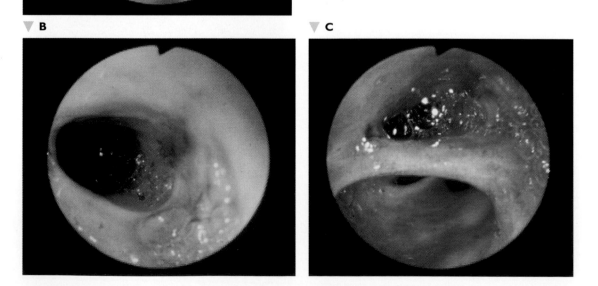

Figure 9.46 *Choledochoscopy.*
*(**A**) A choledochoduodenal anastomosis is seen in the duodenal bulb. (**B**) The common bile duct. (**C**) Bifurcation of the common hepatic duct.*

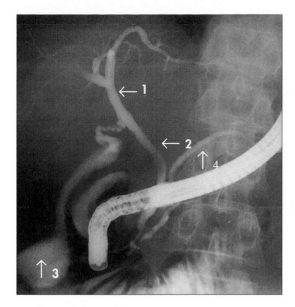

Figure 9.47 *Normal ERCP with diagnostic cannula in common bile duct. Intrahepatic ducts, common hepatic duct (1), common bile duct (2), gall bladder (3) and pancreatic duct (4) are visible.*

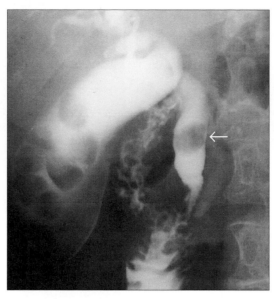

Figure 9.48 *Cholelithiasis with multiple gallstones and a single common bile duct stone (arrow).*

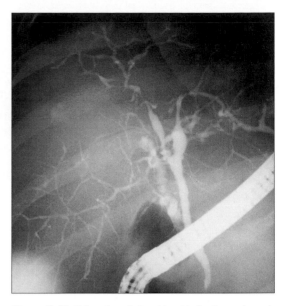

Figure 9.49 *Sclerosing cholangitis with focal ectasia and stenosis of intrahepatic ducts. Area of right hepatic lobe where bile ducts are obliterated is visible in upper left of the x-ray.*

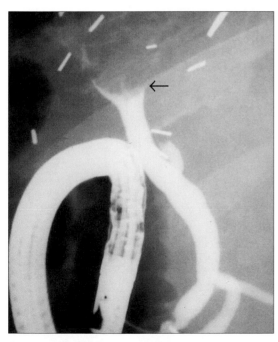

Figure 9.50 *Near total obstruction of common hepatic duct by intraductal colon carcinoma metastasis. Note expansion of duct by growing tumor (arrow), differentiating this lesion from an occluding stone, which does not cause duct enlargement.*

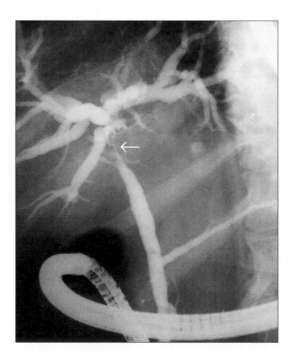

Figure 9.51 *Tight stenosis of common hepatic duct caused by a cholangiocarcinoma at the bifurcation (arrow). The intrahepatic ducts are dilated.*

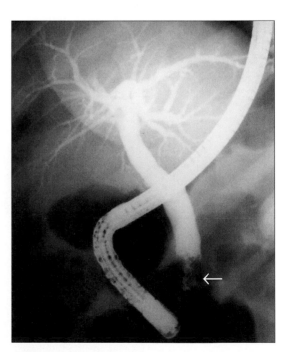

Figure 9.52 *Periampullary carcinoma invading bile duct (arrow). Note destruction of mucosal lining. The extrahepatic ducts are moderately dilated.*

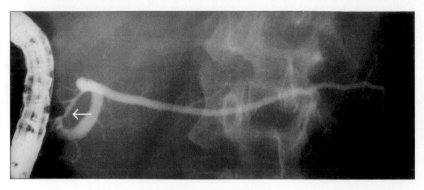

Figure 9.53 *Normal pancreatic duct. The accessory duct of Santorini (arrow) connects the main duct to the accessory papilla.*

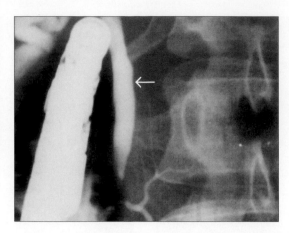

Figure 9.54 *Ventral pancreas with normal thin branching ducts. There is partial filling of the normal common bile duct (arrow).*

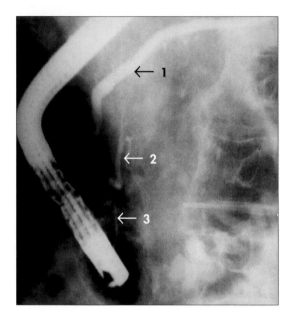

Figure 9.55 *Pancreas divisum with visualization of dorsal (1), and ventral (2) duct system. Each duct was opacified through injection of a separate papilla. The cannula (3) is inserted into the major papilla, which filled the ventral duct system.*

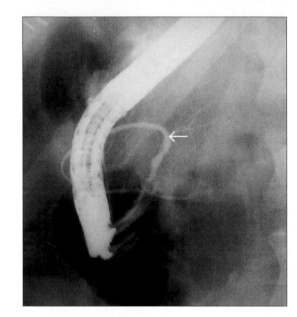

Figure 9.56 *Annular pancreas. Opacification through the major papilla shows annular duct (arrow) encircling the descending duodenum. Note annular pancreas tissue narrowing the descending duodenum.*

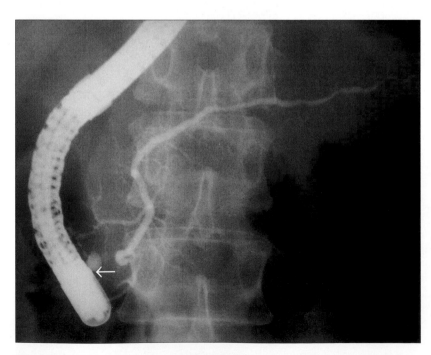

Figure 9.57 *Mild and focal pancreatitis manifested by focal caliber irregularities of the main duct; note ectasia of branches. There is a small pseudocyst in the head of the pancreas (arrow).*

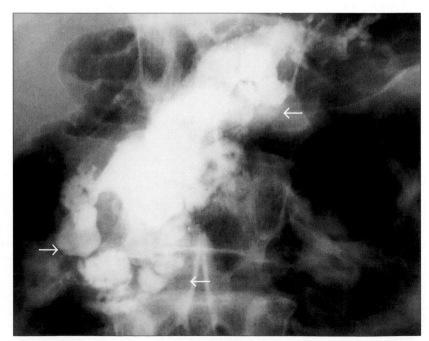

Figure 9.58 *Severe pancreatitis with cystic replacement of the pancreatic duct system. Note marked ectasia of branch ducts (arrows). This condition is also referred to as a pancreatic sac.*

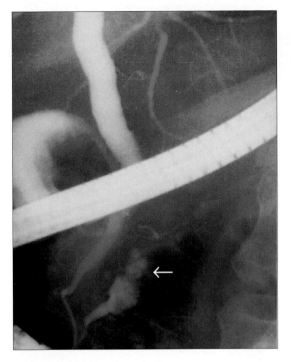

Figure 9.59 *Chronic calcific pancreatitis with obstruction of pancreatic duct by calculus (arrow). The common bile duct is normal.*

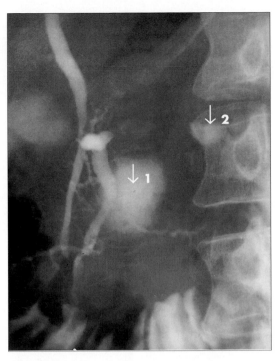

Figure 9.60 *Chronic pancreatitis with pseudocyst formation (1). The pancreatic duct is nearly occluded at the site of the pseudocyst with minimal contrast proximally (2).*

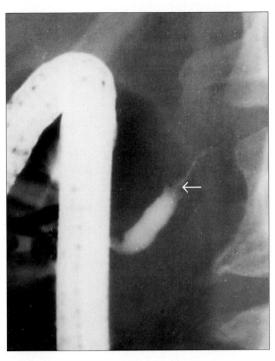

Figure 9.61 *Pancreatic cancer producing an irregular, abrupt tapering with obstruction of the main pancreatic duct (arrow).*

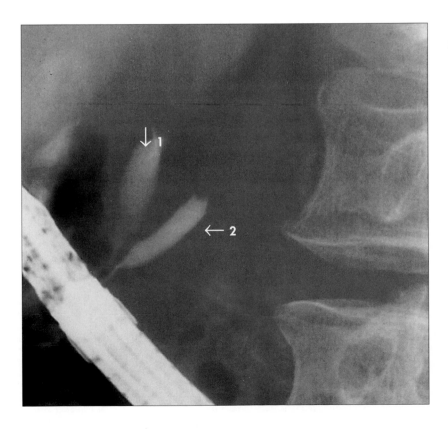

Figure 9.62 *Carcinoma of the pancreas obstructing the common bile duct (1) and pancreatic duct (2). This has been designated as the double duct sign but is not specific for neoplasia and can also be seen in inflammatory processes.*

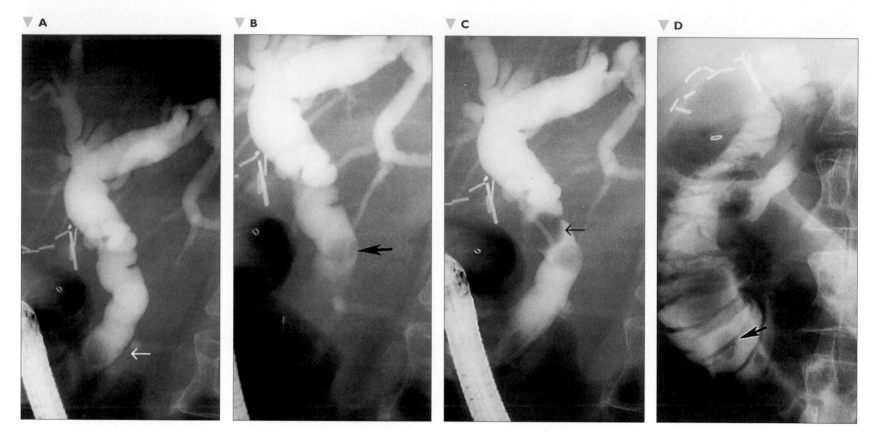

Figure 9.63 **(A)** Single common bile duct calculus (arrow) in a patient after cholecystectomy. **(B)** Papillotome appropriately positioned. Calculus has migrated proximally (arrow). **(C)** A balloon catheter is placed and inflated (arrow) after papillotomy and is used to extract the calculus. **(D)** After extraction the free calculus is seen in the descending duodenum (arrow).

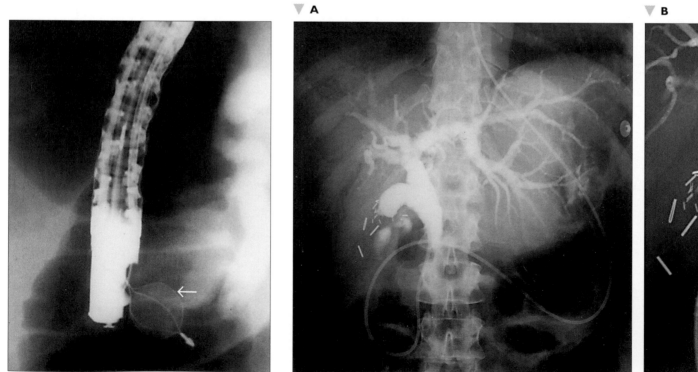

Figure 9.64 Extraction of common bile duct calculus by basket catheter after papillotomy. The calculus and basket (arrow) are in the descending duodenum.

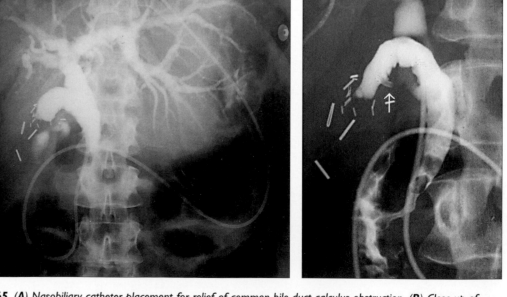

Figure 9.65 **(A)** Nasobiliary catheter placement for relief of common bile duct calculus obstruction. **(B)** Close-up of common bile duct shows position of catheter terminating in cystic duct (arrow) and calculi in the common bile duct.

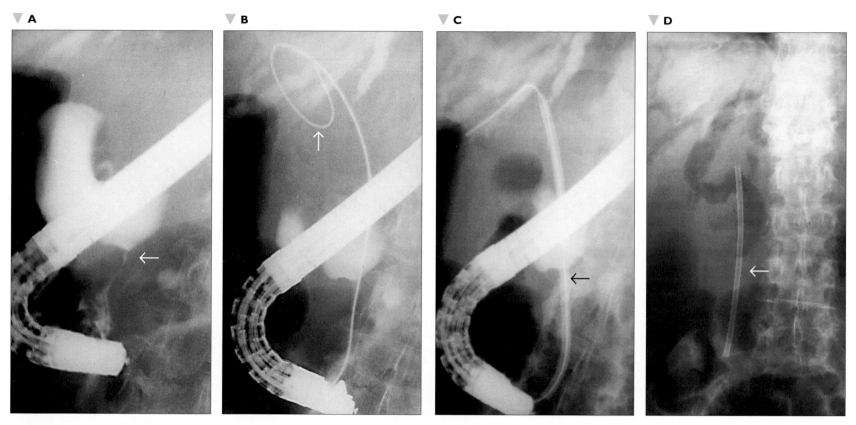

Figure 9.66 (A) Pancreatic cancer producing abrupt narrowing of common bile duct (arrow) typical of neoplastic obstruction. (B) After endoscopic papillotomy, a catheter and guidewire have been placed through the obstruction. The tip of the guidewire loops into the dilated common hepatic duct (arrow). (C) A straight stent has been passed through the obstruction (arrow). (D) Abdominal radiograph after stent placement shows appropriate positioning of stent through the narrowed segment of the common bile duct (arrow). Note air in bile ducts, a normal finding after stent placement.

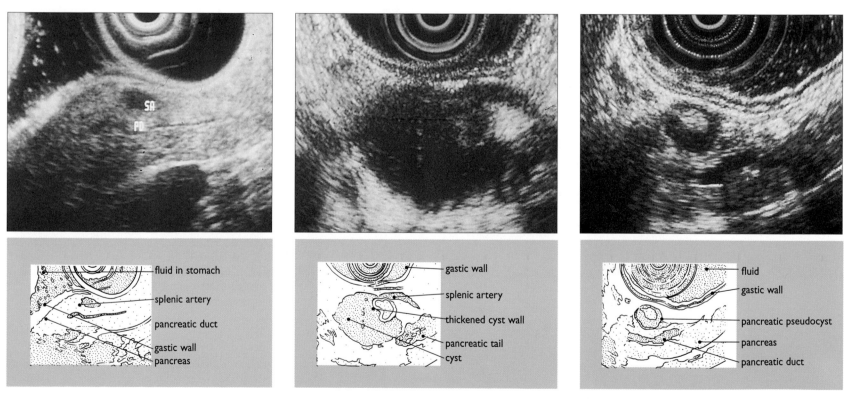

Figure 9.67 Normal pancreas seen through gastric wall. The pancreas has a homogeneous echo pattern and smooth contours. The pancreatic duct is seen and is of normal caliber. (Courtesy of Dr TL Tio)

Figure 9.68 Pseudocyst of the pancreas. The cyst is a hypoechoic inhomogeneous cavity with some evidence of wall thickening. Note calcifications in pancreatic parenchyma. (Courtesy of Dr TL Tio)

Figure 9.69 Small pancreatic pseudocyst (15 mm) with some evidence of wall thickening. The pancreatic duct is slightly dilated. The pancreatic parenchyma has an inhomogeneous pattern with irregularity of the contour. (Courtesy of Dr TL Tio)

biliary ducts (Figs. 9.72 and 9.73), and is proving very effective for delin-eating biliary anatomy, the etiology of dilated ducts and the extent of tumors involving the ducts. Involvement of vascular structures can be determined. As endoscopic biliary and pancreatic therapy continues to develop and improve, the anatomic information provided by endosonography will be invaluable for assisting the physician in selecting appropriate therapy for the patient.

CONCLUSION

Overall, ERCP, ERS, and related therapeutic endoscopic procedures (such as drain and stent placement) are among the most important advances in endo-scopic diagnosis and treatment. These techniques are likely to be the forerunners of other types of endoscopic therapy that will significantly improve the management of difficult medical problems.

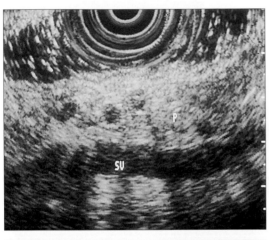

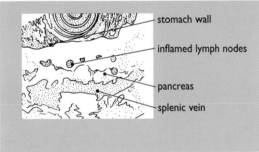

Figure 9.70 *Pancreatitis. The pancreatic parenchyma has an inhomogeneous echo pattern with some irregularity of the contour. The pancreas has a pseudolobule architecture pattern. (Courtesy of Dr TL Tio)*

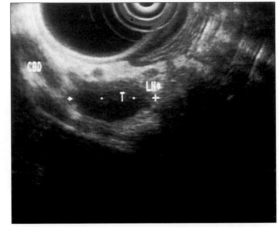

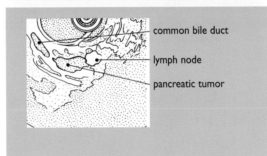

Figure 9.71 *Cancer of the head of the pancreas. The tumor (staged as T_2N_1) is seen adjacent to the common bile duct. An adjacent lymph node is seen and appears to contain tumor metastases. (Courtesy of Dr TL Tio)*

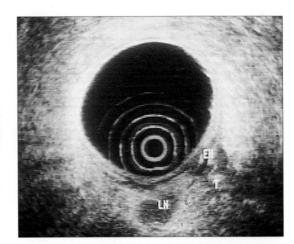

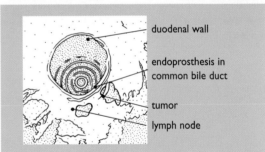

Figure 9.72 *Cholangiocarcinoma of the common bile duct. The tumor is seen surrounding an endoprosthesis in the common bile duct. The tumor is penetrating deeply into the adjacent structures, including the portal vein. This is compatible with a T_3 cholangiocarcinoma. The lymph node seen is suspicious for tumor involvement because of its hypoechoic pattern and distinct boundaries. (Courtesy of Dr TL Tio)*

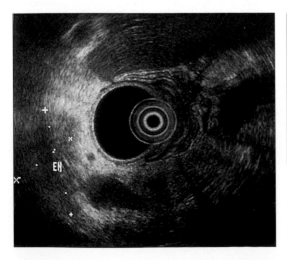

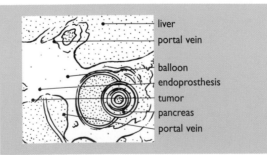

Figure 9.73 *Klatskin tumor of the proximal common bile duct. The hypoechoic tumor is adjacent to the hilum and shows some penetration into the portal vein. This is a pattern consistent with a T_3 Klatskin tumor. An endoprosthesis is in place. (Courtesy of Dr TL Tio)*

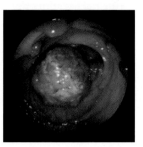

Colon I: Polyps and Tumors

In this chapter we briefly present general techniques for intubation of the colon. With colonoscopy it is possible to detect adenomatous polyps, remove the polyps, and detect colorectal cancers. Laser therapy of colorectal neoplasia is presented. A series of photographs examines Kaposi's sarcoma involving the colon and rectum in patients with AIDS. Each of these entities is discussed in detail later in the chapter.

TECHNIQUE OF COLONOSCOPY

In experienced hands, 80–90% of patients can be colonoscoped to the cecum in 20–30 minutes or less without use of fluoroscopy. Failure to intubate the entire colon is mainly due to anatomical variations such as a long redundant sigmoid colon or transverse colon, fixation of the bowel from prior surgery, or other intra-abdominal problems such as diverticulitis. Fluoroscopy is only necessary in difficult cases requiring special maneuvers (the alpha maneuver, discussed later) or if external overtubes are used to stiffen the colonoscope to reduce formation of loops in the sigmoid colon. Fluoroscopy can also be used to establish the location of the tip of the colonoscope in the cecum, but other indicators are usually adequate to determine that the cecum has been intubated.

Before colonoscopy, most patients are given conscious sedation with a narcotic (meperidine) or a sedative (often a benzodiazepine) or both. An intravenous access line may be used to administer these medications, and in the event of a vasovagal episode, to administer an anticholinergic or other medication. This route can also be used for medications to reverse the effects of the narcotic and sedative, if necessary. In fact, endoscopists are using the benzodiazepine, midazolam, increasingly, partly because its effect can be rapidly reversed by its antagonist, flumazenil.

Patients are examined lying in the left lateral recumbent position with the knees and thighs flexed. The patient may be rotated supine, prone, or onto the right side to assist in passing a difficult bend. In certain circumstances it is valuable to have an assistant press on the patient's abdomen so loops do not reform in the sigmoid colon. This also assists passage through areas such as the proximal transverse colon.

Initially and throughout the procedure a generous amount of lubricating jelly is used at the anus to ease advancement of the endoscope by reducing friction at the anal verge, and also to prevent trauma to the anal canal. This is especially important if anal sphincter tone is high or if large hemorrhoids are present.

Once in the rectum, the instrument is advanced, under direct vision, by gently distending the colonic lumen with air. Most experienced colonoscopists can intubate the entire colon with this technique. Occasionally, blind intubation – called the slide-by technique – is necessary although less desirable. This technique uses gentle pushing pressure so that the mucosa slides past the visual field. The pushing pressure should be discontinued immediately if the tip stops moving or if the color of the mucosa changes, suggesting excessive pressure. Slide-by may be performed for short distances, providing the mucosa does not appear excessively whitened as a result of stretching. In general, advancing with the lumen in view is preferable to slide-by.

Other general principles are to be gentle and not to advance with excessive force. One must try to follow the lumen and be careful not to traumatize a false lumen such as a diverticular orifice. It is also best to keep insufflation to a minimum, and the instrument as straight as possible. The more experienced endoscopist will move the endoscope in and out or 'jiggle' it to reduce the number of bends as the tip is advanced. Unnecessary loops tend to enlarge when the colonoscope is advanced, interfering with progress. The colon is 'accordioned' over the colonoscope, keeping the instrument as straight as possible. The straight position keeps the optimal tip control and allows the colonoscopist to approach flexures (especially at the sigmoid–descending colon junction) at a favorable angle for introducing the tip of the instrument into the descending colon.

If intubation is difficult, lengths of the colonoscope may have to be withdrawn to allow the colon to straighten, thus reducing bends and permitting further intubation. It may be useful to remove as much gas as possible to reduce distension and the chance of loop formation. First, remove some of the colonoscope to see if the colon can be straightened. Next, apply gentle pressure over the area where the loop is forming to prevent further expansion of the loop. Repositioning the patient may facilitate passage into the transverse colon from the descending colon, or into the ascending colon from the transverse colon. This may require the patient to lie on his or her right side or in a prone position. Clockwise rotation may assist passage in several difficult positions by reducing the tendency of the sigmoid colon to form loops.

Special maneuvers, such as the alpha maneuver, can be used to straighten acute angles and permit passage of the colonoscope. In the alpha maneuver, which is performed with fluoroscopy, a loop (which on x-ray resembles the letter alpha) is created in the sigmoid colon (Fig. 10.1). This is accomplished by counterclockwise rotation of the colonoscope. In the alpha

Figure 10.1 *The alpha maneuver.*

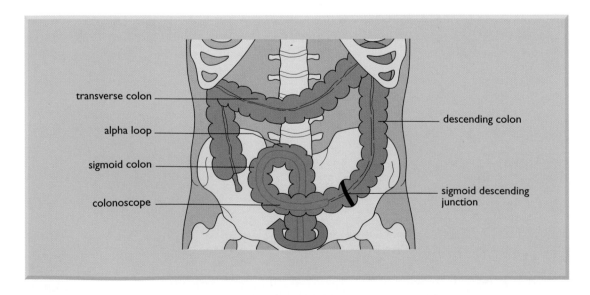

transverse colon

alpha loop

sigmoid colon

colonoscope

descending colon

sigmoid descending junction

configuration it is possible to pass the tip of the colonoscope past the angle at the sigmoid–descending colon junction into the descending colon. When the tip has been advanced to the level of the splenic flexure or the left transverse colon, the alpha loop in the sigmoid colon is removed by gently withdrawing the colonoscope, still under fluoroscopy, with a simultaneous clockwise rotation (Fig. 10.2).

Improvements in the design of colonoscopes have reduced the need for use of a stiffener. The newer models have a flexible tip with a less flexible shaft closer to the controls. This reduces the chance of loop formation when the tip of the colonoscope is up in the colon, for example, at the splenic flexure.

Another technique that assists intubation of the ascending colon is to remove a length of colonoscope to both lift a bow in the transverse colon and to reduce the angulation of the instrument as it approaches the hepatic flexure. Clockwise rotation, aspirating air, and having the patient take a breath will also facilitate passage into the ascending colon.

The cecum has its own distinctive fold pattern, characterized by the appearance of the three converging tenial bands. The orifice of the appendix may be seen at the point of convergence. Light from the endoscopic tip can be seen through the abdominal wall in the right lower quadrant. Other indicators of the cecum include identification of the cecal sling, a circular fold approximately 7 cm proximal to the cecal bottom, representing the frenula valvulae coli, and identification of the ileocecal valve next to the cecal sling. Fluoroscopy can also be used to confirm the position of the tip of the colonoscope.

After documenting depth of penetration of the colonoscope, the instrument is slowly withdrawn. Examination during withdrawal is a critical part of colonoscopy. Each examiner has an individual system for surveying various segments of the colon. Mucosal surfaces should be inspected meticulously. Careful inspection and reinspection of areas behind haustra and around flexures and bends may be required. The instrument may have to be advanced and withdrawn repeatedly over varying distances to ensure that abnormalities have not been overlooked. The examiner should establish a set of survey arcs at intervals of a few centimeters, thus describing a helical configuration as the tip is withdrawn, to optimize inspection of the colonic mucosal surface.

POLYPOID LESIONS

Colonic polypoid lesions are the most common pathology found during colonoscopy. They may be single or multiple, and of epithelial or nonepithelial origin. Within the epithelial polyps, adenomatous, hyperplastic, juvenile, and inflammatory polyps can be distinguished. Neoplastic and non-neoplastic polyposis syndromes are also discussed.

EPITHELIAL POLYPS

Adenomatous Polyps
The characteristic appearance of colonic adenomas varies. It is uncertain why this variation occurs but possibly it relates to the size of the polyp and perhaps to the rapidity of growth. It is impossible to tell endoscopically whether a polyp is an adenoma or a hyperplastic polyp. When dealing with small polyps this distinction is important because we have learned that the presence of an adenoma (even a small one) can be associated with synchronous and metachronous polyps and cancer. Several recent studies suggest that hyperplastic polyps may also be associated with an increased risk of other neoplasia in the colon, although, as yet, the connection is not established absolutely. Most endoscopists, however, currently consider that colonic adenomas are markers for other colonic neoplasia and clearly indicate the need for a full colonic examination.

The smallest or diminutive polyp is typically less than 5 mm, covered with normal-appearing mucosa and rarely large enough to have a stalk. Occasionally, even these small adenomas are red in appearance. Histologically, these adenomas are composed predominantly of branching tubules, packed closely together, surrounded by lamina propria.

As the size of adenomas increases they may be sessile or pedunculated (Figs. 10.3 and 10.4). As with smaller polyps, the covering mucosa may appear normal or slightly erythematous (Fig. 10.5). When the polyp is larger than 1.0 cm diameter, the contour of the surface may vary. The smaller polyps tend to be smooth; as they grow, a lobulated appearance may be noted. These larger polyps usually have been present longer than the smaller polyps, and they are often pedunculated, occasionally with long stalks.

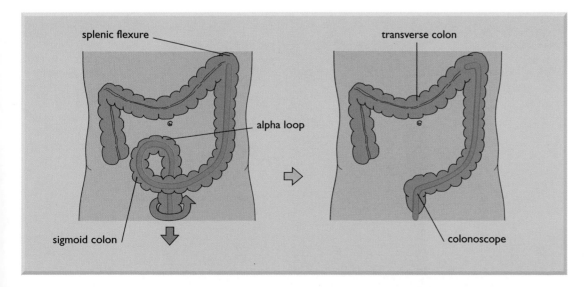

Figure 10.2 Derotating the alpha loop.

Adenomas usually remain pedunculated as they grow and therefore are removable with snare techniques. Most endoscopists are concerned about the potential for immediate or delayed hemorrhage resulting from removal of larger lesions (over 2 cm diameter). Therefore removal as an inpatient is appropriate, if blood for transfusion and observation for delayed hemorrhage is available. In several series, hemorrhage associated with polypectomy may be delayed by as long as 7–12 days. Because of this risk of hemorrhage, most endoscopists discontinue all aspirin, nonsteroidal anti-inflammatory drugs, and anticoagulants sufficiently in advance of the procedure to allow clotting times to return to normal during polypectomy, and if possible for 2 weeks after. Some delayed bleeding is thought to be caused by the eventual sloughing of coagulated tissue, exacerbated by the platelet inhibiting action of aspirin.

There are two predominant histologic forms of adenoma: villous and tubular. In general there is more concern about villous than tubular forms because the villous are generally larger, sessile, and more likely contain a car-

cinoma. It is not unusual to find lesions of greater than 3 cm in diameter. The polyp is frequently sessile, and the surface is often irregular or covered with small nodules several millimeters in height (Figs. 10.6 and 10.7). These polyps are often pale yellow, rather than the typical erythema of tubular adenoma.

There are other common patterns of growth of villous lesions, including where they grow diffusely along the circumference of a segment of colon (Figs. 10.8–10.11). The mucosa at the edge of this type of lesion may have an indistinct vascular pattern referred to as incomplete villous transformation (Fig. 10.12).

Intermediate between tubular and villous forms is the tubulovillous adenoma. These lesions are often moderate in size and pedunculated, with a thicker stalk than a typical tubular adenoma. The surface is often nodular, especially over the area containing villi (Figs. 10.13 and 10.14).

Polyps may disappear spontaneously. Twisting of the stalk of a long polyp or excessive traction due to hypermotility may cause ischemia and autoamputation, characterized clinically by a brief episode of brisk rectal bleeding

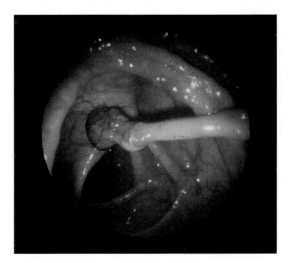

Figure 10.3 *Small tubular adenoma on a long stalk. Note the erythematous mucosa at the polyp tip.*

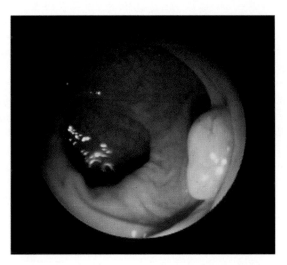

Figure 10.4 *Small, sessile, tubular adenoma in a patient previously operated on for colonic cancer. The mucosa of this polyp appears endoscopically normal.*

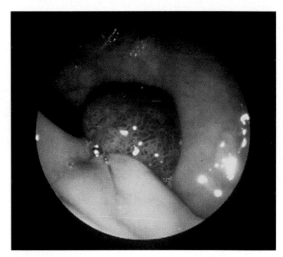

Figure 10.5 *Moderate size tubular adenoma on a short stalk shows conspicuous erythema.*

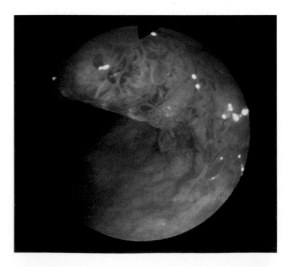

Figure 10.6 *Villous projections on the mucosal surface of an adenoma in the distal rectum show hyperemia.*

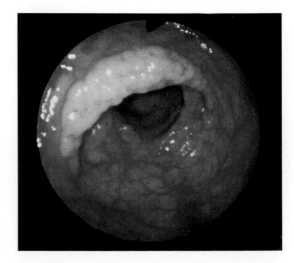

Figure 10.7 *This view shows a flat, sessile, villous polyp, which developed around a valve of Houston in the rectum. The yellow–white color of the multiple tiny nodules is typical of villous adenoma.*

▼ **A**

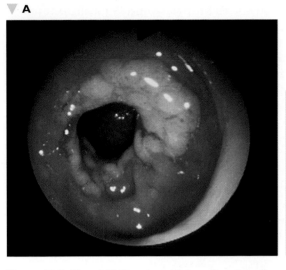

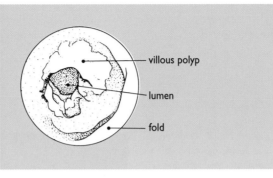

▼ **B**

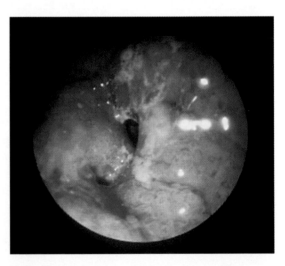

Figure 10.8 (*A* and *B*) *Two views of circumferential, villous adenoma. The surface of the lesion consists of multiple tiny nodules.*

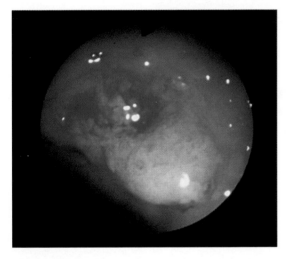

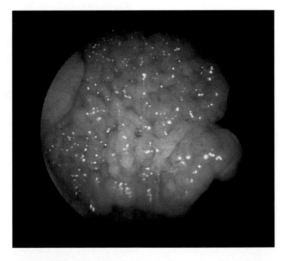

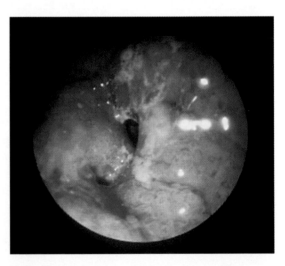

Figure 10.9 *Bleeding sessile villous rectal polyp.*

Figure 10.10 *Extensive villous polyp covers the bowel wall circumferentially in a tapestry-like fashion.*

Figure 10.11 *Extensive villous adenoma extending around the entire colonic circumference and more than 5 cm in length. It may be difficult to exclude the presence of an adenocarcinoma in this type of lesion.*

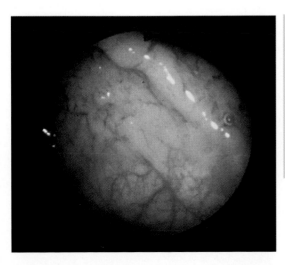

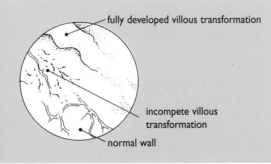

Figure 10.12 *Early villous transformation is characterized by blurring and irregularity of vascular pattern.*

(Figs. 10.15 and 10.16). Endoscopically, a small mucosal defect surrounded by some inflammatory changes may be seen (Fig. 10.17). If the endoscopic examination is delayed, it may be difficult to recognize the site of the lesion. Because autoamputation may occur in adenomatous polyps bearing a focus of malignancy, biopsy of the postamputation ulcer or of the site is essential.

Adenomatous polyps are neoplastic and may undergo cancerous degeneration. Some polypoid structures are composed largely of cancerous tissue with little or no remaining adenomatous elements. These are often sessile or have a short stalk. Characteristic endoscopic features of malignant polyps include subtle changes such as deformity, deep ulceration of the head of the polyp, an excessively granular or friable surface, and bleeding (Figs. 10.18 and 10.19). Sharp, angular edges or a waxy, hard consistency, especially upon biopsy, are also suggestive of malignancy. If the polyp moves easily away from the colonic wall when touched with a catheter or biopsy forceps, invasion of the deeper layers of the wall is unlikely. If the polyp is fixed to the wall such that the polyp and colonic wall move together, invasion into and

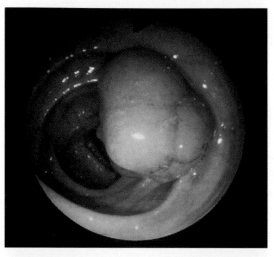

Figure 10.13 Moderate size sessile tubulovillous adenoma. Several lobules are evident.

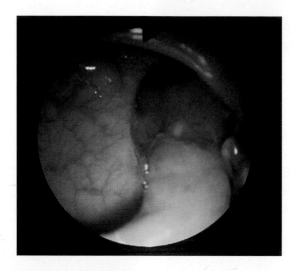

Figure 10.14 Large tubulovillous polyp in the sigmoid colon. Note the wide pedicle and erythematous nodular polyp head.

▼ **A**

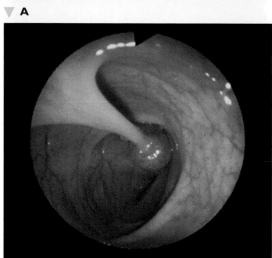

▼ **B**

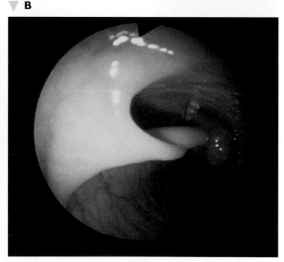

Figure 10.15 Pedunculated adenomatous polyp (**A**) can spontaneously twist on its stalk (**B**). Prolonged or repetitive twisting may cause ischemic damage and lead to autoamputation.

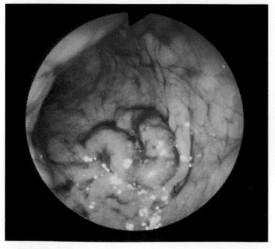

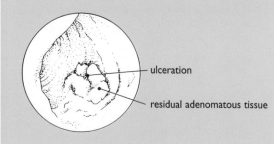

Figure 10.16 Autoamputation of a pedunculated polyp caused sudden massive colonic bleeding. This view shows the residual adenomatous tissue surrounding the central ulcerative defect.

beyond the muscularis propria is likely. Discoloration of the head of the polyp may indicate foci of invasive cancer. Broad-based pedicles or pseudopedicles produced by peristaltic action may also suggest malignant invasion, especially if the pedicle has an ill-defined base.

Endosonography offers a method of examining suspicious polyps for evidence of an invasive lesion. This information assists the endoscopist in making decisions as to whether endoscopic therapy is appropriate.

Hyperplastic Polyps

Hyperplastic polyps are small sessile excrescences, usually less than 5 mm in diameter, most commonly found in the rectum. The tiny mucosal excrescences or slightly larger mammillations are pale or, more commonly, the same color as the surrounding mucosa (Figs. 10.20 and 10.21). In rare cases, hundreds of tiny hyperplastic polyps are visible, especially in the left colon. Giant

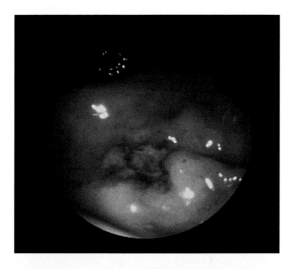

Figure 10.17 Small ulcer in colon surrounded by slight inflammatory changes, caused by autoamputation of a polyp.

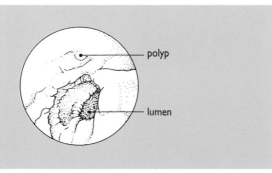

Figure 10.18 This malignant rectal polyp shows a discrete central ulceration and friable surface. After polypectomy, cancer was present in the transection line.

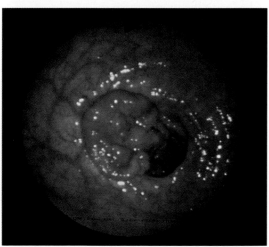

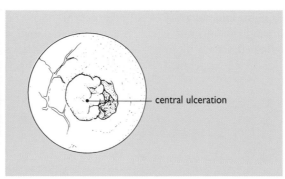

Figure 10.19 Superficial central ulceration in this rectal villous polyp is suggestive of malignancy.

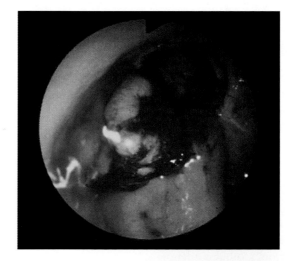

Figure 10.20 Small hyperplastic (metaplastic) polyp on top of a mucosal fold.

Figure 10.21 Tiny hyperplastic (metaplastic) polyp in the sigmoid colon is the same color as the surrounding mucosa.

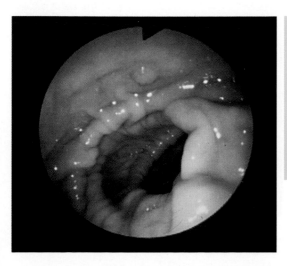

hyperplastic polyps are an exceedingly rare presentation and may simulate carcinoma. Hyperplastic polyps are usually single, but up to 10% of patients may have from five to ten or more in a single segment of bowel.

Although small hyperplastic polyps are invariably sessile, larger lesions may be pedunculated and therefore visually indistinguishable from small adenomatous polyps. If it is not known whether the patient forms adenomatous or hyperplastic polyps, such small polyps should be removed with a diathermy forceps (hot biopsy forceps), especially if the polyps are 4–5 mm diameter and the patient is elderly. This technique destroys the potentially premalignant (adenomatous) tissue and, at the same time, obtains a biopsy for histologic interpretation. (An alternative technique is to take the biopsy first using a standard forceps and then coagulate the remaining tissue using a bipolar forceps.) A small snare can also be used with a coagulating electrosurgical current. Biopsy is essential for future planning, as the need for total colonic surveillance and the timing of follow-up for the patient who forms hyperplastic polyps is different from that for the patient who forms adenomas. This may change in the future if hyperplastic polyps, like adenomatous polyps, come to be regarded as established indicators of other neoplasia in the colon.

Juvenile Polyps

Juvenile polyps, a type of hamartoma, are prevalent in children and adolescents. The typical endoscopic finding is that of a 1.5–3.0 cm diameter sessile lesion with an intensely erythematous friable eroded ulcerated surface (Fig. 10.22). Sometimes the surface is nodular but not ulcerated, making such polyps indistinguishable from a tubular adenoma. When examined histologically, the surface is usually ulcerated. The center of the polyp is composed of cysts with a large mucin component. There is an expansion of the lamina propria and increased number of inflammatory cells.

Inflammatory Polyps

Inflammatory polyps or pseudopolyps occur in the setting of inflammatory changes in the colon. They are nonspecific and indicate prior ulcerative epithelial destruction. They are made up of markedly inflamed, focally ulcerated epithelium with granulation tissue. (See Chapter 11 for a detailed presentation of inflammatory bowel disease.)

NONEPITHELIAL POLYPS AND POLYP-LIKE STRUCTURES

Submucosal tumors are much less common in the colon than in the upper gastrointestinal tract. Lipoma is the most frequently encountered lesion of this type. These are important lesions to recognize endoscopically because they should not be removed with a snare cautery. When one attempts to snare and sever the polyp with radio frequency current, it is difficult to coagulate the fat in the center of the lipoma, and bleeding or deep injury may result. These lesions appear yellow and translucent. They are usually sessile, often over 2 cm in diameter. Although they occur throughout the colon, they are most often found in the right colon. Endoscopically one suspects a lipoma by the color, the smooth surface, and by determining whether the lesion is soft and indents when pressed by an accessory such as a closed biopsy forceps. This indentation is called the 'pillow sign' (Fig. 10.23). If there is doubt concerning the type of lesion, a forceps biopsy may be performed. Fatty tissue may exude from the biopsy site. A biopsy may be necessary when the surface of the lipoma is eroded or irregular rather than smooth. The ileocecal valve may have a large amount of fat, referred to as lipomatous change, and may resemble a lipoma. The endoscopist should be careful to make this distinction and not attempt removal of the lipomatous ileocecal valve.

Leiomyomas are rare submucosal tumors in the colon, ranging in size from 2 mm to 4 cm diameter. At colonoscopy they appear smooth and sessile, and may be covered with a reddish stretched mucosa.

Carcinoid tumors may be found in the rectum but are rare in the colon. Usually a carcinoid appears as a smooth sessile lesion with a glistening surface mucosa, which has a pale yellow color (Fig. 10.24). Generally, such tumors are nonulcerating and of 1–2 cm diameter in size. They often have a firm consistency when touched with the biopsy forceps.

Lymphangiomas are pale smooth round polypoid masses that are usually soft and easily compressible. Overlying mucosa may have a pale yellow coloration somewhat similar to that seen with carcinoids (Fig. 10.25). These cystic lesions in the submucosa are rarely reached by colonic biopsy because of their depth.

An endometrial implant to the serosal layer of the rectum or sigmoid colon occasionally occurs as a submucosal polypoid mass. In addition to the mass there may be central erythematous discoloration, especially at the time of menstruation.

▼ A

▼ B

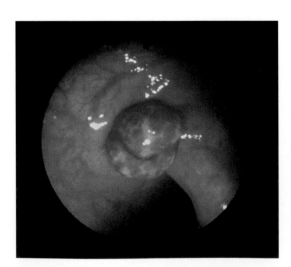

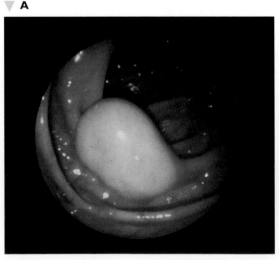

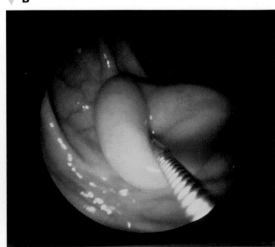

Figure 10.22 *Juvenile polyp. The surface is eroded and erythematous.*

Figure 10.23 *(A) Lipoma of the transverse colon is a soft round sessile lesion with yellow coloration. (B) Easy indentation of the lipoma with a biopsy forceps is termed the 'cushion effect' or 'pillow sign'.*

Pneumatosis cystoides intestinalis is characterized by the presence of gas-filled cysts within the wall of the colon (Fig. 10.26). Cysts may be localized to one segment of the colon or occur throughout, with a predilection for the left side. They appear as submucosal polypoid masses ranging from 2–3 mm to well over 2 cm in diameter. These structures are soft and easily compressible. The overlying mucosa shows nonspecific erythema, especially at the top. Sometimes these masses obliterate the lumen and are mistaken for adenoma or even carcinoma. A forceps biopsy will differentiate a cyst from a carcinoma or adenoma. A small biopsy will not usually penetrate into the cyst but a larger biopsy may. Because the cysts largely contain nitrogen, high-flow or hyperbaric oxygen therapy has been used to stimulate resorption of nitrogen from the cysts. When the cysts disappear, a focal area of brownish discoloration of the mucosa remains.

Other polyp-simulating structures include polyp-like mucosal folds, which are occasionally seen in diverticular disease, especially of the sigmoid colon.

(See Chapter 12 for a detailed presentation of diverticular disease.) Polypoid structures consisting entirely of granulation tissue occasionally develop, especially in the rectosigmoid area. These are caused by breakthrough of inflammatory lesions originating from the pelvic organs, especially chronic salpingitis.

POLYPOSIS SYNDROMES
Neoplastic Polyposis Syndrome

Familial polyposis coli (FPC) is a dominantly inherited disease in which the colon is studded with numerous adenomatous polyps prone to malignant degeneration. Three distinct patterns of FPC may be identified. The most common is the carpet of minute, 1–3 mm diameter, polyps (Fig. 10.27). These polyps are smooth and regular with normal-appearing mucosal coloration; no larger polyps are found (Fig. 10.28). In a less common variant, somewhat larger polyps

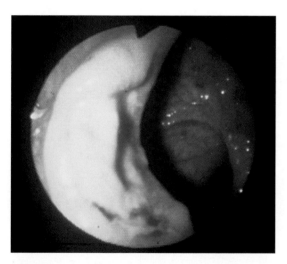

Figure 10.24 *Rectal carcinoid. Note the peculiar yellowish discoloration. The superficial defect is due to prior biopsy.*

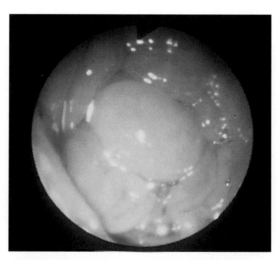

Figure 10.25 *Lymph cyst of the colon. Characteristic transparency and pale yellow color are evident.*

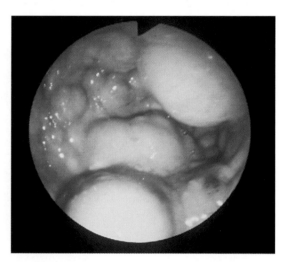

Figure 10.26 *Pneumatosis cystoides intestinalis is characterized by gas-filled cysts within the colonic wall.*

▼ **A**

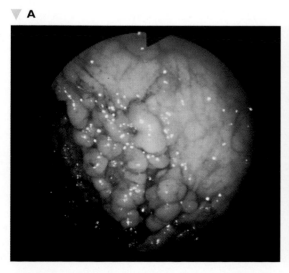

▼ **B**

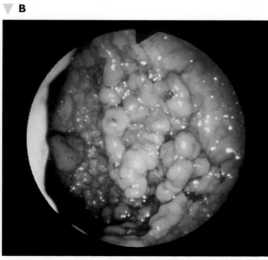

Figure 10.27 *(A and B) Two views from the same patient of a conglomerate of innumerable small polyps that covers the colon wall like a carpet. This is the most common presentation of FPC.*

(4–8 mm in diameter) are distributed throughout the rectum and colon with intervening areas of normal mucosa (Fig. 10.29). These polyps may have a red surface (Fig. 10.30). A third pattern consists of both large and minute polyps (Fig. 10.31). These polyps are sessile and pedunculated (Fig. 10.32).

Patients with adenomatous polyposis are always at risk of malignant transformation (Fig. 10.33). Therefore, a prophylactic proctocolectomy or colectomy with rectal mucosal stripping, along with ileal pouch and ileoanal anastomosis is the best treatment. If colectomy with ileorectal anastomosis is carried out, meticulous follow-up of the rectal stump is necessary to prevent cancer by removing all small adenomas (Fig. 10.34) and to detect early malignancy (Fig. 10.35).

Differentiating FPC from inflammatory, parasitic, or lymphomatous polyposis may occasionally be difficult. Although inflammatory pseudopolyps of ulcerative colitis resemble those of FPC, the intervening mucosa in the latter is normal and the vascular pattern is preserved. In the case of ulcerative colitis, the intervening mucosa is abnormal and a distorted or absent vascular pattern, is expected. Although inflammatory pseudopolyps may be numerous, they rarely carpet the mucosa to the extent of obliterating it.

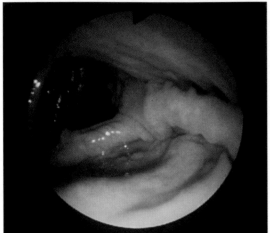

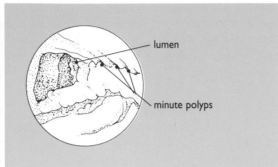

Figure 10.28 FPC. Tenia of the transverse colon studded with minute polyps.

▼ **A** 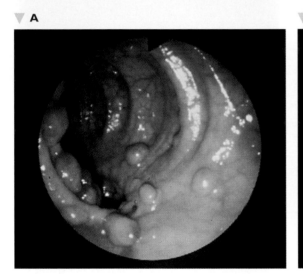 ▼ **B** 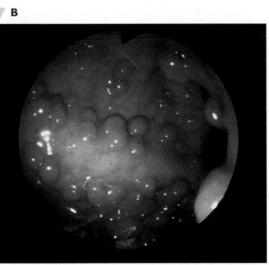 ▼ **C**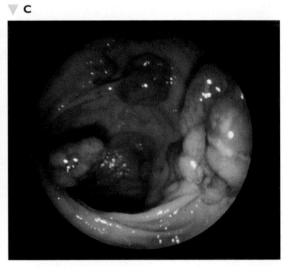

Figure 10.29 (A–C) FPC in three different patients. Small and larger polyps are seen. The lesions are scattered, with normal-looking mucosa in the intervening areas.

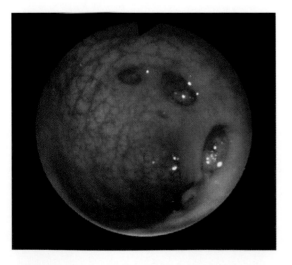

Figure 10.30 FPC with adenomas that appear red.

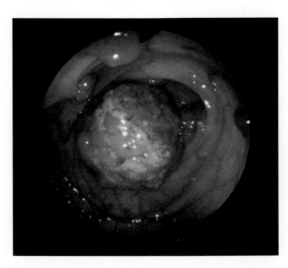

Figure 10.31 FPC with giant polyps. Several smaller adenomas are also seen.

Pseudopolyps tend to vary considerably in size and shape, unlike the monotonous appearance of adenomatous polyposis. In addition, inflammatory polyps often exhibit exudate on the surface. However, biopsy is required to identify with certainty the type of polyp present. Accurate diagnosis is vital, as patient management differs dramatically for each syndrome; consider, for example, the difference between the established therapies for FPC and lymphomatous polyposis.

Non-neoplastic Polyposis Syndromes

Several syndromes involving the intestinal tract are associated with polypoid lesions that are not true neoplasms. These include juvenile polyps, Peutz-Jeghers syndrome, and lymphoid hyperplasia.

The multiple lesions of juvenile polyposis resemble those of single juvenile polyps. These lesions can occur throughout the gastrointestinal tract or be confined to the colon. They may be associated with adenomatous polyps.

▼ **A**
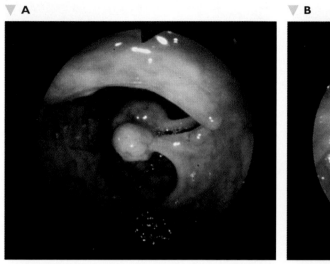

▼ **B**
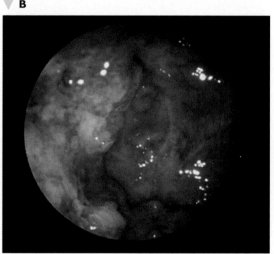

Figure 10.32 (**A** and **B**) Examples of pedunculated adenomas of FPC.

▼ **A**
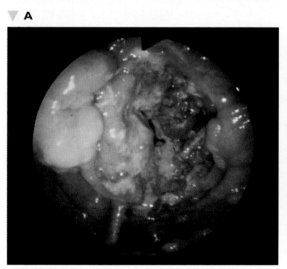

▼ **B**

Figure 10.33 (**A**) FPC with a large irregular multilobed cecal cancer. (**B**) FPC with ulcerating rectal cancer.

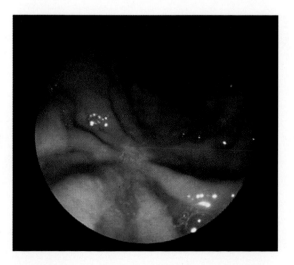

Figure 10.34 Patient with FPC and previous colectomy with ileoanal anastomosis. Prior electrosurgical polypectomy in the rectum produced retracted scar.

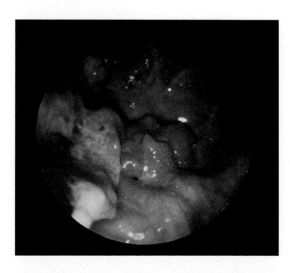

Figure 10.35 Rectal cancer developed after ileorectal anastomosis for FPC.

Peutz-Jeghers syndrome is a problem in gastroenterology in terms of management. Polyps are present throughout the gastrointestinal tract, but especially in the small intestine, where they may be large and cause significant symptoms of obstruction, gastrointestinal bleeding, or intussusception. They are hamartomas with a characteristic histologic appearance of an excessive and redundant muscularis mucosae covered by a non-neoplastic epithelium and lamina propria. Areas of the polyp may show evidence of infarction. The polyps vary in size but may be several centimeters in diameter (Figs. 10.36 to 10.38). They are pedunculated (Fig. 10.39) or sessile and may have an irregular or lobulated surface (Fig. 10.40). Because these polyps tend to recur, endoscopy during surgery may allow the endoscopist to enter the small bowel with guidance from the surgeon, find the polyps, and remove them without opening the bowel wall. This reduces the chance of further adhesion formation, which can be a real problem in these patients who must undergo multiple laparotomies for treatment.

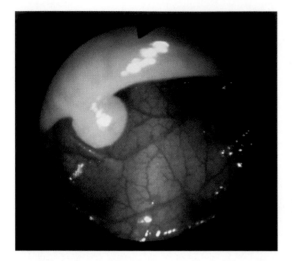

Figure 10.36 Small Peutz-Jeghers polyp.

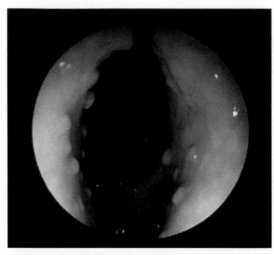

Figure 10.37 Multiple tiny polyps in Peutz-Jeghers syndrome.

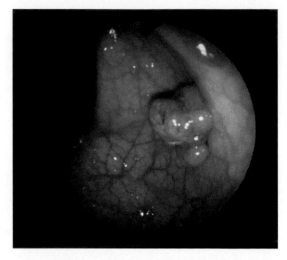

Figure 10.38 Medium-sized polyp in Peutz-Jeghers syndrome with lobulated surface.

▼ **A**

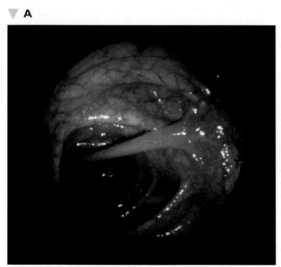

▼ **B**

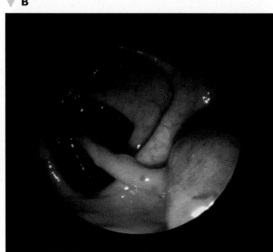

Figure 10.39 Two examples of Peutz-Jeghers polyps with very long stalks. (**A**) The polyp tip is seen in the distance. (**B**) The polyp head is in the foreground.

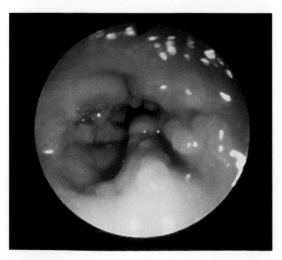

Figure 10.40 Multiple Peutz-Jeghers polyps with lobulated appearance.

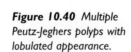

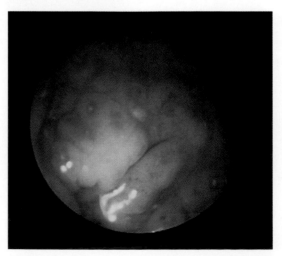

Figure 10.41 Lymphoid hyperplasia caused by follicle enlargement.

Colonic lymphoid hyperplasia consists of lymphoid aggregations seen as slightly raised areas of multiple, 1–2 mm, closely spaced, yellowish-white polyps, similar in appearance to nodular lymphoid hyperplasia of the small bowel (Fig. 10.41). Colonic lymphoid hyperplasia may be noted in children and adolescents. Slightly raised, minute polypoid strictures caused by lymphoid follicle enlargement may be seen occasionally in adults after severe intestinal infection or other colonic disease. The lesions have a central necrotic or slightly hemorrhagic patch. The significance of this finding is unknown.

TECHNIQUE OF ENDOSCOPIC POLYPECTOMY

Polypectomy is used routinely to remove polypoid lesions in the rectocolon. The technique is safe and effective for most colonic polyps, but selection of lesions appropriate for this procedure and performance of polypectomy takes considerable training and experience. The colon must be prepared carefully so that endoscopic visualization is excellent, and to reduce the concentration of potentially explosive gases. Hospitalization may be recommended for patients with respiratory or cardiovascular disease or other significant medical problems, for debilitated patients whose colons are difficult to prepare thoroughly, and for patients with numerous polyps or large sessile polyps.

When an adenomatous polyp is known to be present anywhere in the colon or rectum, a total colonoscopic examination is important because of the increased incidence of synchronous polyps or cancer found at colonoscopy. Whether this is also true of hyperplastic polyps is not yet clear. Some clinicians do not consider hyperplastic polyps to be markers of synchronous neoplasia. Many of these synchronous lesions are small and undetectable radiologically. If a total colonoscopy cannot be achieved at the initial examination, it should be completed within 6–12 months.

The entire polyp and its base or pedicle must be inspected endoscopically before a decision is made on endoscopic removal. Occasionally the lesion must be manipulated with a closed snare to facilitate evaluation. Polyps tend to be located in areas of acute angulation or flexures; patients may have to be repositioned to display the polyp to best advantage. If at all possible, the polyp should be maneuvered around the 5 o'clock position because this facilitates snaring with the polypectomy wire.

Multiple polyps are usually removed at a single session unless they are scattered throughout the colon, in which case they are usually removed in separate right and left excision sessions. In this way, if a problem occurs, such as postpolypectomy bleeding, it can be localized more easily to the right or left colon in a patient with numerous large polyps. In general, the most anatomically proximal polyp is removed first. After retrieval of the specimen, the colonoscope is inserted to the resected polyp and then withdrawn to the next polyp and the procedure repeated until all polyps are removed.

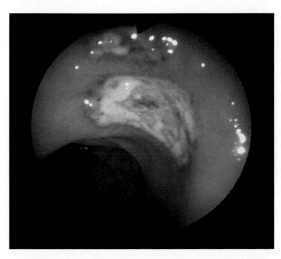

Figure 10.42 One day after colonic polypectomy, an ulcer is seen.

Several sessions may be required. Occasionally India ink is injected into the submucosa to mark a polypectomy site in case of the need for further endoscopic or surgical therapy. Histologic examination of all fragments is essential for correct diagnosis.

After polypectomy an ulcer may be noted at the site of resection (Fig. 10.42).

REMOVAL OF PEDUNCULATED POLYPS

Virtually all pedunculated polyps can and should be removed endoscopically using snare electrosurgical techniques (Figs. 10.43 to 10.46). The plane of transection or coagulation of the stalk is best located near the head of the polyp, rather than close to the normal bowel wall, to minimize the risk of heat penetration and damage. The snare should not be tightened until it is precisely at the proposed plane of transection on the stalk. Grasping the stalk too snugly before application of electrical current can cause premature mechanical transection of the stalk with resulting hemorrhage. One must be certain that the tip of the colonoscope can be controlled so that the polyp does not move out of sight once it is snared, because a complication such as perforation may occur if the polyp is excised blindly.

Once the wire loop is around the polyp, the tip of the snare sheath is advanced to the point of desired separation on the stalk and it is then gently tightened on the stalk. Once the snare has been tightened, it should not be loosened for repositioning, for the partially cut tissue may bleed and impair vision. Instead, that portion should be transected by diathermic current. The snare can then be repositioned to the proper place on the stalk and polypectomy completed. This method of partial or piecemeal polypectomy is often recommended for polyps in which the head is too large for safe, complete encirclement with the snare.

It is essential that the entire thickness of a polyp stalk be adequately coagulated. Ideally, coagulating current is applied as the wire loop is closed around the polyp stalk. Further tightening of the snare is done only after the effect of coagulation is seen to spread a short distance along the pedicle. Higher current power or cutting current modes are used only if resistance to wire closure persists after sufficient coagulation has occurred. If a high power or cutting current is used before adequate coagulation of the stalk, rapid transection may occur and result in hemorrhage. Smoke may be generated while applying current during polypectomy, but can be cleared by suction aspiration.

REMOVAL OF SESSILE POLYPS

The appearance of the sessile polyp is the most important criterion for determining whether it should be removed endoscopically. In general, soft smooth nonulcerated sessile polyps less than 2 cm in diameter are benign and endoscopically excisable. Sessile lesions larger than 2 cm in diameter, especially those containing ulcerations or areas of firm consistency, are usually malignant and therefore not appropriate for endoscopic polypectomy. Endosonographic examination is likely to become an important means of differentiating benign and focally malignant, sessile villous lesions.

Sessile lesions are directly and broadly attached to the rectal or colonic wall. Electrosurgical snare excision is therefore always applied at the level of the bowel wall, making this a delicate and risky procedure. Selected larger lesions can be removed by an experienced endoscopist familiar with the segmental or piecemeal technique.

Small sessile polyps less than 0.5 cm are most easily eradicated using a hot biopsy forceps or a minisnare (Figs. 10.47 and 10.48). The former allows a biopsy specimen to be obtained and, in addition, coagulates the entire base of the lesion. Routine use of the hot biopsy forceps technique is not universally accepted because of the risk of delayed bleeding and perforation.

Another approach is to use a bipolar coagulating forceps. This device causes shallower injury and a more predictable injury pattern than does the standard 'hot biopsy' using monopolar coagulation. However, tissue for histological examination is not as well preserved with the bipolar forceps, so a forceps biopsy before coagulation may be necessary. The bipolar forceps technique is now accepted as effective and safe.

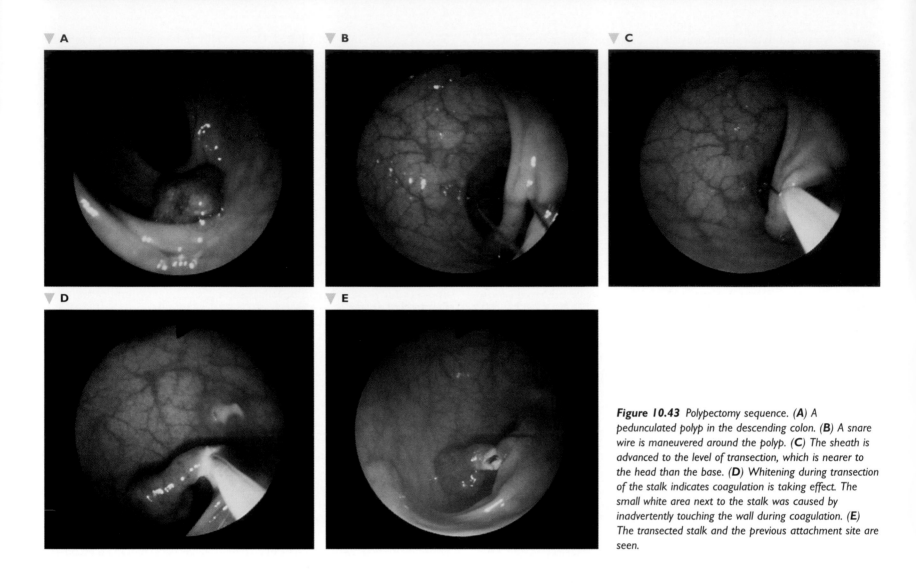

Figure 10.43 Polypectomy sequence. (**A**) A pedunculated polyp in the descending colon. (**B**) A snare wire is maneuvered around the polyp. (**C**) The sheath is advanced to the level of transection, which is nearer to the head than the base. (**D**) Whitening during transection of the stalk indicates coagulation is taking effect. The small white area next to the stalk was caused by inadvertently touching the wall during coagulation. (**E**) The transected stalk and the previous attachment site are seen.

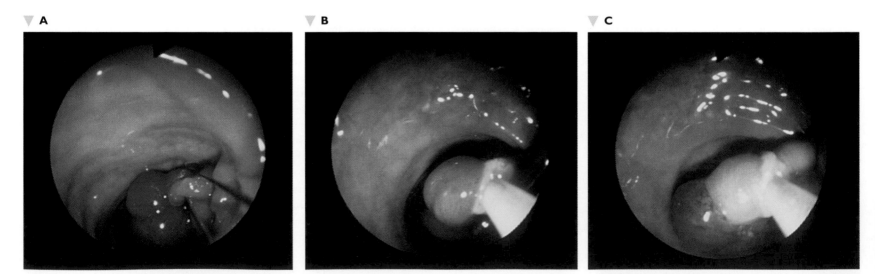

Figure 10.44 Sequence of polypectomy of a multilobulated, peduncular polyp. (**A**) A snare wire is maneuvered around the pedicle. (**B**) During transection, white discoloration indicates coagulation is taking effect. (**C**) Edematous swelling is evident at the transection line.

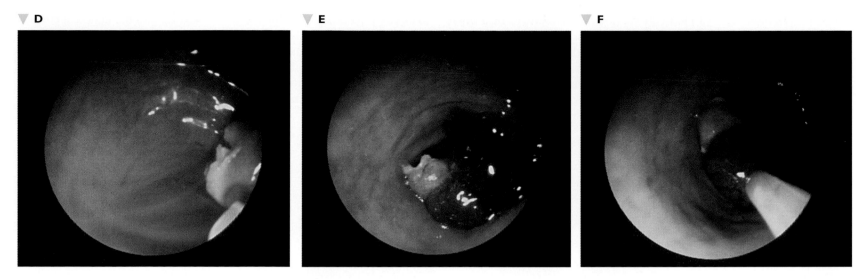

Figure 10.44 *(D) Transected pedicle is seen; faint wisps of smoke generated by application of electrical current are evident. (E) Released polyp lies in the lumen. (F) A grasping device holds the polyp for retrieval as the colonoscope is withdrawn.*

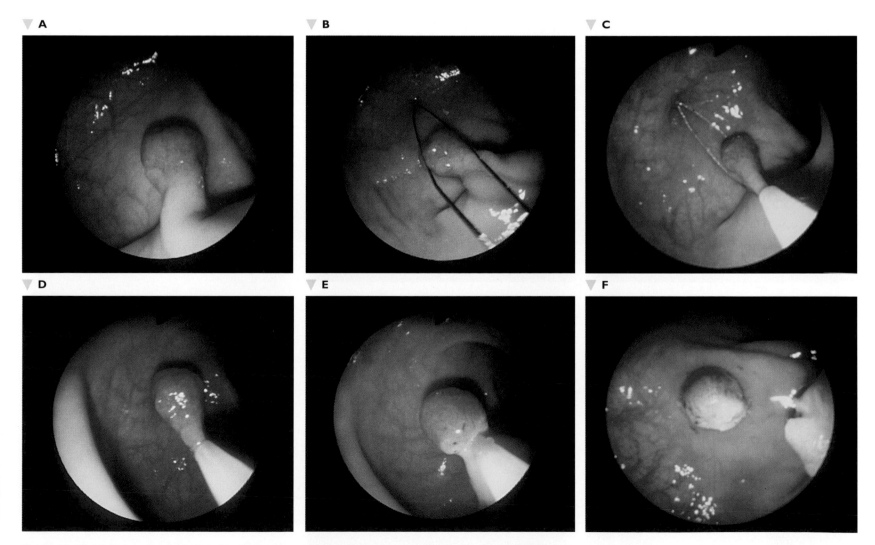

Figure 10.45 *(A) Pedunculated colonic polyp. (B) Snare opened and advanced over polyp. (C) Tip of snare catheter advanced to control where snare closes on polyp. (D) Snare is tightened on stalk in correct position. (E) As coagulating current is applied, snare is tightened. Whitening occurs from coagulating current. (F) Resected polyp is free; coagulated tip of stalk shows excellent hemostasis.*

Sessile polyps in the 0.5–1.0 cm range can usually be removed by a single transection using the snare cautery technique (Figs. 10.49 and 10.50). One side of the wire snare loop is hooked on the edge of the polyp, while the other side of the loop is eased over the widest diameter of the polyp. The wire should be placed at the base of the abnormal tissue to avoid grasping a margin of normal bowel mucosa. With the catheter sheath advanced to the point of transection at the base of the polyp, the snare is tightened gently.

The polyp tissue is then pulled or tented slightly into the lumen. If correctly snared, it moves easily back and forth. If the normal mucosa around the polyp is caught in the snare, the polyp will be difficult to move. After proper placement of the snare, the lumen is distended slightly to prevent the grasped tissue from touching the adjacent or opposite wall. The diathermy current usually coagulates any residual abnormal tissue at the base of the polyp.

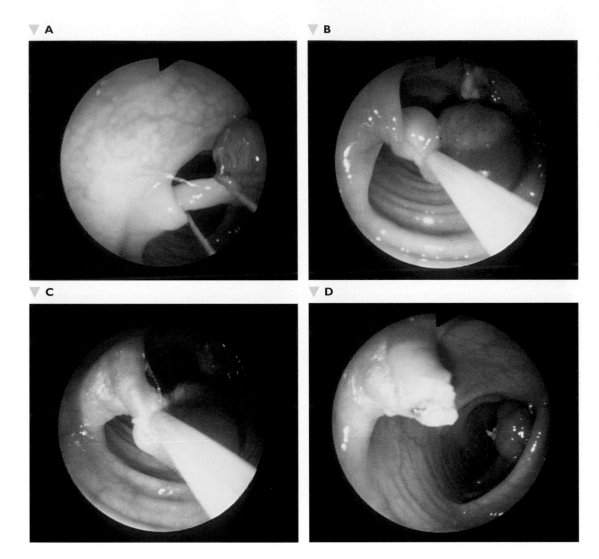

Figure 10.46 Polypectomy sequence (**A**) Snare is placed over stalk of pedunculated polyp. (**B**) Snare is tightened on stalk (**C**) As snare is closed electrocoagulating current causes whitening of stalk under snare. (**D**) Stalk is seen with white tip caused by coagulation. Head of resected polyp is seen in distance.

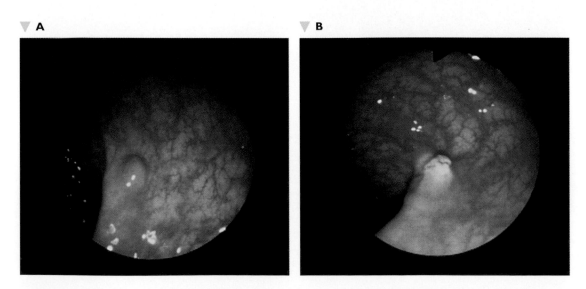

Figure 10.47 (**A**) Small sessile polypoid lesion before removal with a hot biopsy forceps. (**B**) Appearance after removal.

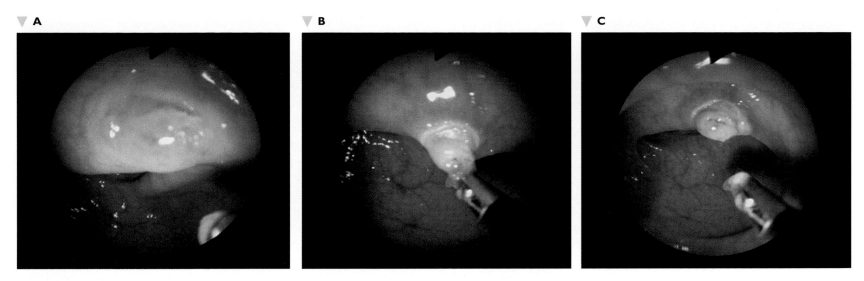

Figure 10.48 (**A**) Small sessile polyp. (**B**) Polyp is grasped with a hot biopsy forceps and coagulated, producing white tissue. (**C**) Biopsy is contained in closed forceps. Residual polyp is coagulated.

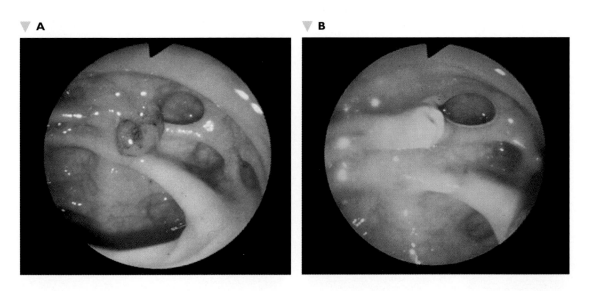

Figure 10.49 Polypectomy of a small sessile polyp at the edge of a diverticulum. (**A**) Appearance of polyp before removal. (**B**) This view shows the appearance of the coagulated insertion base.

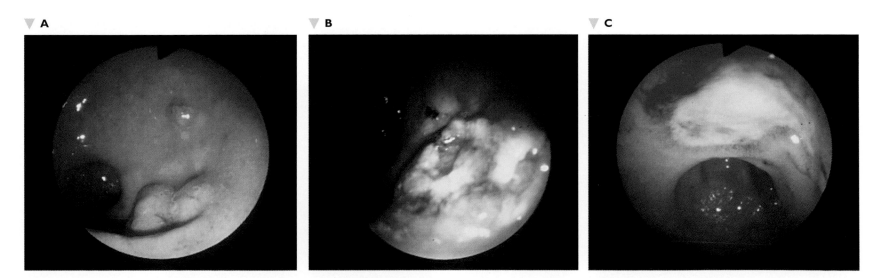

Figure 10.50 (**A**) Sessile polyps before snare resection. (**B**) Snare resection causes a large flat coagulation defect, seen here immediately after polypectomy. (**C**) Two weeks later the ulcer caused by removal of the sessile polyp is beginning to heal.

Sessile polyps larger than 2.5 cm in diameter with a small attachment site should be treated like pedunculated polyps. Those with wide-base attachment are usually removed by segmental transection in several sessions (Fig. 10.51), usually 3–6 weeks apart, with subsequent removal of fragments becoming easier with each attempt. In the segmental transection technique, one end of the wire is hooked at the junction of the polyp and the mucosal surface, and the other flipped over to engage and gently tighten around a large portion of the polyp head. Diathermy current is then applied for a few seconds, followed by simultaneous application of current and closure of the wire snare. The transections are applied obliquely, so that only a portion of the base is cauterized each time. When the approach to a large sessile polyp is poor, one may try to lift the sessile adenoma with submucosal injection of saline or diluted epinephrine. Raising the sessile lesion usually facilitates the piecemeal removal and protects the deeper layers from thermal injury.

Sometimes the cumulative cauterizations injure the bowel wall before the lesion is completely removed. After 4–6 weeks, the cautery effect resolves, allowing resumption of polypectomy and cauterization. Bleeding is rarely a problem in segmental transection as the large blood vessels supplying the polyp branch rapidly, with only small capillary-sized vessels extending into the polyp.

After segmental transection polypectomy, the patient should be examined endoscopically at 3 or 6 month intervals until the polyp site heals completely. The exact site of a large sessile polyp may be difficult to ascertain after removal. Usually an area of whitish discoloration due to fibrosis or telangiectatic vessels may be seen at the re-epithelialized polyp base, or a notch in the colonic wall remains at the site (Figs. 10.52 and 10.53).

If a sessile polyp is wrapped around a fold, the portion of polyp on the distal side of the fold (closest to the anus) should be removed first. Achieving total polypectomy on the proximal side (farthest from the anus) may require considerable manipulation. Delaying until the coagulation ulcer has healed on the distal side may facilitate removal because retraction with healing exposes the proximal side more favorably.

Ideally, the polyp should be shaved so that the base is flat; however, if this cannot be accomplished, it is wise to stop and have the patient return in 4–6 weeks. Upon reinspection, there may be complete healing or an ulcer may be present with minimal polypoid tissue around it. Sometimes the residual polyp may have reformed as several small polypoid excrescences at the site of the polypectomy. The residual polypoid tumor may be removed completely at this time or the piecemeal process may be continued. If tiny foci of adenomatous tissue are still present, a monopolar or bipolar electrocoagulation probe or laser photocoagulation may destroy the remaining neoplastic tissue more easily (Fig. 10.54).

Removal of large 'postage-stamp' or 'tapestry'-type sessile polyps that cover extensive areas of the circumference may be difficult. The recommended method at present combines debulking with the snare wire technique, followed by eradication of remaining polypoid tissue with

▼ A

▼ B

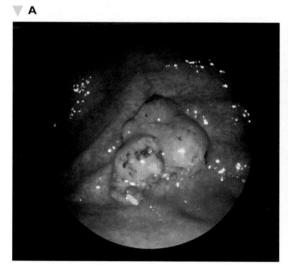
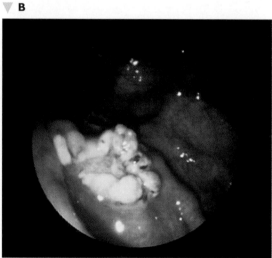
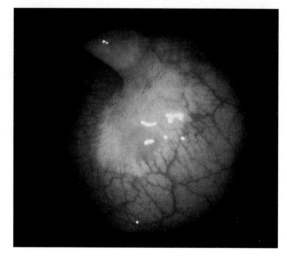

Figure 10.51 (A) Trilobed sessile polyp at base of cecum. (B) After piecemeal removal of several sections, coagulated base is seen.

Figure 10.52 Appearance of the colon wall 3 months after destruction of a villous polyp with Nd:YAG laser. Note an area of whitish scarring and conspicuous telangiectatic vessels at the margin.

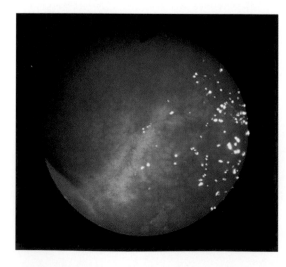

Figure 10.53 Scar in colon several months after laser resection of sessile polyps.

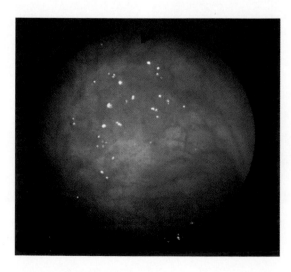

Figure 10.54 In this patient, nearly invisible adenomatous tissue remains after the polyp has been removed.

Nd:YAG laser photocoagulation. Using this elegant technique it is usually possible to eradicate even extensive villous polyps. Destruction with laser requires several sessions to prevent circumferential necrosis and retraction, especially when the entire contour is covered with polypoid tissue.

An alternative technique is to use monopolar or bipolar electrocoagulation devices. To reduce the risk of a perforation, the tip of the device must be moved continuously and steadily across the mucosa, and the endoscopist must be careful to avoid exerting undue pressure against the wall.

RETRIEVAL OF POLYPECTOMY SPECIMENS

Retrieval of all polypectomy tissue is extremely important to assure accurate histologic diagnosis. Single polyps or polyp fragments in the 0.5–1.5 cm diameter range can be retrieved by suctioning the fragment to the tip of the scope and maintaining the suction power as the scope is removed. However, larger polyps may fall loose while maneuvering the scope through the narrow and angulated sigmoid colon, especially in patients with diverticular disease. Therefore, for polyps larger than 1.5 cm, it may be easier to grasp the specimen by the stalk with the snare (Fig. 10.55). In patients with severe disease, this method serves a dual purpose; by keeping the grasped specimen 3–4 cm from the tip of the scope, other polyps can be detected during withdrawal. In withdrawing a large snared polyp, it is wise to bring the specimen flush to the tip of the scope just before bringing it through the anal canal.

If a polyp specimen is lost from sight and cannot be relocated, it can often be retrieved by using the endoscope to flush the area with 50–100 ml tap water or saline. This fluid can then be aspirated and the polyp can often be found and retrieved. An enema can also be used as a retrieval technique, but this is uncomfortable for the patient. Specimens retrieved 10–12 hours or more after polypectomy are often too autolysed for accurate histologic examination.

Several passes of the instrument may be necessary to remove all fragments of a large sessile polyp. It is important to orient the resected fragments for pathologic and histologic examination. Retrieval of the resected portion from closest to the base of the polyp is especially important for histologic examination to determine the depth of invasion, if cancer is detected.

COMPLICATIONS OF ENDOSCOPIC POLYPECTOMY

Errors in identifying or labeling the site of a malignant polyp could lead to surgical resection of the wrong colonic segment. Exacting technique is especially critical in patients with a high risk of malignancy, such as those from families in which one or more members have colon or breast cancer. This familial aggregation is referred to as the cancer family syndrome.

In several large series of colonoscopic polypectomy complications, the most common serious complication is that of hemorrhage (Fig. 10.56). Although this complication may occur with an endoscopist of any degree of experience, it is more common with inexperienced examiners. Bleeding after polypectomy may be immediate or delayed by up to 14 days. Immediate hemorrhage occurs when the stalk of a polyp is severed before sufficient coagulation has occurred to thrombose the arterial vessels in the stalk (Fig. 10.57). This may occur by premature mechanical transection or by the application of cutting radio frequency current before adequate coagulation has been accomplished.

Serious postpolypectomy bleeding requires the immediate application of standard emergency measures, volume replacement, continuous monitoring of the patient, endoscopic attempts to control the bleeding, and angiographic treatment in selected cases. Surgical intervention is a last resort. If immediate bleeding occurs after the stalk is transected, it may be possible to place the snare over the stalk and gently close the snare to achieve hemostasis. If the snare is held closed for approximately 10 minutes, hemostasis may be achieved. To check the area for further bleeding, the snare is released just slightly. If there is any oozing or bleeding, additional coagulation may need to be attempted cautiously. Alternative methods to control hemorrhage include local injection of epinephrine or a sclerosing agent to induce vasospasm and mechanically compress the bleeding vessel. Laser photocoagulation can also be applied to the bleeding spot.

If blood obscures the polypectomy site, the patient's position should be shifted to drain blood away from the area. Aspiration of blood and clots through a standard colonoscope is usually unsuccessful and nearly always plugs the suction channel. Ice water lavage or enema of the bleeding polypectomy site is probably not effective and may perhaps activate the bleeding during reactive hyperemia.

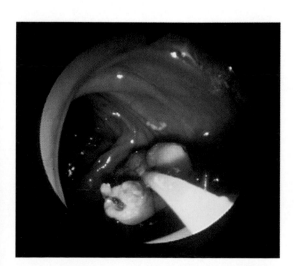

Figure 10.55 A snare is used to remove the resected polyp by grasping the stalk of the specimen.

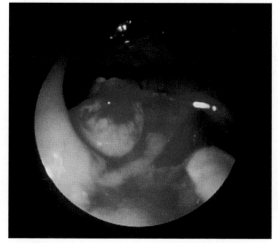

Figure 10.56 Spurting arterial hemorrhage after polypectomy.

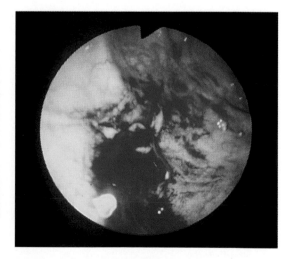

Figure 10.57 Profuse bleeding results from premature mechanical transection with polypectomy snare.

The colonic wall opposite the lesion may be damaged, especially during resection of large polyps in contact with the wall, during application of diathermy current. Damage may be avoided or minimized by moving the polyp slightly during transection to prevent overheating of a narrow segment of colonic wall. On occasion, some damage is unavoidable (Fig. 10.58).

Transmural damage may lead to serosal irritation or outright perforation. Perforation is encountered mainly with resection of sessile polyps. Pain and signs of peritoneal irritation should lead to prompt investigation and, if necessary, surgical exploration.

The endoscopist should be aware of the endoscopic changes brought about by application of diathermy current or laser photocoagulation. The base of a recently coagulated polyp may rapidly take on a peculiar, edematous appearance (Fig. 10.59). This is followed by sloughing of the necrotic tissue, causing an ulcerative defect that gradually forms granulation tissue (Fig. 10.60). After re-epithelialization and healing, the area retains some whitish discoloration due to subepithelial scarring. In the early phases of healing, neocapillaries can be seen, especially at the rim between the coagulated base and surrounding mucosa. After extensive and deep coagulation, widespread scarring may cause convergence of folds and retraction (Fig. 10.61). Occasionally, excessive granulation occurs and a granulation polyp forms. These small polyps are highly vascularized and easily traumatized.

ENDOSCOPIC REMOVAL OF MALIGNANT POLYPS

Correct orientation of the excised polyp is the most crucial aspect of endoscopic removal of malignant polyps. The pathologist must identify the coagulation site to evaluate the depth of invasion of the cancer. In this way it can be determined whether endoscopic excision is adequate therapy. Orientation may be aided by placing a small needle into the coagulated polyp base before fixation of the tissue in formalin. Multiple tissue sections are examined.

Risk of malignant transformation increases with the size of the polyp, the villous character of the adenomatous proliferation, and the degree of dysplasia. The relationship of the malignant focus to the level of the muscularis mucosae is crucial. When malignancy crosses the muscularis mucosae, there is potential for lymphatic spread, and surgical resection may be required. A focus of malignant tissue at the top of a polypoid structure, well above the level of the muscularis mucosae, is best referred to as severe dysplasia rather than intramucosal cancer or carcinoma *in situ* (Fig. 10.62). Such very superficial lesions have negligible capacity for lymphatic spread.

When cancer cells invade into or through the muscularis mucosae of a polyp, the lesion must be regarded as a true cancer. For pedunculated polyps, the depth of penetration of malignancy into the stalk or insertion base of the polyp can usually be precisely delineated (Fig. 10.63). This is more difficult for large villous polyps (Fig. 10.64) removed by multiple transection as it

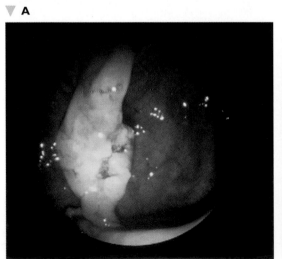

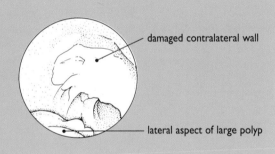

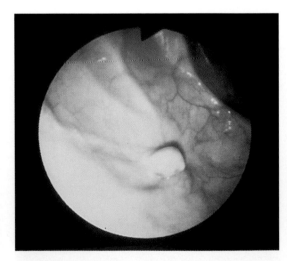

Figure 10.58 *Damage to the contralateral wall after endoscopic transection of a large polyp.*

damaged contralateral wall

lateral aspect of large polyp

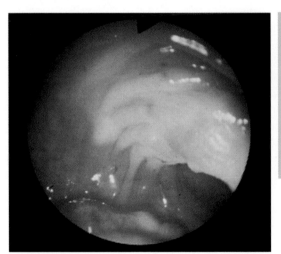

▼ **A**   ▼ **B**

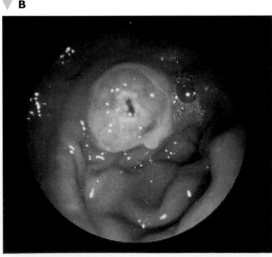

Figure 10.59 *After polyp transection. (A) Whitish discoloration and swelling of insertion site. (B) Peculiar appearance with marked edema.*

Figure 10.60 *Granulation tissue developed at the site of a previous polypectomy.*

is virtually impossible to orient all the tissue fragments correctly (Fig. 10.65). The risk of a noncurative endoscopic excision of a sessile or pedunculated polyp appears to be greatest if the cancer is poorly differentiated, comes close to or is within the margin of the transection, or if malignant cells are present in blood vessels or lymphatics of the polyp stroma.

There is a debate as to whether malignant polyps should be removed endoscopically or surgically. The decision depends in part on the age and health of the patient. Some physicians do not recommend surgical bowel resection in the area of a cancer if there is adequate clearance between the level of cancer invasion and the line of cautery, especially if the tumor does not invade

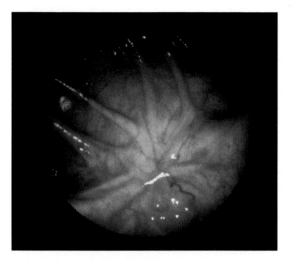

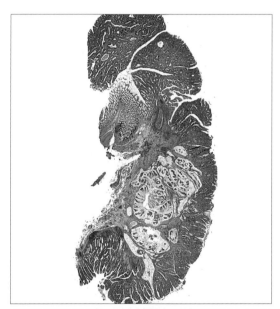

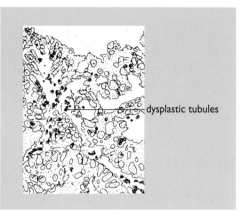

Figure 10.62 Detail of a focus of severe dysplasia located at the top of adenomatous polyp. Note irregular, hyperchromatic nuclei, loss of polarity, and absence of mucous secretion.

dysplastic tubules

Figure 10.61 Scarring and retraction 1 year after snare polypectomy with deep intramural burn.

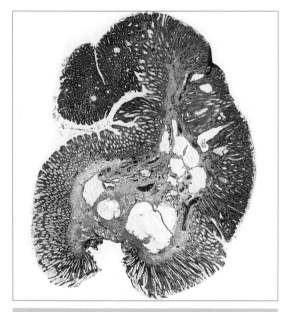

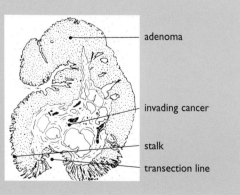

adenoma

invading cancer

stalk

transection line

Figure 10.63 Pedunculated malignant polyp with deep infiltration of the stalk near the transection line. Note the precise orientation of the polyp, allowing histologic interpretation.

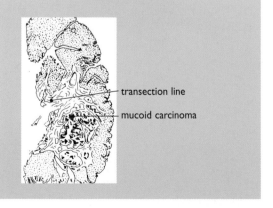

transection line

mucoid carcinoma

Figure 10.64 Sessile tubulovillous adenoma with mucoid carcinoma invading the submucosal layer close to the line of transection.

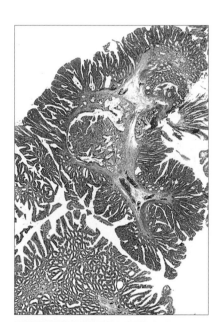

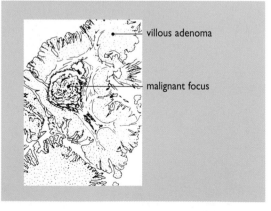

villous adenoma

malignant focus

Figure 10.65 Fragment of a large villous polyp removed with piecemeal polypectomy technique. Because of poor orientation, it is impossible to analyze the depth of penetration of the malignant focus.

the submucosa of the colonic wall at the site of attachment of the polyp. In these cases, the risk of lymph node metastasis is low, unless the malignancy is poorly differentiated or there is evidence of vascular or lymphatic invasion. When the malignant growth is at or near the line of transection, surgical removal is recommended because of the risk of residual cancerous tissue at the polypectomy site, and of lymph node metastases.

For patients in whom surgical risk might approach or exceed the risk of cancer or metastases, the therapeutic approach is different. If cancer invades or approaches the line of transection, the next step is usually endoscopic removal of any remaining stalk. Multiple biopsies are then obtained from the base and edges of the coagulation ulcer. If positive for cancer, additional coagulation of the gut wall, preferably with laser, is carried out until there is no further histologic evidence of malignant tissue. Transmural endosonographic examination is useful to document the potential presence and depth of remaining malignant tissue.

COLONIC MALIGNANCY

Most adenocarcinomas of the rectocolon follow the adenoma-dysplasia-carcinoma sequence. *De novo* carcinomas are rare, as are nonepithelial malignancies such as lymphomas and metastatic tumors of the colon. Yet increasingly, Japanese authors stress the importance of the flat adenoma and the flat adenocarcinoma in which malignancy develops in the colonic wall without the formation of a macroscopically recognizable polyp.

EPITHELIAL MALIGNANCIES
Adenocarcinoma

Adenocarcinoma, the second most common cancer in the USA, accounts for about 13% of cancer-associated deaths. The adenomatous polyp is a premalignant condition associated with colorectal adenocarcinoma. With early detection and removal of such polyps, the incidence of adenocarcinoma is reduced. In addition, colonoscopy helps the physician diagnose and treat colorectal cancer at an early pathologic stage, before patients become symptomatic. Screening and early detection reduce mortality from these cancers, and early-stage tumors have higher 5-year survival rates than later stage tumors.

Adenocarcinomas may occur throughout the rectocolon but are most common within the distal 40 cm. An ulcerated mass is a commonly encountered configuration of adenocarcinoma (Fig. 10.66). The ulcer is irregular, deep, and gray or pink, with a necrotic appearance (Fig. 10.67). The surrounding mucosa is heaped-up, red, and friable, which accounts for the bleeding that occurs in the majority of these lesions. The lesion is hard when touched with the biopsy forceps. Sharp angles occur where the tumor tissue meets the adjacent colon wall.

About one-third of colorectal malignancies occur as polypoid, nonexcavating masses of variable dimensions (Figs. 10.68 and 10.69). The raised, sessile mass typically has nodular surface distortion, with sharply angulated borders showing focally eroded surface area and, occasionally, striking friability. The mass is obviously fixed to the bowel wall.

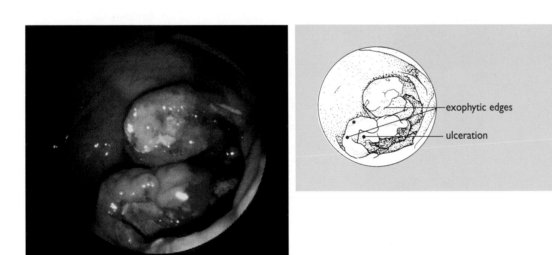

exophytic edges

ulceration

Figure 10.66 *Adenocarcinoma of the cecum appearing as a centrally excavated mass with exophytic overhanging edges.*

▼ **A**　　　▼ **B**

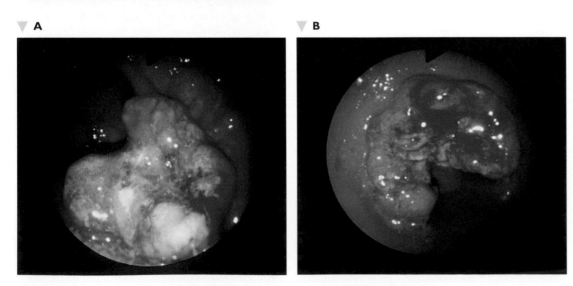

Figure 10.67 *(A and B) Two examples of exophytic rectal cancer with central necrotic ulcer.*

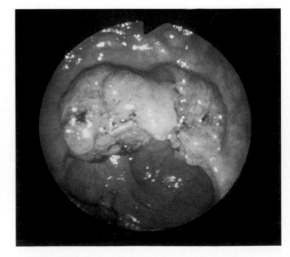

Figure 10.68 *Polypoid mass without excavation developed around a valve of Houston.*

An annular mass is a third presentation. A large ulcerated mass spreads circumferentially, enveloping and penetrating the colonic wall. Generally only the distal margin of the mass can be seen, although a glimpse of the central ulcerated area is possible (Figs. 10.70 and 10.71).

A distinctly uncommon appearance is that of a plaque-like, slightly raised, flat, or discoid mass with a central depression or ulceration. Also uncommon is the stricturing type, seen as an abrupt termination of the lumen without an obvious mass. In this type the growth pattern is infiltrative and linitis plastica-like; no tumor rim is apparent. The stricturing or stenotic appearance also occurs where the lumen has been narrowed by extension of the tumor into the pericolic fat, causing distal compression and obscuring the exophytic mass (Fig. 10.72).

Synchronous polyps and carcinoma are also common: a second carcinoma occurs in approximately 5% of patients with one cancer, and polyps in up to 25%. Therefore, it is important to perform total colonoscopy to rule out a synchronous lesion before surgery because the findings may change the surgical approach (Figs. 10.73 and 10.74). If the tumor is obstructing, the examination of the total colon may have to be performed 1–2 months after surgery, but it is essential to examine the entire colon. The same is true for polyps – the entire colon must be surveyed for other polyps or carcinomas. A lifelong screening program is essential for those patients with adenocarcinomas and adenomatous polyps to detect metachronous lesions.

Several lesions may be confused with colon cancer. A sessile adenomatous polyp of the sigmoid colon may be mistaken for carcinoma if the lesion is obscured by associated diverticular disease and luminal narrowing. Large villous adenomas may show enough surface irregularity and friability to suggest malignancy.

The distinction between a diverticular stricture and underlying malignancy can be difficult. In contrast to diverticular stricturing, carcinomatous narrowing is usually characterized by the distinctly irregular and heaped-up appearance of the folds, together with some discoloration or destruction of the mucosa at the level of the narrowing. When a strictured area cannot be passed even with a small caliber colonoscope, the endoscopist should be reluctant to make a macroscopic diagnosis, even if the visible mucosa appears normal. If, on the other hand, the strictured area is passed with a small caliber colonoscope and no macroscopically suspicious tissue is recognized upon slow withdrawal, the lesion most likely represents benign diverticular disease. Endoscopic ultrasound may prove useful in this situation. The image generated by passing a probe through the narrowed area can assist in the differential diagnosis of cancer versus diverticular disease as the cause of stenosis. Abnormal-appearing tissue should be biopsied to confirm the macroscopic suspicion.

The endoscopist should also be familiar with the appearance of recurrent cancer at a resection line, as this occurs in up to 10% of operated patients (Fig. 10.75). Most recurrences are found at sites outside the colon, such as lymph nodes or liver. In lymph node recurrences, the narrowed area usually shows marked nodularity, but is lined with normal-looking mucosa. Mucosal breakthrough is seen in the case of suture line recurrences.

▼ A ▼ B

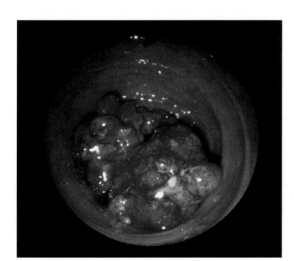

Figure 10.69 *This polypoid, nonulcerated, exophytic mass obstructs the transverse colon.*

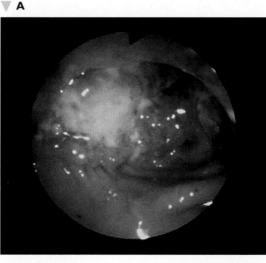

Figure 10.70 *(A) This annular circumferential rectal mass in a young patient was missed for over 6 months in another institution. (B) This view shows details of circumferential infiltration and ulceration.*

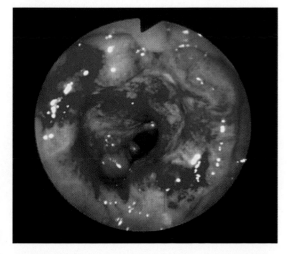

Figure 10.71 *Rectal cancer involving the entire bowel circumference. The lesion is nodular and friable.*

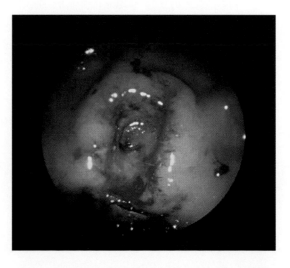

Figure 10.72 *Stenosing type of adenocarcinoma with complete luminal cancerous obstruction.*

After operation and anastomosis, examination with the colonoscope may be undertaken to rule out a suture line recurrence. The distinction may be difficult because of deformity caused by the suture line and the occurrence of nodules at the suture line resulting from suture granulomas. When a recurrent tumor is encountered, the mass is usually hard, friable, and may be ulcerated, presenting a different appearance from that of a granuloma. Endoscopic ultrasound imaging of this area may be important in the future to distinguish a small granuloma from a recurrent tumor with a large extracolonic mass.

Patients treated for colonic cancer should be seen at regular intervals to screen for metachronous polyps and cancer (Fig. 10.76). The timing of follow-up is not yet established; however, colonoscopic re-examination at 6 and 12 months is recommended. A schedule for lifelong screening must then be planned. This includes combinations of testing for carcinoembryonic antigen, occult blood testing, and full colonoscopy. The frequency of colonoscopy is suggested as yearly initially, gradually extending to every 2 or 3 years if no lesions are found on several subsequent colonoscopic examinations.

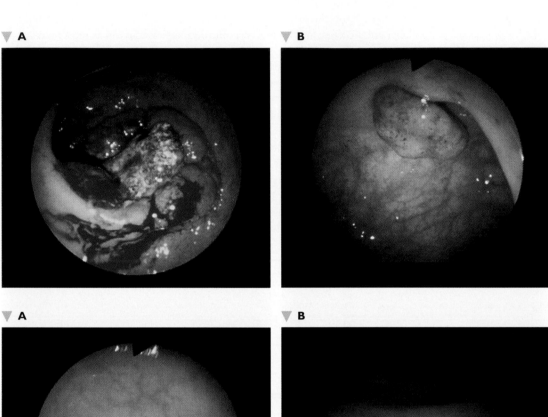

Figure 10.73 (**A**) A large excavated bleeding cancer in the midrectum was found in conjunction with a second, synchronous, smaller polypoid malignancy (**B**) at the rectosigmoid junction.

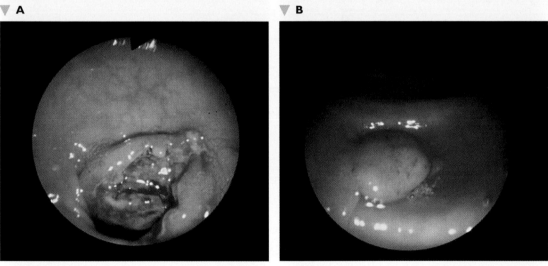

Figure 10.74 (**A**) Colon cancer. (**B**) Synchronous sentinel polyps.

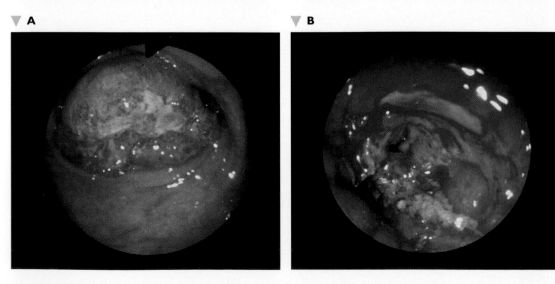

Figure 10.75 (**A** and **B**) Two examples of recurrent carcinoma at level of anastomosis after resection of rectal cancer. Recurrences occurred at the level of anastomosis.

Extrinsic Mass

Rectal wall masses covered by normal mucosa may be caused by lesions such as prostate cancer (Fig. 10.77).

Epidermoid Cancer

Epidermoid or squamous cell carcinoma originating from the anal verge may occasionally invade the distal rectum (Fig. 10.78) as may a cloacogenic cancer originating from transitional epithelium (Fig. 10.79).

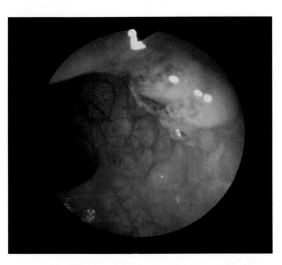

▼ **A**

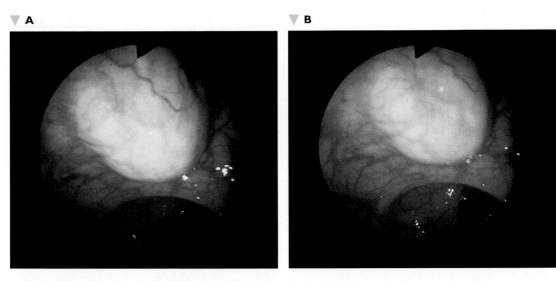

▼ **B**

Figure 10.76 *Metachronous cancer at the rectosigmoid junction in a young patient with familial colon cancer syndrome. The patient had been treated for cecal cancer 2 years previously.*

Figure 10.77 *(A and B) Two examples of extrinsic compression of the rectum caused by prostate cancer.*

▼ **A**

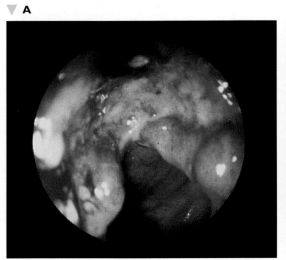

▼ **B**

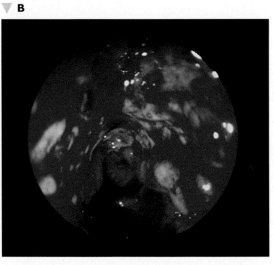

Figure 10.78 *(A) Large, ulcerating epidermal carcinoma invading the distal rectum. (B) Diffuse bleeding after a single pass of the colonoscope.*

▼ **A**

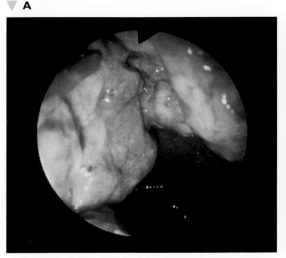

▼ **B**

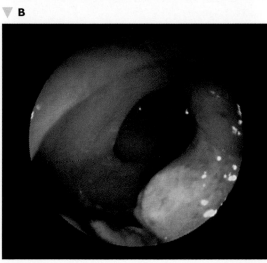

Figure 10.79 *(A) Cloacogenic tumor invades the distal rectum. (B) This view shows the proximal extent of the cancer.*

NONEPITHELIAL MALIGNANCIES
Lymphoma

The colon may be involved with lymphoma in two ways: first, with a primary lymphoma and second, as part of a generalized lymphoma. With primary disease the cecal area is usually involved. On occasion, multiple areas are affected such as the cecum and transverse colon. Generalized lymphoma typically involves the left colon and rectum.

In the primary type of involvement, the lesion appears as polypoid masses of various sizes (Fig. 10.80). The masses may be multiple and large enough to obstruct the lumen. They also may bleed (Fig. 10.81). These masses are firm, indurated, and may be friable. When the colon is involved as part of a generalized process, the findings are less specific and may occur as a friable, indurated, erythematous mucosa. Rarely, an exophytic malignant annular stricture develops, indistinguishable from that seen in adenocarcinoma. The occurrence of multiple tiny flat or slightly raised polypoid lesions is rare and easily overlooked unless dye-scattering techniques are used (Figs. 10.82 and 10.83). These lesions can be confused with those of FPC. Biopsy is essential in this differential diagnosis.

Kaposi's Sarcoma

Kaposi's sarcoma, a tumor seen with increasing frequency mainly in the population with AIDS, may involve any segment of the intestine, including the esophagus, stomach, small intestine, and colon. When Kaposi's sarcoma involves the gastrointestinal tract, the colon is involved in approximately one-half of the cases.

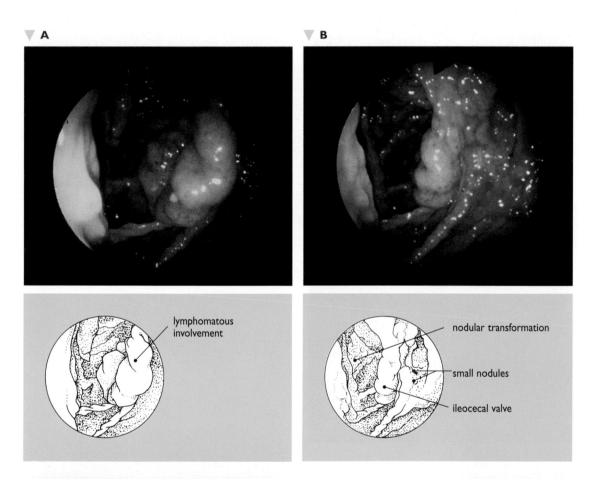

Figure 10.80 *Lymphomatous invasion of the ileocecal area appears as mild erythema of the enlarged ileocecal valve (**A**) and nodular irregularity of the surrounding mucosa (**B**).*

lymphomatous involvement

nodular transformation

small nodules

ileocecal valve

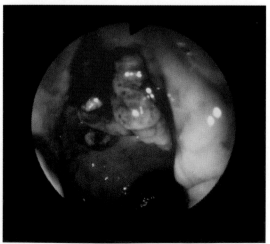

Figure 10.81 *Bleeding lymphoma of the sigmoid colon in a patient diagnosed with AIDS.*

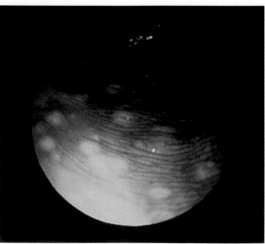

Figure 10.82 *Monotonous lymphomatous invasion mimics FPC. The numerous, slightly raised, whitish structures are easily overlooked without dye-scattering.*

The most common appearance is an intensely red, raised macule (Fig. 10.84). The surface is often slightly irregular. Other appearances are less common. The lesions may be multiple and resemble small polyps of an inflammatory nature (Fig. 10.85). The early Kaposi's sarcoma lesion may be very small (Fig. 10.86). The lesions may also occur with a configuration of a dense cluster of polyps with destruction of long segments of the colonic wall (Fig. 10.87). Biopsies of these lesions show the typical elongated cells with increased blood vessel components.

Metastases of the colon

Involvement of the colon with carcinoma of other organs occurs in two forms: direct extension and distant metastases to the colonic wall. Both are rare.

When an adjacent organ invades the colon it may produce a submucosal mass or a narrowed segment. The tumor often spreads submucosally so the overlying mucosa is normal or minimally abnormal with slight erythema (Fig. 10.88). This pattern may occur with cancer of the pelvic organs. In the future, echo endoscopy may help to define the presence of a mass and the extent of the involvement.

The second type of spread is that of metastases to the wall. These lesions may grow in the wall and then extend through the mucosa so that the appearance from inside the bowel lumen is that of an abnormal mucosa covering a small polyp up to 2 cm in diameter. These tumors can outgrow their blood supply and present with a depression or ulceration on the tip. The tumors that commonly metastasize in this manner include gastric, renal, pancreatic, breast, and melanoma. When the tumor is a melanoma, as in the upper gastrointestinal tract, it may be pigmented with brown or black coloration or, if large, it may be amelanotic.

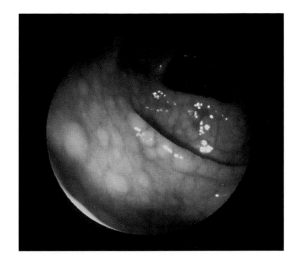

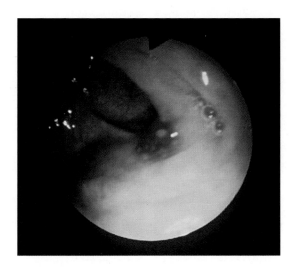

Figure 10.83 *Numerous, minute, whitish lymphomatous foci are easily overlooked.*

Figure 10.84 *Solitary Kaposi's sarcoma lesion in the colon is visible as a slightly raised, purple–red macule.*

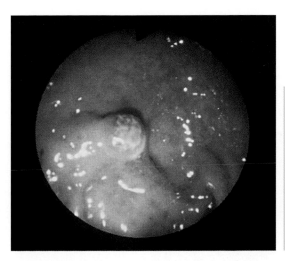

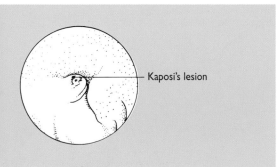

Kaposi's lesion

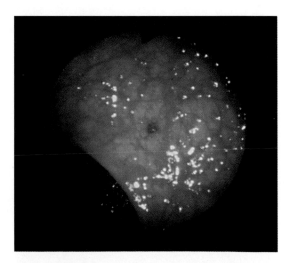

Figure 10.85 *Early Kaposi's sarcoma lesion in the colon of a patient diagnosed with AIDS. The lesion mimics an inflammatory pseudopolyp.*

Figure 10.86 *Early Kaposi's sarcoma in an AIDS patient with a single small red macule.*

BIOPSY OF COLONIC MALIGNANCIES

Any suspicious abnormality of the rectocolon should be extensively biopsied to establish a diagnosis and to direct therapy. In general, necrotic tumor tissue should not be biopsied. Biopsy of fresh, nonulcerated, malignant tissue or tissue from the edges between the exophytic overhanging borders and the ulcerative defects increases the likelihood of obtaining a positive specimen (Fig. 10.89).

Simple forceps biopsy is a relatively high yielding procedure in most cases of exophytic growth pattern cancer. Low yield, even for exophytic lesions, may be related to inability to position the instrument *en face* to the lesion. When the lesion is seen tangentially, it may not be possible to sample the surface of the cancer where it has broken through the mucosa. Moreover, biopsy forceps may fail to penetrate deeply enough to allow diagnosis of invasive cancer.

Sampling normal-looking mucosa at the edge of a malignant stricture is not usually productive. Even biopsies taken blindly from within the strictured area may not reveal malignancy. Brush cytology is most valuable in this situation, as brushing deep within the stenotic segment of a lesion may recover neoplastic cells.

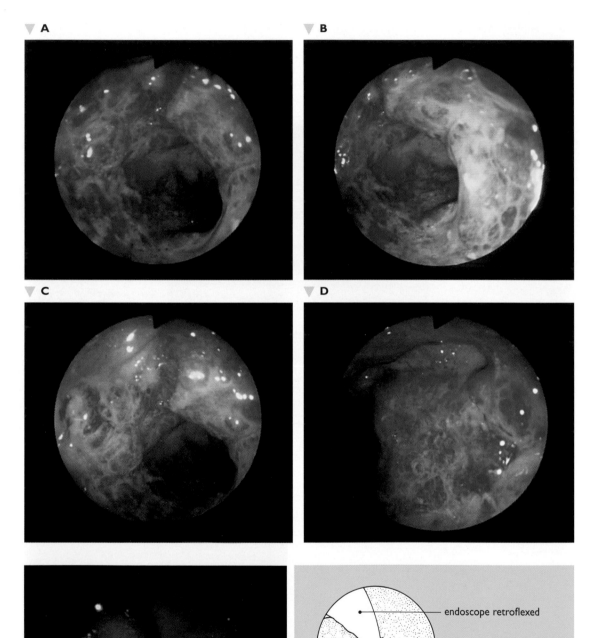

▼ **A**

▼ **B**

▼ **C**

▼ **D**

Figure 10.87 (**A–D**) *Extensive Kaposi's sarcoma of the rectum in AIDS patients. This is rarely seen.*

endoscope retroflexed

bulge caused by metastasis

Figure 10.88 *Extramucosal impression caused by submucosal bladder carcinoma metastasis.*

PALLIATIVE TREATMENT OF COLONIC NEOPLASIA

High grade obstruction of the colon must be relieved by proximal diversion, resection, or endoscopic palliation. Ultimately, therapy depends on the cause of the obstruction. Palliative tumor destruction may be carried out with electrocoagulation, freezing, or with Nd:YAG laser energy. Laser photodestruction is especially indicated for chronically bleeding tumors or to open up obstruct-

ing colorectal malignancies (Fig. 10.90). This palliative approach is especially useful in elderly patients to avoid emergency colostomy in an unprepared colon. Usually one or two sessions are sufficient to reopen the bowel (Figs. 10.91 to 10.93). Laser treatment may not be possible for tortuous lesions or lesions located at acute bends. Occasionally complete eradication of bulky exophytic malignancies can be obtained with laser photocoagulation.

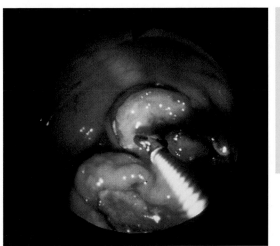

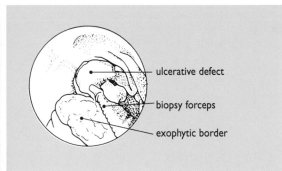

Figure 10.89 Guided biopsy from rim between overhanging border and excavated area.

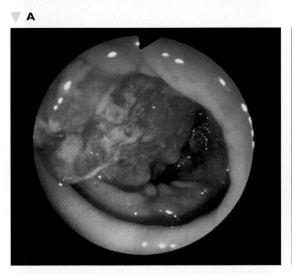

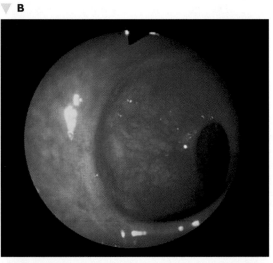

Figure 10.90 (A) A bulky exophytic rectal cancer before laser treatment. **(B)** Full eradication of the cancerous mass is apparent after four Nd:YAG applications.

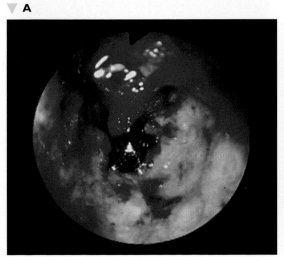

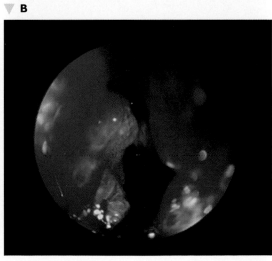

Figure 10.91 (A) Total colonic obstruction by carcinoma. **(B)** The lumen is re-established after laser therapy.

Ulceration may be noted after laser therapy of colonic neoplasia (Fig. 10.94), as may scarring (Fig. 10.95), which may be circumferential (Fig. 10.96). The neoplasm may recur and a carcinoma may be encountered where a villous adenoma was previously treated (Fig. 10.97). This underlines the real need for lifetime follow-up of these patients. Palliative therapy can dramatically improve a patient's symptoms and quality of life.

ENDOSONOGRAPHY OF COLORECTAL ADENOCARCINOMA

Endosonography can be used to image carcinomas of the colon and rectum. Imaging can be accomplished using blind transrectal probes (passed without visual endoscopic guidance) to image the rectum and surrounding structures, or ultrasound devices (attached to the endoscope tip or passed via the biopsy channel) to image the colon or rectum. The depth of tumor penetration into the wall can be seen, as can any involvement of adjacent structures. This information is important for the accurate staging of tumors and the planning of subsequent therapy (Figs. 10.98 to 10.100).

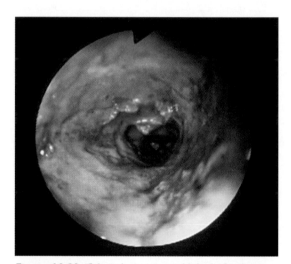

Figure 10.92 *Colonic lumen re-established after laser therapy of obstructing circumferential cancer.*

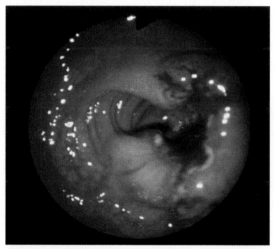

Figure 10.93 *A carcinoma obstructing the colon has been treated with a laser to reopen the lumen. The white mucosa at the tumor rim is coagulated tissue.*

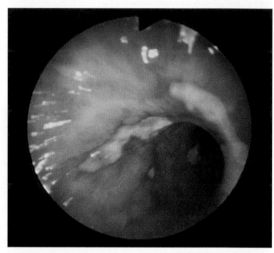

Figure 10.94 *Large colonic ulcers after laser treatment of a villous polyp.*

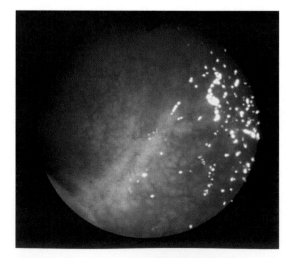

Figure 10.95 *Scarring of colon wall after laser therapy.*

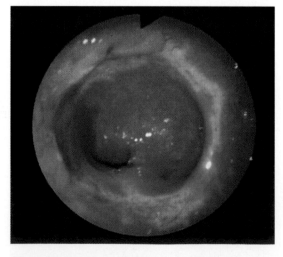

Figure 10.96 *Circular fibrosis of colon after laser therapy of circumferential villous adenoma.*

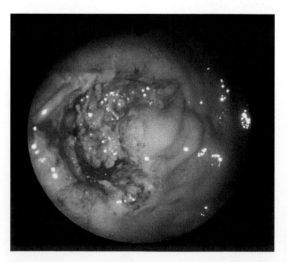

Figure 10.97 *This infiltrating colon cancer occurred after prior laser therapy of a villous adenoma in the same area.*

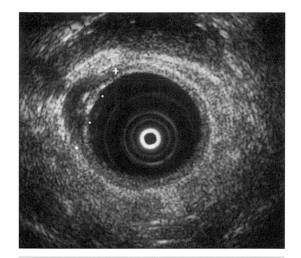

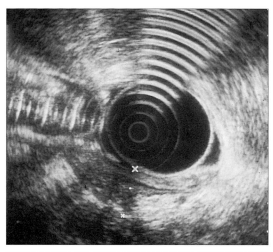

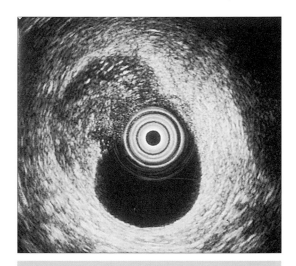

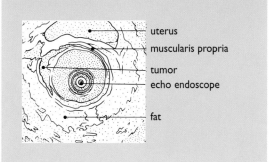

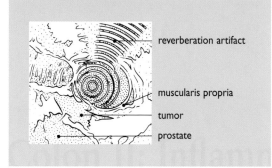

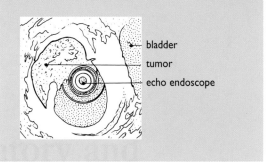

Figure 10.98 *Rectal cancer. The tumor is seen penetrating the muscularis propria and into the adjacent fat tissue.*

Figure 10.99 *Rectal cancer. The tumor is seen deeply penetrating the muscularis propria with some invasion of the capsule of the prostate. The reverberation artifact is caused by an adjacent biopsy channel.*

Figure 10.100 *Carcinoma of sigmoid colon imaged with a 10 MHz prototype echo endoscope. The tumor is polypoid and hypoechoic, and can be seen to penetrate the subserosal layer of the sigmoid colon.*

IDIOPATHIC INFLAMMATORY BOWEL DISEASE

Ulcerative colitis and Crohn's disease are called idiopathic because neither their etiology nor pathogenesis is completely understood. The basic features indicating inflammation are swelling, erythema, mucoid or purulent exudation, mild or severe epithelial destruction (ranging from tiny superficial erosive defects to serpiginous, linear, or deep ulcers), fine or coarse granular deformity of the mucosa, pseudopolyp formation, retraction, and stricturing.

Colonoscopy is an established procedure for evaluating patients with inflammatory disorders of the large bowel. Direct inspection of the mucosa and the ability to obtain mucosal biopsies provide high diagnostic accuracy. Few endoscopic changes, when considered separately, are specific. In addition, the range of abnormalities produced by the mucosal lining in response to injury is limited.

Despite the lack of specificity, a presumptive diagnosis of idiopathic inflammatory bowel disease is usually possible by a compilation of the relevant findings. Idiopathic disease must be differentiated from the various forms of infectious colitis, antibiotic-associated colitis, and ischemic damage of the colon. In a vast majority of patients, colonoscopy may enable precise determination of the distribution of the abnormalities and the extent and severity of involvement. Consideration of previous topical or systemic therapy is essential because this may obscure or interfere with the more characteristic elements of the inflammatory features.

Endoscopy also provides a route for obtaining mucosal biopsies, which are required for differential diagnosis, detection of dysplasia, and diagnosis of carcinoma. Tissue for flow cytometry and other diagnostic tests can also be obtained. These procedures are all important to the diagnosis and surveillance of patients with colitis.

ULCERATIVE COLITIS

Active ulcerative colitis inflames the mucosa in a continuous symmetrical fashion. The colitis may extend throughout the colon or may involve only part of it; characteristically, the rectal mucosa is affected. The diagnosis is usually made by history and proctosigmoidoscopy, but colonoscopy may provide a more exact evaluation. An accurate determination of extent depends upon total intubation to the cecum, which is usually relatively easy because of the foreshortening and tubularization of the colon.

Endoscopic Appearance

There is no unique macroscopic, mucosal abnormality pathognomonic for the endoscopic diagnosis of ulcerative colitis. Copious amounts of mucoid discharge seen as white creamy material covering the mucosa may be the most conspicuous sign of early disease or flare-up (Fig. 11.1).

With minimal inflammation, the mucosal vascular pattern may disappear or look blunted or blurred. The obliteration is caused by edema and inflammation of the lamina propria. The vascular appearance is abnormal in that the branching pattern is markedly irregular and distorted in contrast to the normally smooth gradual tapering and arcading of the vessels (Fig. 11.2). Abnormal vascular patterns are partially caused by the loss of mucosal transparency, which may be the only visible abnormality in the quiescent or healing stage of ulcerative colitis.

Erythema is caused by mucosal capillary dilation and is usually diffuse (Fig. 11.3). The erythematous mucosa is friable and bleeds easily after trivial amounts of pressure (Fig. 11.4). Erythema indicates active mucosal involvement, especially when associated with granularity and a distorted or absent vascular pattern. The presence of loosely adherent yellow–brown mucopurulent exudate indicates even more active disease than does erythema (Fig. 11.5).

Granularity is a visual manifestation of fine or coarse surface irregularity. The normally homogeneous light reflex disappears, indicative of the granular change in the normally smooth mucosa (Figs. 11.2 and 11.6).

Superficial or deep epithelial necrosis or ulceration results from extensive epithelial destruction and crypt abscess formation. Single or multiple ulcerations, varying from a few millimeters to several centimeters in diameter, are to be expected in active ulcerative colitis. They may be linear (Fig. 11.7), serpiginous, circular, or oval. Whatever the form or shape, the ulcers' most common characteristic feature is the erythematous and friable mucosa in which they are located (Fig. 11.8).

Ulceration may be very severe with little mucosa remaining (Fig. 11.9). Deep ulcers may show submucosa or muscularis propria at the base (Fig. 11.10). Severe ulcerative colitis may be associated with spontaneous bleeding (Fig. 11.11).

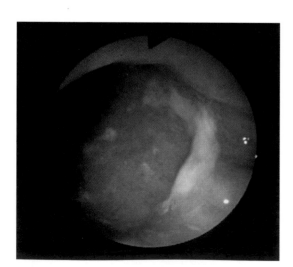

Figure 11.1 Abundant mucous discharge is an early sign of acute flare-up of ulcerative colitis.

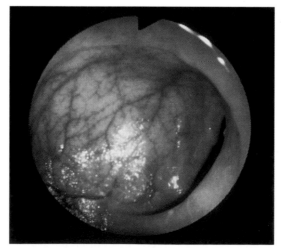

Figure 11.2 Ulcerative colitis in remission. Fine granular appearance is shown by multiple tiny dots of reflecting light. Note mild blurring of vascular pattern.

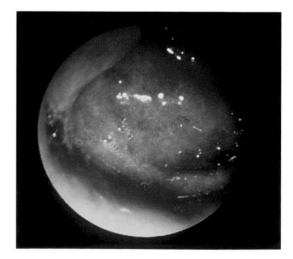

Figure 11.3 Chronic mild ulcerative colitis with mucosal erythema and friability.

Inflammatory Pseudopolyps

Inflammatory polypoid structures or pseudopolyps are thought to develop from epithelial buds that remain in areas of extensive ulceration or at margins of ulceration. As the ulcerations heal and the acute inflammation subsides, focally nodular areas of remaining mucosa protrude, resulting in the formation of inflammatory polyps or pseudopolyps. These are usually multiple, and range from little more than mucosal excrescences of a few millimeters up to 1 cm diameter. Occasionally single lesions may exceed 1.5 cm (Fig. 11.12).

Inflammatory polyps may be broad-based, sessile, or pedunculated. They have a soft texture, and are easily compressible and friable. Often, they are covered with a whitish cap of exudate (Fig. 11.13). The larger pseudopolyps

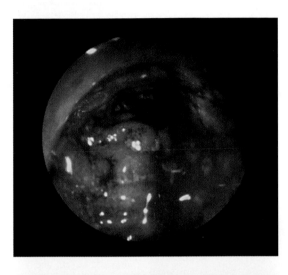

Figure 11.4 *Active ulcerative colitis. Markedly friable mucosa, which bled after one pass with the colonoscope.*

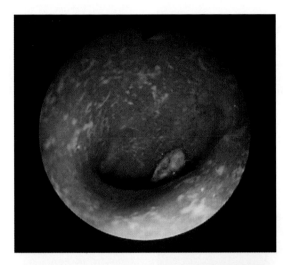

Figure 11.5 *Scattered mucopurulent exudate with obvious erythema and blurring of vascular pattern in active ulcerative colitis.*

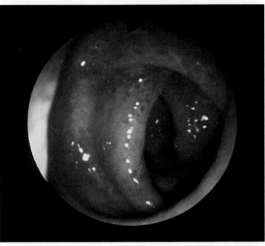

Figure 11.6 *Early ulcerative colitis with petechiae and dull or granular appearance of folds.*

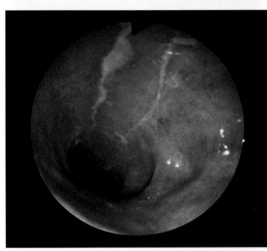

Figure 11.7 *Linear, longitudinal ulceration in the descending colon of a patient with ulcerative colitis. Diffuse erythema, friability, and hemorrhage are also evident.*

▼ **A** ▼ **B** ▼ **C**

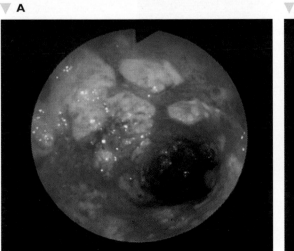 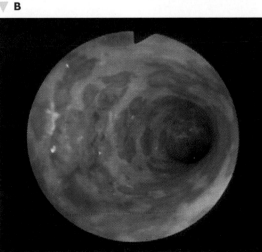 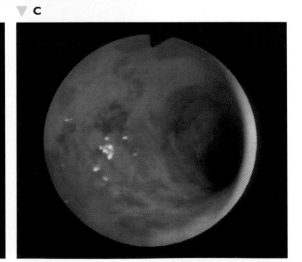

Figure 11.8 (A–C) *Examples of ulceration in active ulcerative colitis. Background mucosa shows marked erythema and friability.*

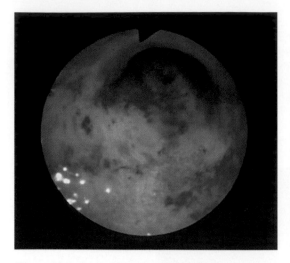

Figure 11.9 *Severe ulcerative colitis with extensive ulceration and little remaining mucosa.*

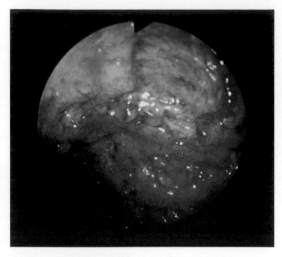

Figure 11.10 *Severe chronic ulcerative colitis with deep ulcer thought to be impending perforation. Muscularis propria seen in base of deep ulcer.*

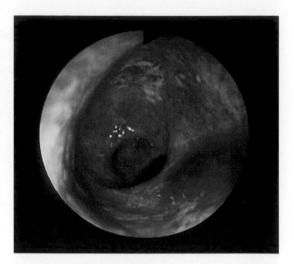

Figure 11.11 *Patient with severe ulcerative colitis with profuse spontaneous bleeding.*

▼ **A**

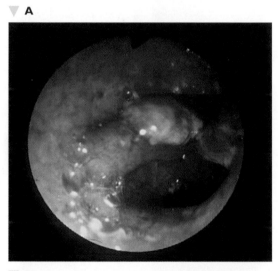

Figure 11.12 *Large pseudopolyps in chronic ulcerative colitis (A) give a characteristic x-ray appearance (B).*

▼ **A**

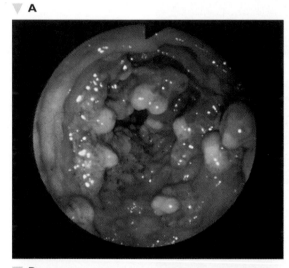

Figure 11.13 *(A and B) Multiple pseudopolyps in ulcerative colitis. Their surface is smooth and glistening. Exudate creates the whitish caps.*

▼ **B**

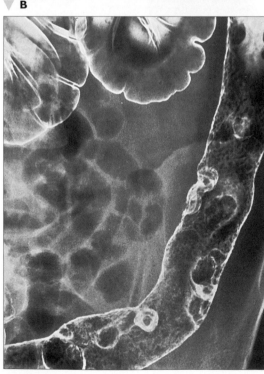

▼ **B**

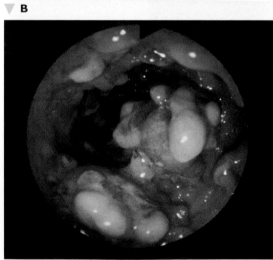

in particular may be eroded or ulcerated on the surface. Sometimes the pseudopolypoid bulges show a striking erythema, contrasting with the pale surrounding mucosa seen in the remission phase of the disease (Fig. 11.14).

A less common finding is that of many clusters of flimsy finger-like mucosal projections (Fig. 11.15). Such long filamentous pseudopolyps, especially those arising in grape-like clusters, are characteristic of ulcerative colitis. Rarely, the pseudopolypoid structures are interconnected by bridging mucosal folds (Fig. 11.16). These probably form as a consequence of undermining ulcers that leave a latticework appearance (Figs. 11.17 and 11.18).

▼ A   ▼ B

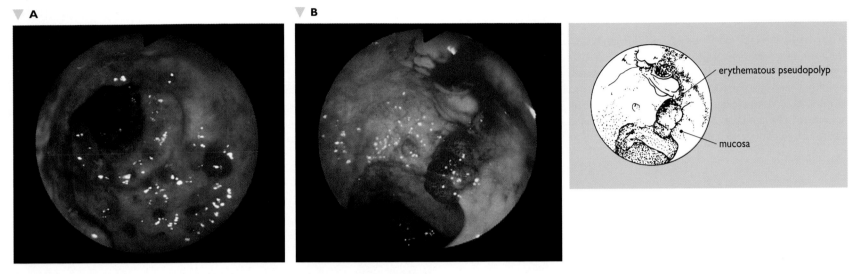

Figure 11.14 **A)** *Pseudopolyps in ulcerative colitis occur here as cherry red spheres.* **(B)** *Larger pseudopolyp shows striking erythema, which contrasts with the paler mucosa. Ulcerative colitis is in the quiescent phase.*

▼ A   ▼ B

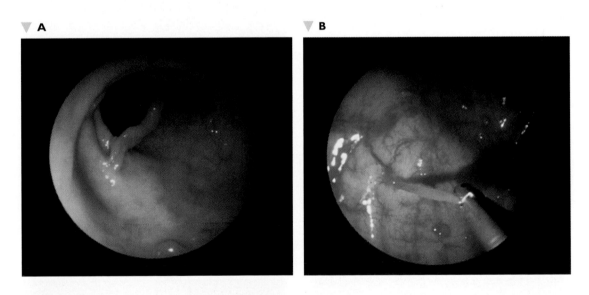

Figure 11.15 *Filiform polyps.* **(A)** *Filiform polyp.* **(B)** *A biopsy forceps demonstrates their filamentous nature.*

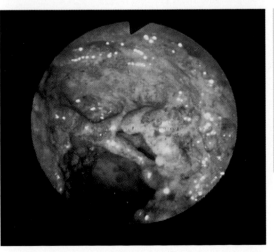

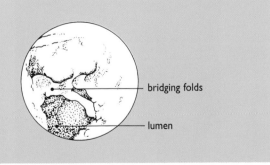

Figure 11.16 *Active ulcerative colitis with bridging mucosal folds.*

In cases of severe ulceration with intervening large inflammatory pseudo-polyps, coarse nodular deformity of the mucosal contour occurs. Typically, the mucosa surrounding the ulcerations is abnormal with pronounced erythema and friability (Fig. 11.19). This is in contrast to the cobblestone-like appearance in Crohn's disease, in which the mucosa surrounding ulcers is only slightly erythematous or even looks normal with a preserved mucosal vascular pattern.

Anatomic Variations Caused by Ulcerative Colitis

Inflammatory changes within the mucosa may produce structural abnormalities. Many of the structural changes are primarily the result of edematous swelling, inflammatory infiltration, muscle contraction, and muscle hypertrophy. Loss of sharpness of the interhaustral folds or valvulae is an early structural change (Fig. 11.20). The thickened and blunted appearance is caused by swelling and inflammation, and is most noticeable in the transverse colon where the expected sharp, thin, triangular folds become rounded and appear broader. Disappearance of the interhaustral fold pattern, which is generally thought to result from hypertrophy and contraction of the teniae coli, suggests chronic disease.

Ongoing muscle hypertrophy and retraction may substantially decrease the width of the colonic lumen. Sometimes the lumen contracts to less than 13 mm in diameter, barely admitting a standard colonoscope. Loss of the haustral pattern and narrowing of the lumen create a tubular appearance (Fig. 11.21).

Strictures may form in ulcerative colitis, mainly due to focal muscle hypertrophy and retraction. They tend to be composed of thickened smooth muscle; by contrast, strictures in Crohn's disease are fibrotic. At the area of narrowing, one characteristically sees superficial or deep ulceration with markedly erythematous and friable intervening mucosa (Fig. 11.22). The presence of intact nodular indurated mucosa without ulceration is atypical and suggests possible malignancy.

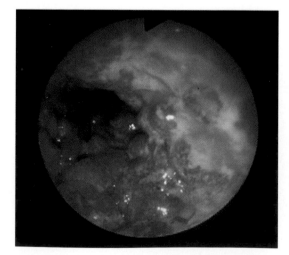
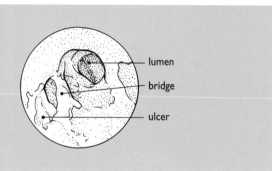
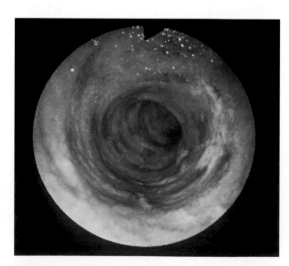

Figure 11.17 *Ulcerative colitis and bridging associated with ulceration.*

Figure 11.18 *Ulcerative colitis with pseudopolyps and bridging.*

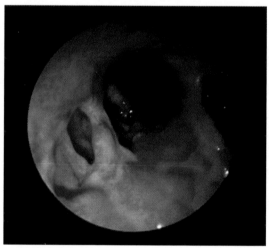
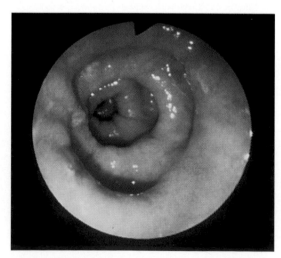
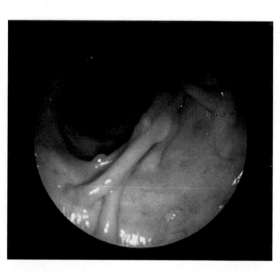

Figure 11.19 *Coarsely nodular deformity of mucosal contour in ulcerative colitis. Mucosa is intensely erythematous and friable.*

Figure 11.20 *Thick and blunt interhaustral folds in the distal transverse colon are an early structural abnormality in ulcerative colitis.*

Figure 11.21 *Tubularization of the colon occurs in longstanding ulcerative colitis. Plaques of exudate and punctiform petechial hemorrhages are also apparent.*

Strictures resulting from inflammation are relatively short; as they are distensible, they can be entered using a narrow caliber endoscope. Strictures longer than 5 cm should raise suspicion of malignancy. Benign strictures are easily distensible. However, all strictures must be biopsied because a smooth contour does not exclude dysplasia or underlying malignancy. Strictures too narrow for an endoscope are usually surgically removed as future surveillance would be impossible.

Chronic, long-standing, ulcerative colitis may lead to effacement of the ileocecal valve, usually associated with a narrowing in caliber of the right colon (Fig. 11.23). The valve appears patulous with a diameter approximating that of the terminal ileum. Because the ileocecal valve is effaced and patulous, the colonoscope can enter the terminal ileum easily. Often there is evidence of back-wash ileitis – tubularization of the terminal ileum with disappearance of the mucosal fold pattern. This occurs in patients with total colonic involvement. The smooth mucosa may show evidence of inflammatory activity such as patchy or diffuse erythema and friability. Mucosal ulceration is not part of this entity except in severe cases of backwash (Fig. 11.24).

Distribution of Lesions

Before treatment, a conspicuous gradient in disease activity is usually apparent, with more severe disease located towards the rectum. There is often a sharp transition from normal to diseased intestine (Fig. 11.25). In some instances, however, the abnormalities at the anatomically proximal extent of the disease may appear patchy (Fig. 11.26). In severe disease there may be

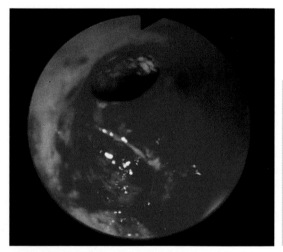
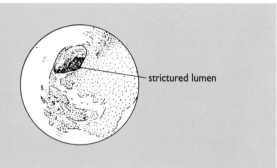

Figure 11.22 *Ulcerative colitis with stricturing. Attempts to pass the stricture caused bleeding. Ulceration is present around the mouth of the stricture.*

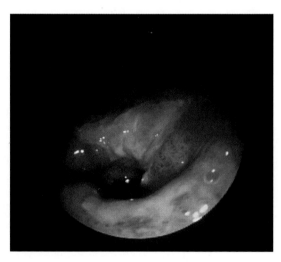

Figure 11.23 *Severe, unhealed ulcerative colitis resulted in this ulcerated and incompetent ileocecal valve.*

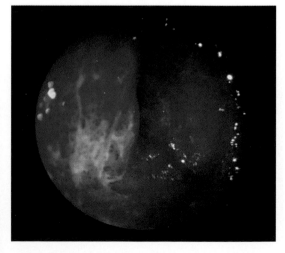

Figure 11.24 *Severe inflammation and ulceration of the distal terminal ileum are due to backwash or reflux ileitis.*

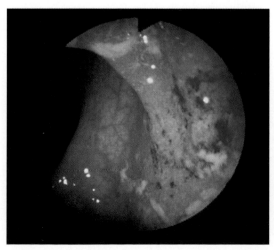
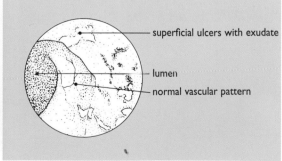

Figure 11.25 *Sharp transition from normal to inflamed bowel is discernible at the rectosigmoid junction. Erythema and superficial ulceration of diseased mucosa contrast with the normal vascular pattern above the transition.*

rectal sparing or less pronounced rectal involvement, with deep ulceration starting at or beyond the rectosigmoid junction. A continuous symmetrical involvement from the rectum to the point of the highest extent of involvement is characteristic.

Distinct patterns of involvement may be recognized based on the extent of the disease. Total colitis is diagnosed when the entire colon is involved. Usually the activity is more severe distally, especially in the distal descending colon, sigmoid colon, and rectum. In less than total involvement, the disease usually terminates at the hepatic flexure. In left-sided involvement, the disease stops at or just proximal to the splenic flexure, where a relatively sharp demarcation usually can be seen. An occasional patient may have predominantly right-sided involvement of the colon in a diffuse manner with ulceration and pseudopolyp formation, whereas the left side of the colon shows only minimal or discrete abnormalities.

In rectosigmoid colitis, the disease is confined to the rectum and sigmoid colon. When only the rectum is involved, this is termed proctitis. As a rule, there is a sharp inflammatory demarcation between the rectum and the sigmoid colon.

Levels of Activity

In nonactive or quiescent ulcerative colitis, the colitic mucosa appears normal except for some alteration of the vascular pattern or the presence of fine granularity. There may also be slight friability and a few petechiae.

There is no widely accepted system for determining activity of ulcerative colitis, but it can be divided into three stages.

- Mildly active colitis: unequivocal erythema, either diffuse or focal. The mucosal vascular pattern may be either distorted or absent.
- Moderately active colitis: single or scattered small ulcerations in a limited section of the colon. In addition, there is erythema, friability, granularity, and mucopurulent exudate.
- Severe colitis: deeper, larger, more numerous ulcers, often with spontaneous bleeding, marked friability, and excessive amounts of mucopurulent exudate.

The severity of the colitis may be underestimated if only the rectum is evaluated and if topical therapy with corticosteroids or 5-aminosalicylic acid, delivered rectally, has already been given. The rectal mucosa may even look normal despite unequivocal edema, erythema, and friability in the more anatomically proximal colon (Fig. 11.27). Reappearance of inflammatory

changes during flare-up may be more obvious in the more proximal colon than in the distal (previously topically treated) segment. Therefore, evaluation of the severity of a flare-up may be misleading if only the rectum is inspected.

The loss of the rectal indicator function after topical therapy is unfortunate because many clinicians use the macroscopic appearance of the rectum to titrate therapy. Increasingly, flexible sigmoidoscopy is used to visualize the sigmoid colon. This should more precisely mirror overall disease activity.

Frequent inspection of the inflamed mucosa using a small caliber endoscope without bowel preparation may improve clinical evaluation during severe attacks and may be helpful in deciding whether medical therapy should be continued. Healing through re-epithelialization may occur even after extensive ulceration, provided that medical therapy controls the inflammatory process (Fig. 11.28). Occasionally the appearance of the healing stage is bizarre (Fig. 11.29).

As the mucosa responds to medical therapy, the symmetrical diffuse pattern of involvement may be lost or may become less evident. Such inequality of involvement may occasionally lead to error in diagnosis. As a rule, the endoscopic aspect before therapy is always more informative for the differential diagnosis than the appearance during or after medical therapy.

Risk of Dysplasia or Malignancy

Patients with universal, subtotal, or possibly even left-sided, ulcerative colitis are considered to have an enhanced cancer risk after 10-years. The magnitude of the increased risk is not definitively established. Colonoscopy can be used to identify patients particularly at risk by looking for histologic evidence of severe dysplasia, and by obtaining tissue for flow cytometric analysis to detect abnormalities in DNA. Surveillance is important in individual patients, but will have little impact on overall colon cancer mortality rates because only 1% of colorectal cancer is associated with a history of previous ulcerative colitis.

During screening colonoscopy, as much of the surface as possible should be inspected for the macroscopic appearance of colonic cancer and dysplasia-associated lesions or masses. Some investigators recommend that four-quadrant biopsies should be taken at approximately 10 cm intervals for histologic evidence of dysplasia. Additional biopsies should be obtained from areas showing surface irregularity and from large polypoid lesions. Areas that differ in appearance from the small, shiny or worm-like benign inflammatory pseudopolyps, frequently seen after a severe attack of colitis, should also be sampled.

▼ A   ▼ B

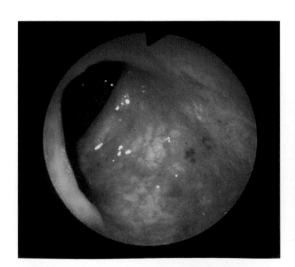

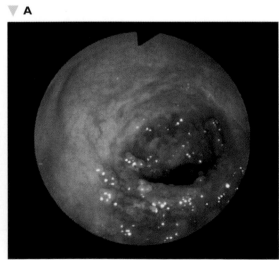

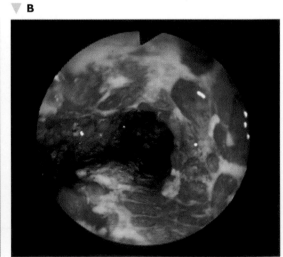

Figure 11.26 *Distal transverse colon of an ulcerative colitis patient displays patchy distribution of erythema and blurring of vascular pattern.*

Figure 11.27 *Topical therapy causes obvious improvement of rectal disease with reappearance of a vascular pattern. Notice the transition to the markedly abnormal sigmoid colon (**A**). Above this transition there is ongoing severe disease with marked ulceration in the sigmoid colon (**B**).*

Dysplasia may be identified as an unequivocal neoplastic alteration of the colonic epithelium. Dysplastic mucosa is arbitrarily divided into low-grade and high-grade, the latter including carcinoma *in situ*. The presence of high-grade dysplasia, especially if present on more than one examination or in several locations, carries a high risk of a coexisting cancer or impending cancer formation. Because these cancers may still be intramural, they could easily escape endoscopic detection.

Flat dysplasia and macroscopic dysplasia can be studied by colonoscopy. There may be no macroscopic feature to suggest flat dysplasia. Rather, abnormal tissue is detected in routine random biopsies. Occasionally, dysplasia will occur with a flat, focal, villous-like or wart-like appearance that can be recognized as different from the granular-type mucosal unevenness common to quiescent ulcerative colitis (Fig. 11.30).

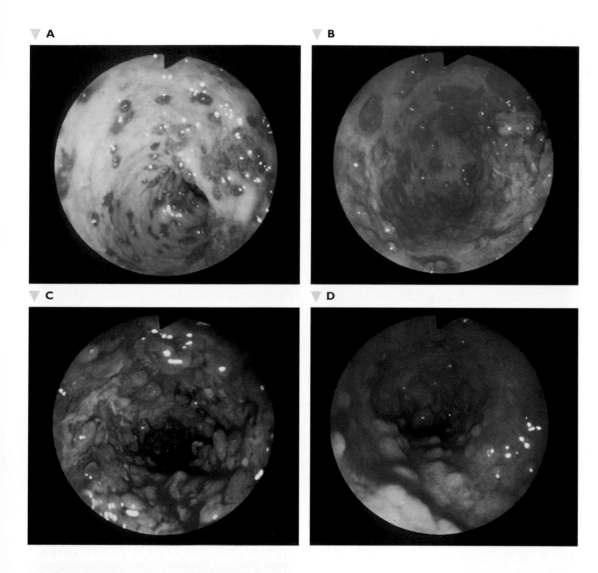

A

B

C

D

Figure 11.28 *Sequential study of severe pancolitis. Massive ulceration of the colon was studied at intervals of 4–6 weeks after institution of medical therapy. (**A**) This view of the proximal sigmoid colon shows extensive ulceration before therapy. Some islands of remaining mucosa are visible. (**B**) Regression of inflammation and early re-epithelialization are noted here. (**C**) In this view ulcers are regressing with pseudopolypoid elevation of nonulcerated mucosal islands. (**D**) Full re-epithelialization and pseudopolypoid transformation characterize healing.*

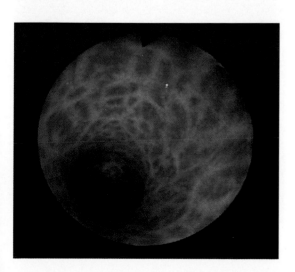

Figure 11.29 *Healing stage after extensive ulceration of rectum. Interconnecting, lace-like whitish stripes correspond to areas of previous ulceration.*

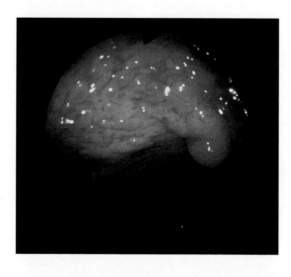

Figure 11.30 *Irregular wart-like deformity of the mucosal lining due to severe dysplasia. Small nodular elevations are also present.*

Macroscopic dysplasia is associated with polypoid masses or other macroscopic appearances termed dysplasia-associated lesions or masses (DALM). The appearance of DALM may be variable (Fig. 11.31). Occasionally, one may see a single, 2–4 cm in diameter, sessile polypoid mass with a slightly irregular nonulcerated surface. Sometimes multiple 5–15 mm polypoid bulges of firm consistency are clustered together; these usually present with ill defined borders. DALM may also appear as slightly elevated nodular, plaque-like areas extending over a finite distance. Hence, any irregular or elevated area or polyp should be carefully inspected; biopsies should be taken of the apex and in particular of any nodularity surrounding the lesion.

It may be impossible in chronic ulcerative colitis to distinguish an isolated adenoma from a polypoid area of dysplasia as both are composed of identical-looking neoplastic epithelium (Fig. 11.32). There is an arbitrary tendency to regard such lesions as examples of dysplasia in younger patients,

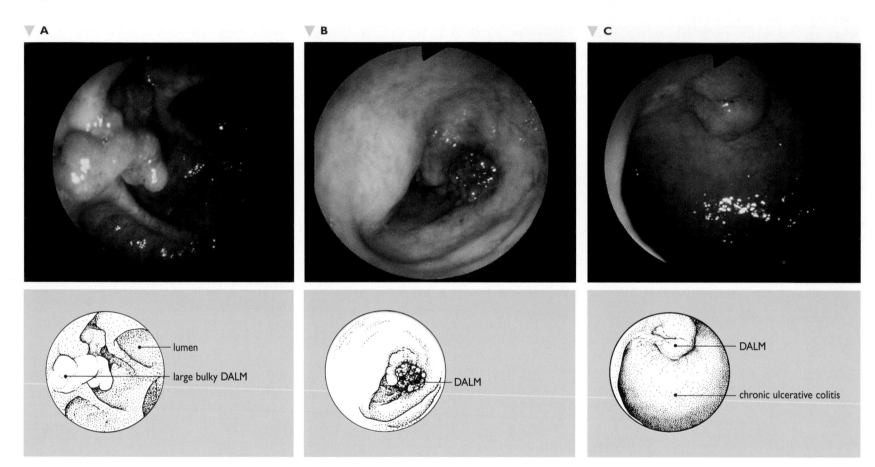

Figure 11.31 (**A–C**) Examples of DALM in long-standing inactive ulcerative colitis.

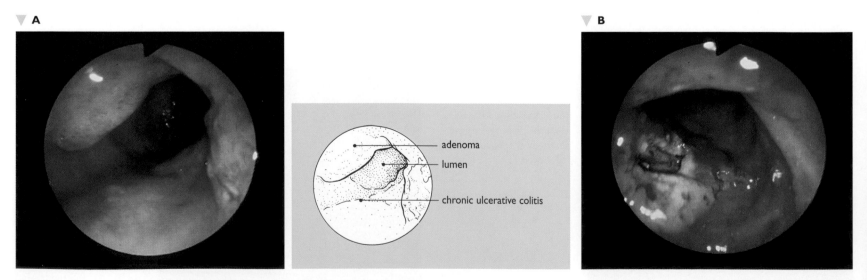

Figure 11.32 (**A**) Chronic ulcerative colitis with an adenoma. (**B**) After polypectomy of this sessile adenoma a wide coagulation defect is seen.

with the implication of an impending need for colectomy, whereas in older patients they are usually considered unrelated to the colitis and treated simply by polypectomy. However, it is best in all cases to seek further evidence of dysplasia in the mucosa immediately adjacent to the polyp or along its stalk because the polyp may prove to be part of a larger area of dysplasia. Polypectomy may not be curative if dysplasia is present in these other sites. When in doubt, any nonstalked adenoma, as reported by the pathologist, should be assumed to be a local area of precancerous dysplasia.

Biopsy

During endoscopic examinations, biopsies should be taken from plaques; from nodular, thickened, or villous-appearing areas; from slightly elevated areas; from areas that appear velvety or show minor roughness; and from other unusual polypoid lesions and stenotic regions. Polypoid lesions should be especially biopsied when they show irregularities and friability of the mucosal surface, and when they are large and of firm consistency.

If no suspicious areas are visible, multiple random biopsies of otherwise flat or uninvolved mucosa should be taken from all regions of the colon at 10*cm intervals so that a total of eight or nine sets of biopsies are taken. Ordinary-appearing inflammatory pseudopolyps and small areas of active inflammation are best avoided as histopathologic interpretation may be difficult and such areas are rarely dysplastic. Because of the difficulties of histologic interpretation during the active phases of colitis, patients should be examined preferentially during a quiescent phase of their disease. Mucosal biopsies should be separately labeled by colonic segment to permit return to a specific area in the event of a suspicious or positive finding.

Although a high proportion of patients with dysplasia in colonoscopic biopsies also have dysplasia in rectosigmoidoscopic biopsies, most experts agree than multiple biopsies from various parts of the colon are desirable. The frequency of colonoscopy with biopsies is a matter of opinion, logistics, patient acceptance, and results of previous examinations. Most large centers are making annual colonoscopy examinations of patients with a 10-year or longer history of chronic ulcerative colitis involving the whole colon. The procedure may be performed more often in patients with suspicious findings on previous examination. It may be necessary to repeat the colonoscopy after several weeks to rebiopsy if high-grade dysplasia is noted on the first examination. Other patients with normal findings may have colonoscopy with biopsies every 2 years. Whether patients with colitis confined to the left half of the colon should be submitted to a surveillance program is a matter of debate.

Biopsies yielding high-grade dysplasia justify serious consideration of colectomy in view of the high rate of synchronous occult carcinoma. This recommendation must be weighed against the immediate and long-term morbidity and mortality of the operation and sequelae. It is always wise to have an experienced pathologist confirm the diagnosis by demonstrating dysplasia in more than one biopsy specimen taken at the same colonoscopy, and in biopsies from the same area during repeat colonoscopy. A second pathologist should review the biopsy findings.

Because repeat colonoscopy is occasionally needed, the examination must be carried out with minimal discomfort to the patient. As the colon in extensive colitis is sometimes shortened and tubular, the endoscopic procedure is often relatively easy and may be done comfortably without sedation. If the colon is tortuous and difficult to examine, patients should be sedated to encourage compliance for repeat examinations.

Cancer in Ulcerative Colitis

The overall risk of cancer in patients with long-standing ulcerative colitis is increased, particularly for patients with universal involvement. The risk is felt to be significantly increased with disease of more than 8–10 years and especially with disease in excess of 20 years. The exact risk, however, is uncertain, as most published reports are from special centers whose patient populations are often skewed towards the most severe cases. As 50% or more of early cancers in ulcerative colitis are located proximal to the splenic flexure area, screening colonoscopy is a means for detecting cancer while it is still curable; sigmoidoscopy alone is not adequate.

The predominant growth pattern in colitic cancers is intramural and infiltrating, presenting a variety of endoscopic findings (Fig. 11.33). A local infiltrating malignancy may give rise to a flat or slightly elevated plaque-like mass with ill defined edges (Fig. 11.34). Colitic cancer may also appear as an ulcerated exophytic mass, indistinguishable from noncolitic cancer (Fig. 11.35). In the case of infiltrating colitic cancer, biopsy may fail to show malignancy. However, biopsies usually reveal high-grade dysplasia.

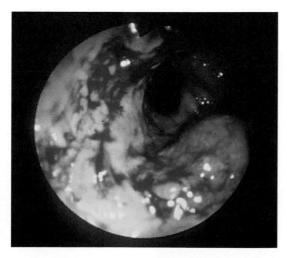

Figure 11.33 *Advanced infiltrating ulcerated cancer in ulcerative colitis.*

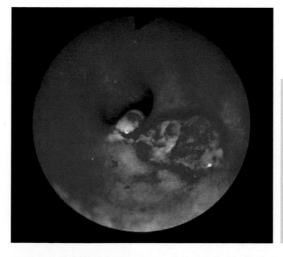

Figure 11.34 *Chronic ulcerative colitis with early plaque-like cancer adjacent to an inflammatory polyp.*

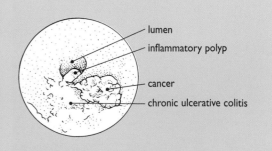

lumen
inflammatory polyp
cancer
chronic ulcerative colitis

A malignant stricture appears at endoscopy as an abrupt narrowing of the lumen. The mouth of the stricture appears nodular and friable but is usually nonulcerative. Biopsies from the mouth of the stricture give the endoscopic impression of a firm surface. Occasionally brush cytology may be a useful procedure for detecting malignancy in stricturing lesions.

Cancer may also present as a single, 2–4 cm diameter, nonulcerated sessile polypoid mass (Fig. 11.36), with a smooth or slightly irregular covering mucosa. Only about one-third of the cancers in ulcerative colitis are of this protuberant variety and may appear similar to polypoid cancer. Less often, cancer may occur as multiple, 1–2 cm diameter sessile polypoid masses with a friable but nonulcerated surface lining. The absence of ulceration and exudation, along with the hard rubbery consistency appreciated on biopsy, distinguishes this lesion from clustering inflammatory pseudopolyps.

CROHN'S DISEASE

Crohn's disease is a chronic inflammatory disease, usually involving the terminal ileum and segments of the colon. Ileocecal or ileocolonic involvement is present in up to 50% of cases. Overall, some colonic involvement is expected in two-thirds of the patients. The focal asymmetrical patchy discontinuous distribution of the lesions contrasts with the diffuse symmetrical continuous involvement in ulcerative colitis.

Endoscopic Appearance

Occasionally, the only endoscopic abnormality in Crohn's disease is diffuse or patchy erythema and mild friability of the mucosa, more or less indistinguishable from that seen in ulcerative colitis (Fig. 11.37). Sometimes zones of redder color alternate with patches manifesting a peculiar, whitish opaqueness. Tiny erythematous spots may also occur during the early phase or early flare-up of Crohn's disease.

Spotty reddening with localized edema is a dominant abnormality during the pre-aphthoid phase of Crohn's disease. Such erythematous mucosal spots or plaques presumably consist of intramucosal hemorrhage, associated with focal crypt abscesses and destruction of crypt epithelium. This spotty erythema may distort the vascular pattern (Fig. 11.38).

Aphthoid erosions are generally regarded as an early specific endoscopic finding in Crohn's disease. They are flat or just slightly depressed and usually less than 5 mm in diameter. They have a characteristic small rim of erythema in the absence of a raised margin, and usually a grayish or yellowish central crater (Fig. 11.39). Often occurring in groups, aphthoid erosions may develop from pre-aphthoid erythematous spots or plaques. They presumably result from partial or total destruction of crypts and surrounding surface epithelium in areas of previous focal inflammation.

Aphthoid erosions may be seen in otherwise normal-appearing mucosa at some distance from more severe lesions (Fig. 11.40). This discontinuity, often termed skip areas, is a key finding. Segments of normal bowel are interspersed between abnormal areas, or one wall will be normal with the opposite or adjacent wall abnormal.

Using dye-scattering techniques, very small aphthoid erosions (microerosions) have a worm-eaten appearance. Such lesions are probably caused by distortion and destruction of the surface epithelium covering lymphoid

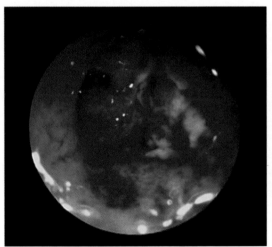

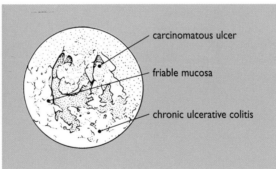

carcinomatous ulcer

friable mucosa

chronic ulcerative colitis

Figure 11.35 *Mass with an ulcer in chronic ulcerative colitis, which proved to be a carcinoma.*

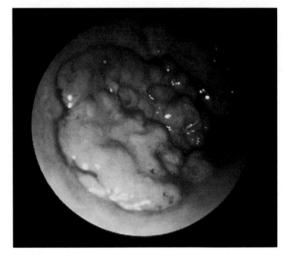

Figure 11.36 *A single nonulcerative sessile cancerous mass present in the sigmoid colon of a patient with long-standing inactive ulcerative colitis.*

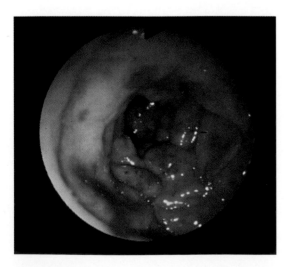

Figure 11.37 *Focal erythema occurring in early flare-up of Crohn's disease.*

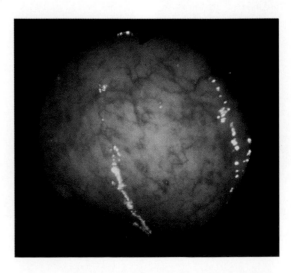

Figure 11.38 *Distortion of vascular pattern with spotty reddening is common in early Crohn's disease.*

aggregates, and are often rich in granulomas. The normal honeycomb pattern becomes distorted and the mucosa fails to take up the dye (Fig. 11.41). In some patients, larger lesions may be seen that resemble white spots. These are probably more advanced lesions than microerosions as they are larger and very slightly raised because of local edema.

From an endoscopic viewpoint, ulceration is a dominant abnormality in Crohn's disease. Between tiny aphthoid erosions and large deep longitudinal ulcers, there is a progression of intermediate forms, varying greatly in shape and depth (Figs. 11.42 to 11.46). Characteristically, such epithelial defects are sharply outlined and abruptly surrounded by normal or only slightly diseased mucosa.

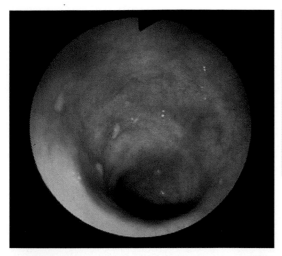

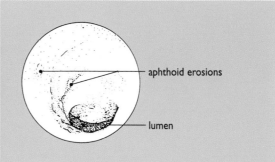

Figure 11.39 *Characteristic superficial aphthoid erosions in Crohn's disease have erythematous rings.*

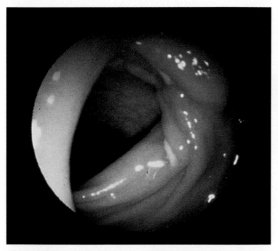

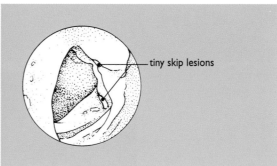

Figure 11.40 *This view shows an example of skip erosions. The entire colon appears normal, except for a tiny patch of aphthoid abnormality in the sigmoid colon.*

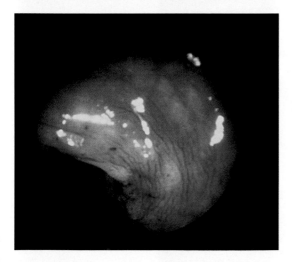

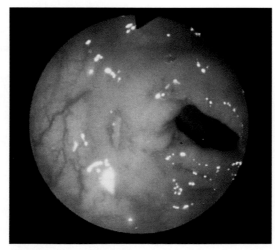

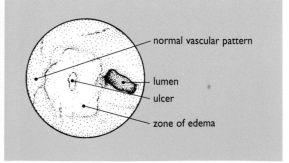

Figure 11.41 *Microerosions are seen as tiny white spots amidst normal mucosa stained with methylene blue. Failure to absorb dye is due to distorted architecture of the gland pits.*

Figure 11.42 *Small flat ulcer in Crohn's disease is surrounded by a zone of edema. Blurring of vascular pattern is also evident.*

The most common ulcers in Crohn's disease measure more than 5 mm in diameter. They vary from flat to deep, and often are irregular and tortuous in shape. There is a distinct margin to such ulcers because of their depth. Some ulcers look serpiginous, presumably as a result of coalescence of several smaller ulcers (Fig. 11.47). Deep serpiginous ulcers, greater than 1 cm in length, are most characteristic of Crohn's disease.

There is a peculiar tendency for linear ulcers to align longitudinally, creating a 'railroad-track' appearance (Figs. 11.48 and 11.49). This appearance is more typical of Crohn's disease than of ulcerative colitis. Such linear ulcers are easily seen in smooth even mucosa but are sometimes difficult to detect in coarsely nodular mucosa.

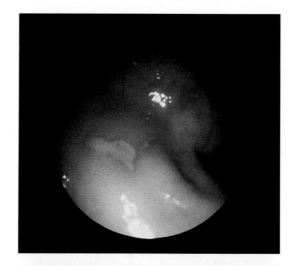

Figure 11.43 Early Crohn's ulcer.

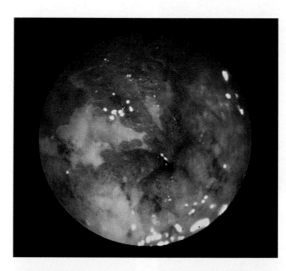

Figure 11.44 Irregular superficial serpiginous ulcer in Crohn's disease.

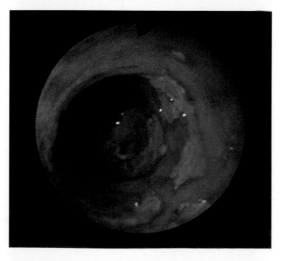

Figure 11.45 Multiple large deep excavated ulcers in severe ulcerating Crohn's disease show distinct margins. This patient has concomitant sclerosing cholangitis.

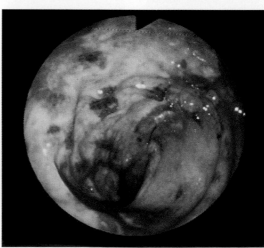

Figure 11.46 Extensive confluent ulceration in Crohn's disease involves one-half of the circumference of the bowel wall, whereas the other half appears fairly normal.

Severe hemorrhage may occur when a large ulcer penetrates into blood vessels deep in the submucosa. In contrast, more diffuse bleeding is associated with acute exacerbations of Crohn's disease that are characterized by marked ulceration. The bleeding may be worsened by medicines given for arthritis or arthralgias, which disturb platelet function (Fig. 11.50).

Cobblestoning – a rough irregular nodular mucosal relief pattern with or without intersecting depressions or ulcerations – is characteristic and perhaps pathognomonic for Crohn's disease. The cobblestone pattern is usually created by the interplay of parallel, longitudinal ulceration and transverse, fissuring-type ulceration. Thickened, slightly edematous, mucosal bumps occur between intersecting ulcerations (Figs. 11.51 and 11.52). The mucosa of the cobblestone area between ulcerations may be pinker than the surrounding epithelium, but it is not typically friable. In contrast with pseudopolyps, the base of the cobblestones is usually wider than their height. Because focal involvement in Crohn's disease is common, the cobblestone appearance is often contained in segments of less than 5 cm in length. Cobblestoning is particularly prevalent at the mouth of inflammatory strictures.

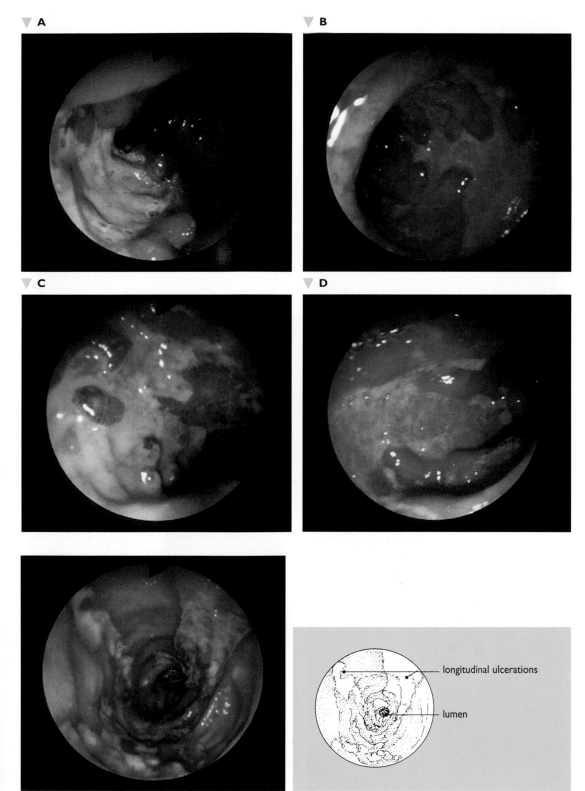

▼ A

▼ B

▼ C

▼ D

Figure 11.47 (**A–D**) Four examples of extensive deep confluent ulceration in Crohn's disease.

longitudinal ulcerations

lumen

Figure 11.48 Longitudinal alignment of ulceration causes a 'railroad-track' appearance in Crohn's disease.

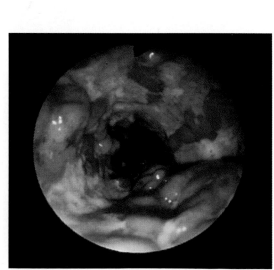

Figure 11.49 Severe longitudinal ulceration in Crohn's disease.

Inflammatory Pseudopolyps

Inflammatory pseudopolyps are found somewhat less frequently in Crohn's disease than in ulcerative colitis. They tend to be focal and localized to one distinct portion of the colon, although within any single area more than one may be noted. Generally, inflammatory pseudopolyps are less than 1.5 cm in greatest dimension (Figs. 11.53 to 11.55). Coarse nodular deformity of the mucosal contours may occur in long-standing severe disease through the combination of cobblestoning and pseudopolyp formation.

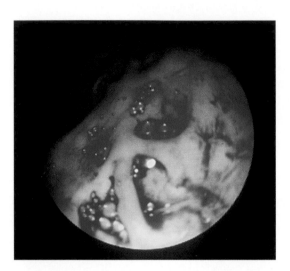

Figure 11.50 *Severe flare-up of Crohn's disease with concomitant arthritis. Platelet dysfunction due to antiphlogistic medication is responsible for diffuse bleeding from ulcer margins.*

▼ **A**   ▼ **B**

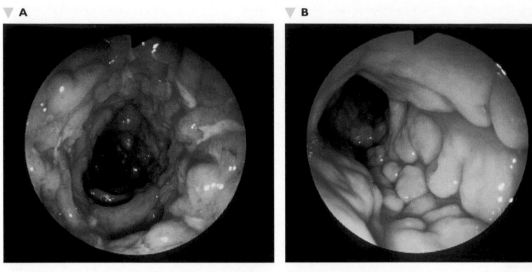

Figure 11.51 *(A) Active phase of Crohn's disease shows cobblestoning, caused by interconnecting ulcerations. (B) Area of cobblestoning after therapy.*

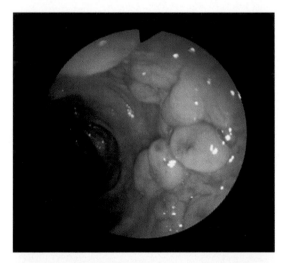

Figure 11.52 *Crohn's colitis with large pseudopolyps.*

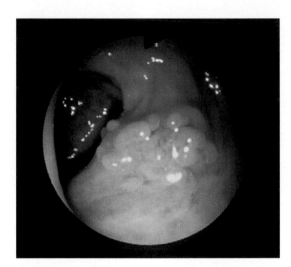

Figure 11.53 *Cluster of small smooth shiny pseudopolyps with a transparent appearance is seen in quiescent Crohn's disease.*

▼ **A**   ▼ **B**

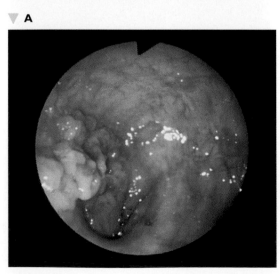   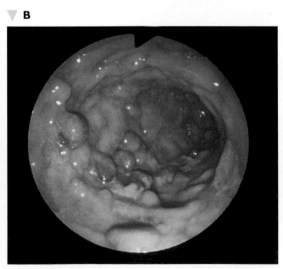

Figure 11.54 *(A and B) Two examples of pseudopolyps in Crohn's disease.*

Anatomic Variations Caused by Crohn's Disease

Structural alterations often accompany changes in the mucosal lining as a consequence of fibrosis and scarring after deep ulceration and transmural fissuring. Thickening and blunting of the interhaustral folds may often be seen in segments in which there is ulceration and occur as a consequence of submucosal edema and fibrosis. Occasionally, there is a striking predilection for ulcers to cluster in and around areas of convergence of the interhaustral folds. In severe cases, the haustral pattern may be completely lost due to major architectural derangements.

The thickened interhaustral folds and muscularis retraction may decrease the luminal diameter of the colon. Extensive underlying ulceration may result in the creation of mucosal bridges across the lumen once the acute phase has subsided and re-epithelialization has occurred (Fig. 11.56).

Fibrotic strictures, more than several centimeters long, are common in Crohn's disease and are a consequence of intense, deep ulceration and fissuring into the submucosa. The lumen is compromised to varying degrees; diameters after stricturing may range from 10–15 mm to less than 5 mm. Low-grade and moderately severe strictures can be examined with a small caliber colonoscope but not with the standard 13 mm colonoscope. Strictures are often irregular, with evidence of inflammation and focal epithelial destruction (Figs. 11.57 and 11.58). Ulcerations are generally found within the strictured area, especially at the opening. Cobblestoning is common in the area leading to the stricture. Strictures caused by active inflammation are lined by edematous, erythematous, friable, and ulcerated mucosa. Smooth, inactive-looking strictures are usually lined by fairly normal-appearing mucosa.

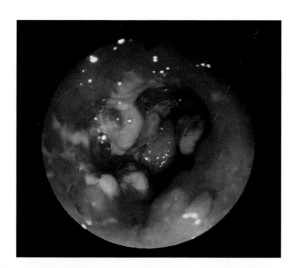

Figure 11.55 Cluster of pseudopolyps in Crohn's disease.

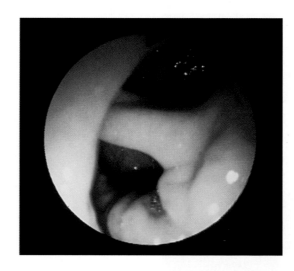

Figure 11.56 Crohn's disease with bridging and pseudopolyps.

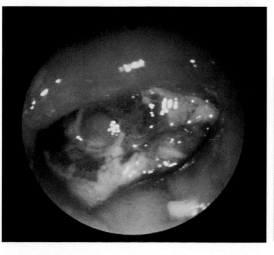

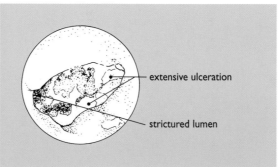

extensive ulceration

strictured lumen

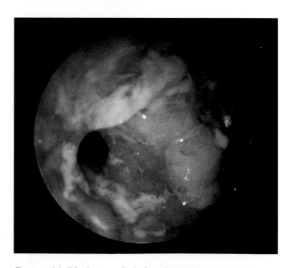

Figure 11.57 Moderately severe, irregular stricture in Crohn's disease. Interconnected ulcers are visible around the mouth of the stricture.

Figure 11.58 Severe Crohn's colitis with stricture.

Healing of deep ulceration may result in thick bands of scar tissue in the small and large bowel. Between these bands, diverticular outpouchings of the wall may occur (Fig. 11.59). Such extensive scarring that dissects the mucosal lining is always indicative of severe previous damage (Figs. 11.60 and 11.61).

Fistula formation is a well known complication of Crohn's disease. A variety of fistulas may occur, such as colocutaneous, colocolonic, coloenteric, and colovesical. Usually a focal area of edema and erythema surrounds the fistulous opening, which itself may not be readily apparent. In other instances, the orifice of the fistula is a deep rounded ulcer-like cavity. The presence of epithelial defects adjacent to and at a distance from the fistulous opening is an indication that the fistula-bearing bowel segment is intrinsically involved in Crohn's disease (Figs. 11.62 to 11.65). When the inflammatory activity subsides and the epithelial lesions heal, the mucosal aspect of the fistulous opening may appear inactive (Figs. 11.66 and 11.67). When fistulas develop between the small bowel and colon, it is important to determine whether they are a manifestation of small bowel disease only or whether the large bowel is also involved. In the former case, there is only edematous swelling and some reddening around the fistulous opening in the colon. In the latter case, there is usually evidence of ulceration in the region of the colonic fistulous opening.

Often mucosal and structural abnormalities are spread out over the colon, in combination. The variability and severity of the defects are important elements in the differential diagnosis. Early lesions may be subtle, requiring careful inspection of the mucosal lining (Fig. 11.68). New lesions superimposed on older abnormalities occasionally produce bizarre appearances (Fig. 11.69). The characteristic finding is of focal lesions with normal intervening mucosa (Fig. 11.70).

Examination of the Terminal Ileum

Involvement of the ileocecal valve in Crohn's disease is often associated with stenosis resulting from ulceration and fibrosis. This inflammatory narrowing may prevent entry of the colonoscope tip into the terminal ileum (Fig. 11.71). Nevertheless, the terminal ileum should be inspected whenever possible. Because the terminal ileum and ileocecal valve are usually involved simultaneously, patchy inflammation or ulceration of the valve alone can be sufficient to make a correct diagnosis, even if the endoscope cannot be passed into the terminal ileum.

The abnormalities described for the colon can also be seen in the terminal ileum. A characteristic finding is the presence of either aphthoid erosions or ulcers, ranging from small superficial defects to large lesions measuring

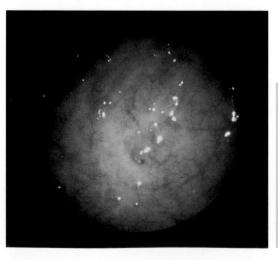

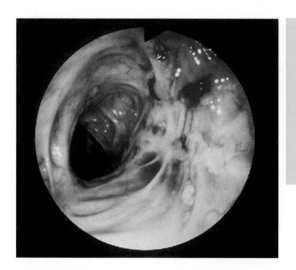

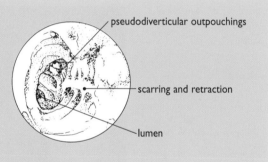

pseudodiverticular outpouchings

scarring and retraction

lumen

Figure 11.59 *Severe longitudinal scarring and retraction lead to the formation of pseudodiverticular outpouchings.*

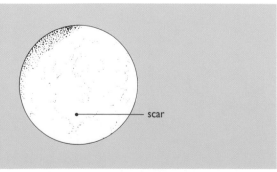

scar

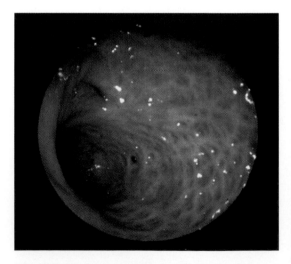

Figure 11.60 *Broad longitudinal scar is seen as a white band interrupting the vascular pattern.*

Figure 11.61 *Extensive confluent scarring gives the bowel wall a bizarre appearance.*

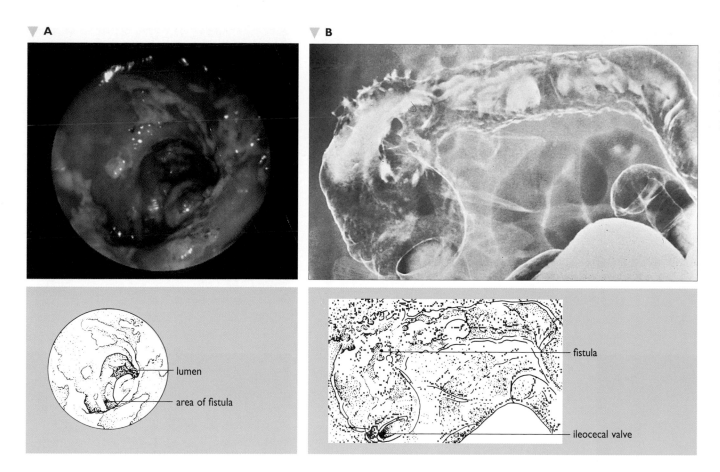

Figure 11.62 (**A**) Colocolonic fistula in Crohn's disease. Mucosa also shows evidence of ulceration. (**B**) Corresponding x-ray shows fistula at hepatic flexure.

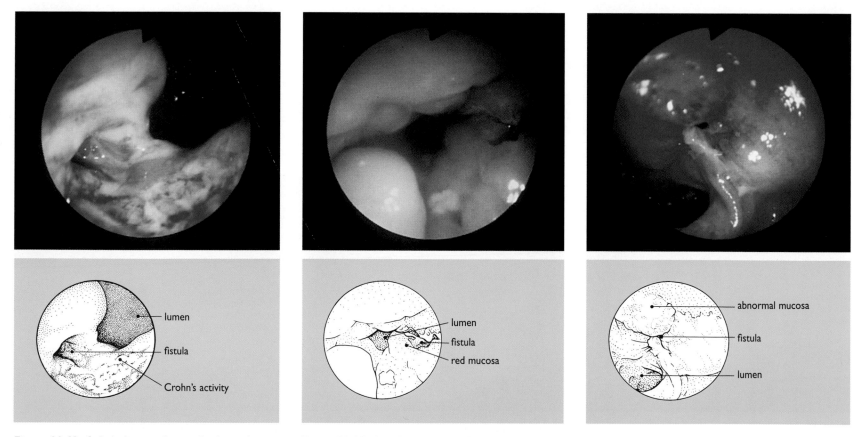

Figure 11.63 Crohn's disease of sigmoid colon with fistulous tract (drawing).

Figure 11.64 Crohn's disease with fistula in the rectum. The surrounding mucosa is erythematous and edematous.

Figure 11.65 Fistula in ileoanal anastomosis in Crohn's disease.

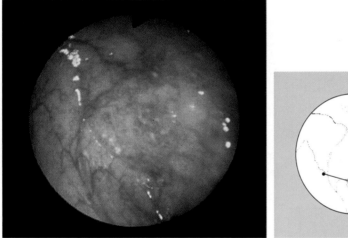

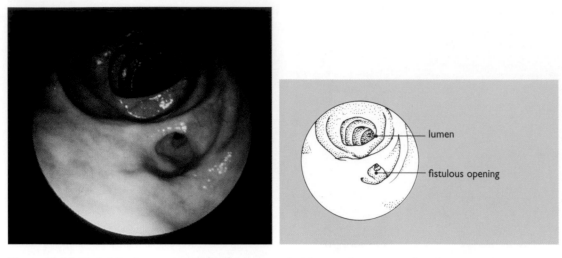

lumen

fistulous opening

Figure 11.66 *Healed fistulous communication between terminal ileum and transverse colon shows normal mucosa.*

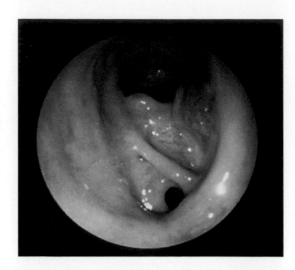

Figure 11.67 *Crohn's disease with colocolonic fistula. Crohn's disease is inactive.*

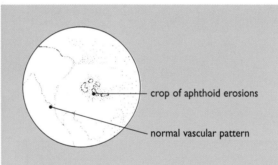

crop of aphthoid erosions

normal vascular pattern

Figure 11.68 *Crohn's disease may take on a subtle appearance. This area of patchy aphthoid erosions in the cecum is barely visible.*

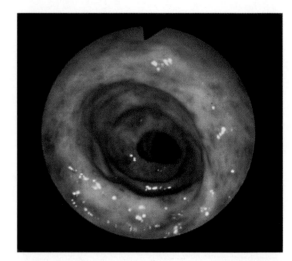

Figure 11.69 *Spectrum of new lesions is superimposed on older abnormalities in Crohn's disease. Red spots and tiny aphthoid erosions appear on a whitish background due to scarring.*

▼ **A**

▼ **B**

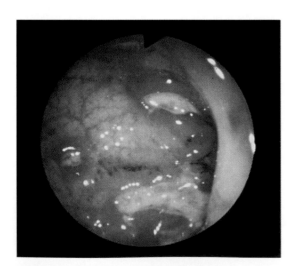

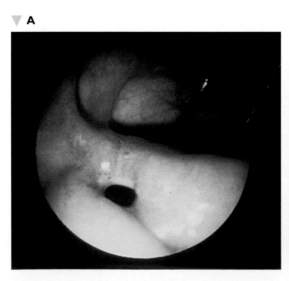

Figure 11.70 *Characteristic focal lesions in Crohn's disease. The discontinuous abnormalities have intervening normal-appearing mucosa.*

Figure 11.71 *Involvement of the ileocecal valve in Crohn's disease can occur as stenosis (**A**) or ulceration (**B**).*

up to 1 cm in diameter. The larger ulcers may be associated with stricture formation. Long longitudinal parallel ulcers may result through coalescence of smaller lesions. There may be evidence of inflammation surrounding the ulcers, shown by the presence of erythematous spots or punctiform hemorrhage. Between ulcerations, there may be areas of normal-looking mucosa. In general, the inflammatory changes tend to involve the entire circumference in the distal terminal ileum (Fig. 11.72), but are patchy and focal in the more proximal ileal segment (Fig. 11.73).

Crohn's disease may affect younger patients, and nodular lymphoid hyperplasia of the terminal ileum is not uncommon in that age group. The typically nonfriable excrescences of lymphoid hyperplasia in the ileal mucosa should not be confused with cobblestoning of Crohn's disease.

Recrudescence of Crohn's disease after extirpation of diseased elements of the terminal ileum is common. In the majority of patients, tiny aphthoid or small superficial ulcers are left behind in the neoterminal ileum (Fig. 11.74). Progression of such lesions presumably leads to clinically manifest

▼ A

▼ B

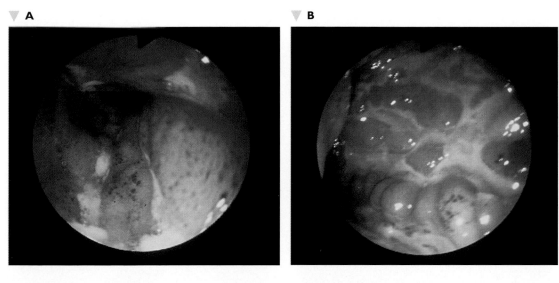

Figure 11.72 (A) Diffuse, concentric involvement of the distal terminal ileum in Crohn's disease occurs as swelling, erythema, punctiform bleeding, and ulceration. **(B)** Circumferential involvement of the distal terminal ileum with longitudinal ulcers and cobblestoning.

▼ A

▼ B

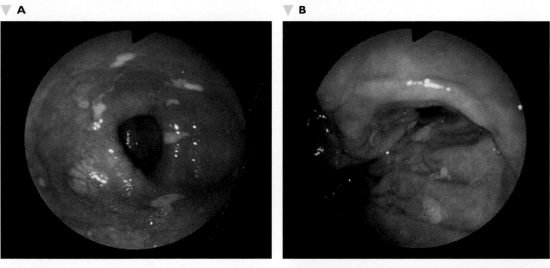

Figure 11.73 In contrast to the distal portion close to the ileocecal valve **(A)** the more proximal segment of the terminal ileum **(B)** shows smaller, patchy ulcerative lesions, with normal-appearing intervening mucosa.

▼ A

▼ B

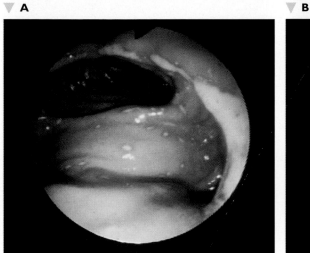
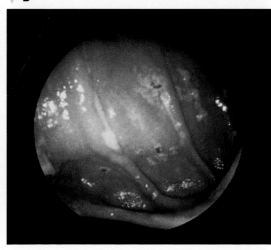

Figure 11.74 Recrudescent Crohn's disease. **(A)** Postsurgically, tiny aphthoid erosions are discernible scattered throughout the neoterminal ileum. In addition, the margin of a larger ulcer is seen. **(B)** In this case, a hemorrhagic spot is seen in the center of small superficial ulcers.

recurrent disease (Fig. 11.75). Recrudescent disease is nearly always within 20 cm of the anastomotic line, although not necessarily involving the anastomosis. When examining patients in the symptomatic stage after recurrence, one should carefully inspect the anastomosis itself before entering the neoterminal ileum (Figs. 11.76 and 11.77). It is by using colonoscopy to examine the anastomotic line and to inspect the neoterminal ileum that we have learned about the form that recurrent disease takes in this clinical circumstance.

Ulcerative defects are most often seen just at and proximal to the anastomosis. When the terminal ileum is involved in recurrent disease, the ulcers tend initially to be circumferential and located preferentially on the ridge of Kerckring's folds. They are apt to be superficial and may be accompanied by aphthoid erosions. Not uncommonly, normal mucosa may be present between areas of active disease. When the ulcerations are deep, the intervening mucosa may be edematous and appear thickened, accentuating the

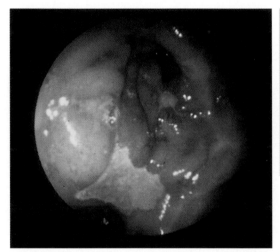
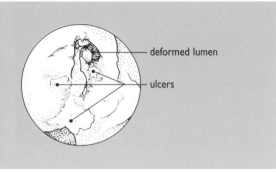

Figure 11.75 *Recrudescent Crohn's disease in the neoterminal ileum with large ulcers. Note the luminal deformity.*

▼ **A**

▼ **B**

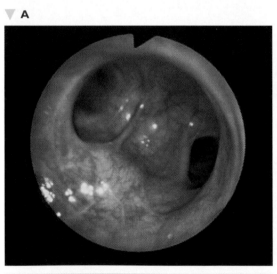
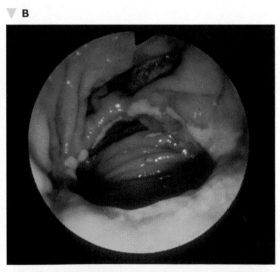

Figure 11.76 *(A) The normal appearance of a side-to-end ileocolonic anastomosis after resection for Crohn's disease. (B) Early recrudescence at side-to-end anastomosis is seen 3 months after resection. Ulcers appear at the anastomotic site. Aphthoid erosions are visible in the neoterminal ileum.*

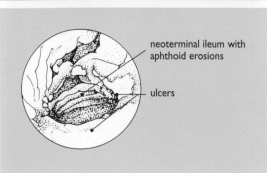

basic nodular character of the anastomotic line that results from its construction with interrupted sutures. Occasionally, deep ulcerations at the anastomosis seem to follow the lines of previous sutures. With extensive ulceration, the intervening mucosa may disappear altogether, with the anastomotic line resembling one continuous area of ulceration. This type of ulceration ultimately leads to a high-grade strictured anastomosis. Adjacent to such areas of deep ulceration, the segment may show cobblestoning.

A tight stricture can occur after resection in Crohn's disease. An endoscopic balloon can be used to dilate the stricture, effectively reducing symptoms and avoiding further surgery (Fig. 11.78).

Distribution of Lesions

One of the hallmarks of Crohn's disease is the focal patchy discontinuous distribution of the lesions. Although Crohn's disease is probably panenteric, predilection for certain areas of the bowel occurs sufficiently often to allow some patterns to be distinguished.

- Right-sided involvement: the ileocecal area is the most common site of involvement in up to 60% of all cases. In an additional 20–30%, the right colon is involved exclusively. Thus, in the majority of cases, the disease tends to be right-sided. Overall, nearly 70% of patients have largely, if not exclusively, right-sided involvement, which includes the ileocecal valve and terminal ileum.
- Rectal sparing: often disease begins at the rectosigmoid junction. Deep ulceration and strictures are characteristic. In some cases the anus and 3–4 cm of the distal rectum are involved, but the rectum above this point is normal.
- Segmental involvement: skip lesions are the rule in the majority of the cases. Areas of normal bowel appear preserved between areas of obvious disease. Segmental involvement may be seen in any area of the gut, including the anal canal and the appendix (Figs. 11.79 and 11.80). In some cases ulcerations are seen on only one side of the colonic mucosal surface.

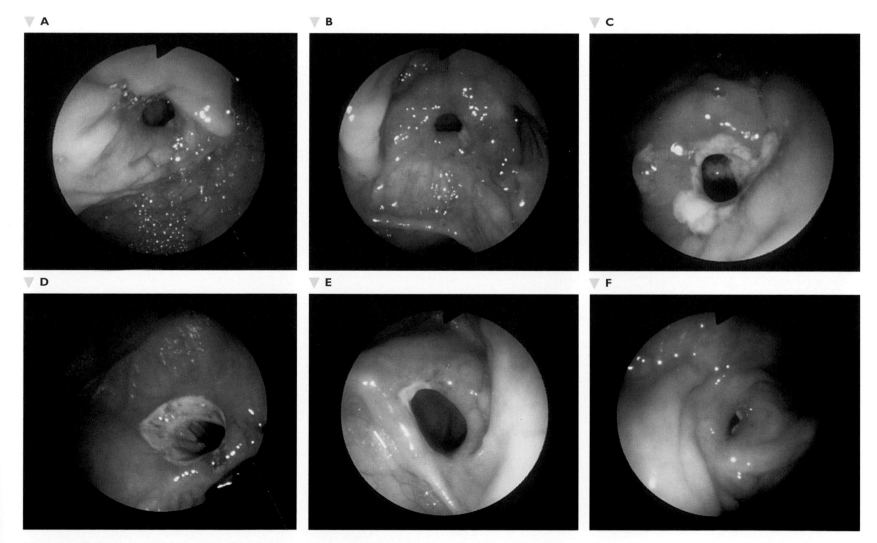

Figure 11.77 (**A**) *The normal appearance of ileocolonic anastomosis.* (**B–F**) *Examples of severely strictured ileocolonic anastomosis, some with adjacent ulceration.*

Levels of Activity

Crohn's disease is called inactive when the vascular pattern is only slightly distorted and there is fine granularity without obvious friability or epithelial defects. There is no standardized system for staging the activity of Crohn's disease. The term mildly active is used when there is unequivocal erythema, either focal or confluent, and some friability without epithelial necrosis. Arbitrarily, the stage is moderately active when a few aphthoid erosions or small ulcers are noted. Cases are described as severe when ulcers are larger and more numerous. Complications of Crohn's disease such as stricturing, fistula formation, and massive bleeding usually indicate severe disease.

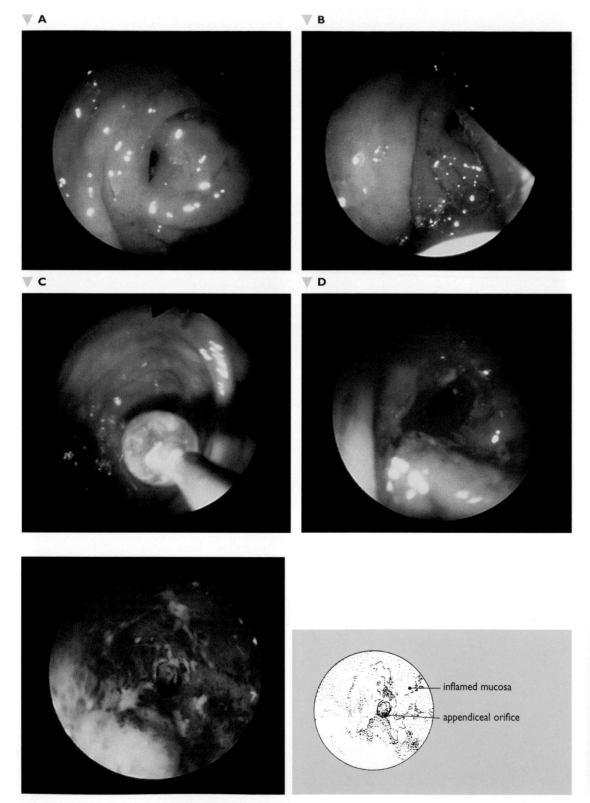

▼ A

▼ B

▼ C

▼ D

Figure 11.78 (*A*) *Colonic anastomotic stricture after resection for Crohn's disease.* (*B*) *A balloon is passed through the endoscope and into the stricture.* (*C*) *The balloon is inflated, dilating the stricture.* (*D*) *The anastomosis is widened and symptoms of obstruction are relieved.*

inflamed mucosa

appendiceal orifice

Figure 11.79 *Crohn's disease with obvious involvement of appendix and cecum.*

Figure 11.80 *Distal colon has a normal appearance except for patchy involvement.*

Risk of Dysplasia or Malignancy

There may be a slightly increased incidence of cancer in Crohn's disease patients, especially in cases of extensive colonic involvement with early onset, and after previous surgery and bypass. Tumors may occur in the excluded intestinal loop. The cancers occur in relatively young patients, tend to locate on the right side and in areas of fistula formation, and are often infiltrative in nature. A variety of gross morphologic appearances may be encountered, for example polypoid or sessile nodular masses, or flat plaque-like cancers. In Crohn's disease, the appearance of such infiltrating cancer may be obscured by the endoscopic findings of Crohn's disease itself, including strictures, cobblestoning and ulceration.

DIFFERENTIAL DIAGNOSIS OF ULCERATIVE COLITIS, CROHN'S DISEASE, AND ACUTE SELF-LIMITED COLITIS

The main differential diagnosis of idiopathic inflammatory bowel disease centers around ulcerative colitis and Crohn's disease. Colonoscopy is useful in the differential diagnosis and to assess the extent and severity of the disease. Despite increased experience, the diagnosis remains difficult for 5–10% of patients and changes back and forth over the years. Differential aspects of ulcerative colitis and Crohn's disease are summarized in Figure 11.81.

Factors Favoring Diagnosis of Ulcerative Colitis

Diffuse involvement of the rectum is almost a prerequisite for the diagnosis of ulcerative colitis. Most often, some evidence of rectal involvement is present initially. Conversely, a normal rectal appearance favors a diagnosis of Crohn's disease.

A continuous symmetrical diffuse pattern of mucosal involvement strongly favors ulcerative colitis. Although there may be some variability in activity, the mucosa will always be abnormal over the segment involved. Occasionally the endoscopic abnormalities may be subtle and consist of only minor loss of shininess. In this case, even with a visible, sharply demarcated, vascular pattern, one is often surprised by the heavy amount of mononuclear infiltration seen at biopsy.

Ulceration seen in a background of diffuse mucosal abnormality is the most important indicator of ulcerative colitis. This acute mucosal inflammation may consist of erythema, friability, or mucopurulent exudate. A patulous or effaced ileocecal valve with a patent opening favors the diagnosis of ulcerative colitis. (In contrast, the presence of extensive ulceration around a closed or stenotic ileocecal valve favors the diagnosis of Crohn's disease.)

Factors Favoring Diagnosis of Crohn's Disease

Patchy, discontinuous, and segmental distribution of lesions is a key finding in support of the diagnosis of Crohn's disease. Areas of apparently normal mucosa alternate with ulcerations, or there may be asymmetrical distribution of ulceration within a given segment.

Absence of rectal involvement, which may occur in 30% of cases of colonic involvement, strongly favors Crohn's disease. When the rectum is involved in Crohn's disease, it is usually in the rectosigmoid or perianal areas.

Ulcers set in relatively normal mucosa with a preserved vascular pattern or a least without evidence of acute inflammation strongly suggest Crohn's disease. Deep extensive ulceration seems to be more characteristic of Crohn's disease. The adjacent mucosa may appear cobblestoned, heaped-up, nodular, and perhaps slightly pink, but it is not friable. Ulceration, stenosis, or distortion of the ileocecal valve along with a predominantly right-sided involvement strongly favors the diagnosis of Crohn's disease.

BIOPSY

Colonoscopic biopsies of abnormal and normal mucosa are always advisable to supplement any visual impression that tends to differentiate between ulcerative colitis and Crohn's disease. Colonoscopic biopsies are usually taken with a standard 7 Fr forceps with round cups or oval jaws, with or without a central spike. Such biopsies are usually small and superficial, and contain only the mucosa and fragments of the muscularis mucosae, with an occasional small bit of submucosa. Biopsy forceps with larger cups are available for use with large channel colonoscopes.

Figure 11.81 Differential diagnosis of ulcerative colitis and Crohn's disease.

Differential Diagnosis of Ulcerative Colitis and Crohn's Disease

Characteristics	Ulcerative Colitis	Crohn's Disease
Distribution	Symmetrical	Asymmetrical
Continuous involvement	Always	Exceptional
Patchiness	Absent	Frequent
Rectal involvement	Almost always	Often absent
Vascular pattern	Blurred or lost	Often normal
Profuse bleeding	Common	Rare
Granularity (fine/coarse)	Common	Less common
Cobblestoning	Absent	Characteristic
Erythema	Characteristic	Less pronounced
Edema (blunting of septa)	Present	Present
Friability	Common	Uncommon
Spontaneous petechiae	Common	Rare
Superficial to small ulcerations	Occasional	Frequent
Large (>1cm) ulceration	Severe disease	Common
Deep longitudinal ulceration	Rare	Common
Linear ulceration	Rare	Common
Aphthoid ulceration	Absent	Characteristic
Serpiginous ulceration	Rare	Common
Pseudopolyps	Occasional	Occasional
Bridging	Occasional	Occasional
Mucosa surrounding ulcer	Abnormal	Normal

Nonspecific histologic findings include mucosal ulceration, fibrinous purulent exudate, infiltration by inflammatory cells, crypt abscesses, and lymphoid aggregates. In general, the biopsy finding of multiple basal crypt abscesses in the presence of epithelial cells, with a diminished mucus content and a continuous pattern of activity, favors a diagnosis of ulcerative colitis. The most important histologic feature of Crohn's disease is the presence of focal granulomas or microgranulomas. Other criteria include discontinuity of the inflammatory infiltrate, disproportionate infiltration and transmural extension of the inflammatory infiltrate, marked lymphoid hyperplasia, fissuring, ulceration, and lymphangiectasia. The histologic diagnosis of Crohn's disease varies substantially depending on the number of biopsies and the number of sections of each biopsy examined. However, it should be possible to obtain granulomas in at least 30% of Crohn's cases.

Acute Self-Limited Colitis vs. Idiopathic Inflammatory Bowel Disease

When a patient presents with acute bloody diarrhea, one must consider the possibility that this is the onset of inflammatory bowel disease, either ulcerative colitis or Crohn's disease. On the other hand this may be an episode of acute self-limited colitis. This is not a simple differential diagnosis when the patient first presents. In time the acute self-limited colitis disappears, gradually resolving over a few weeks. Idiopathic inflammatory bowel disease may also resolve in a period of weeks but the course is usually one of recurrent episodes.

Biopsies of the rectal mucosa may assist in the differential diagnosis between self-limited colitis and idiopathic inflammatory bowel disease. In self-limited colitis, the histology appears fairly normal with normal crypt architecture, scattered polymorphs, and few mononuclear cells. Crypt abscesses, if they occur,

are superficial, and the main location of the inflammation is the upper half of the mucosa. In idiopathic inflammatory bowel disease the crypts are abnormal with distortion of the crypt architecture, including abnormal branching of the crypts. The infiltrate is often predominantly mononuclear. Granulomas may be seen as may lymphoid aggregates. There may be crypt atrophy. In some patients (approximately 1 in 5) biopsy may not distinguish acute self-limited colitis from inflammatory bowel disease.

OTHER INFLAMMATORY BOWEL DISORDERS

INFECTIOUS COLITIS
Acute and chronic infectious diseases involving the colon may mimic features of idiopathic inflammatory bowel disease to the point where they cannot be differentiated endoscopically. Thus, endoscopy should not be the prime diagnostic tool in infectious colitis, but used only when problems of differential diagnosis occur. There are many different organisms that cause colitis; they vary in the degree to which the presenting features mimic ulcerative colitis or Crohn's disease (Fig. 11.82).

Campylobacter fetus, subspecies jejuni is recognized as the etiologic agent in episodes of acute watery diarrhea and acute mucoid bloody diarrhea in otherwise healthy individuals. The endoscopic findings may vary. Occasionally, zones of edema, patchy erythema, and friability with some scattered ulcers alternate with areas of relatively normal mucosa, thus giving the appearance of Crohn's disease (Fig. 11.83). Also, the presence of tiny aphthoid erosions is increasingly recognized. In other patients, erythema, hyperemia, edema, friability, and some superficial ulceration may create an endoscopic appearance similar to ulcerative colitis (Fig. 11.84). Deep ulceration is unusual, although

Figure 11.82 *Types of infectious colitis.*

Types of Infectious Colitis

Disorder	Similarity to * Ulcerative Colitis	Similarity to * Crohn's Disease
Campylobacter colitis	2	1
Yersinia enterocolitica colitis	1	3
Salmonellosis	3	1
Shigellosis	3	1
Tuberculosis	1	3
Mycobacterium avium-intracellulare	1	–
Gonorrhea	1	–
Syphilis	2	1
Amebiasis	2	2
Schistosomiasis	–	–
Vibrio parahaemolyticus	1	–
Cytomegalovirus colitis	3	1
LVG-Chlamydia proctitis	1	3
Non-LVG Chlamydia proctitis	2	–
Herpes simplex	–	1
Antibiotic-associated colitis	2	–

Similarity ranked from 1 to 3, 3 being most similar.

large shaggy ulcers with markedly friable mucosa at the margins have been observed. In some patients, abundant mucopurulent exudate rather than ulceration may be noted. Although the rectum is usually involved, occasionally only the more proximal areas of the colon are affected. All these abnormalities disappear in time. On biopsy, the lamina propria contains a variety of inflammatory cells (most of which are polymorphonuclear leukocytes) and crypt abscesses, but shows little crypt distortion.

Yersinia enterocolitica may cause acute and chronic diarrhea and colitis. The characteristic endoscopic feature is that of multiple small shallow or punched-out aphthoid erosions or small ulcers, surrounded by a small zone of erythema and then normal-looking adjacent mucosa. The lesions in yersin-iosis tend to be small and uniform, although larger ulcers may develop occasionally (Fig. 11.85). The lesions observed in Yersinia colitis almost always have a segmental or patchy distribution. Quite regularly, the lesions may be confined to the terminal ileum, cecum, and ascending colon, but in about 50% of patients the entire colon, including the rectum, may be involved. Because of the appearance of the lesions and the distribution, yersiniosis may mimic Crohn's disease. Much less commonly, *Y. enterocolitica* colitis may be associated with more uniform edematous, erythematous, and friable mucosa, compatible with the appearance of ulcerative colitis.

Salmonellosis may involve the small or large bowel. Involvement is preferentially on the right side but may include the entire colon; rectal sparing is

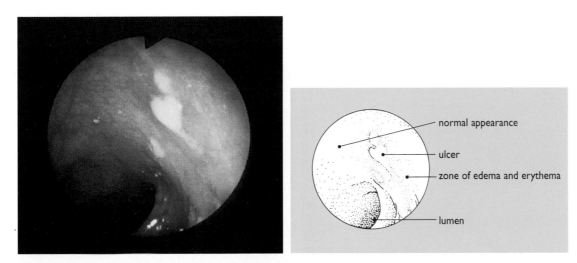

Figure 11.83 *Campylobacter colitis. A zone of edema and erythema includes a superficial ulcer with exudate resembling Crohn's disease.*

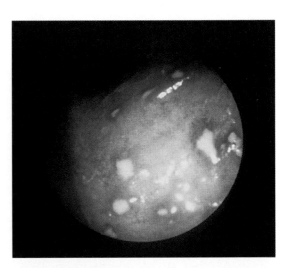

Figure 11.84 *Several discrete, small ulcers with pronounced erythematous rims are set in a background of abnormal mucosa in this case of Campylobacter colitis, mimicking ulcerative colitis.*

▼ **A**   ▼ **B**

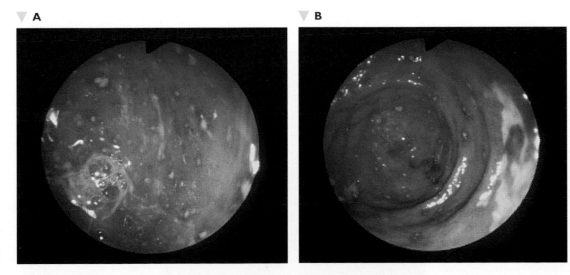

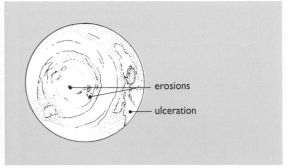

Figure 11.85 *(A and B) Yersiniosis of the terminal ileum, with small aphthoid-like erosions and ulceration.*

common. The endoscopic findings vary from relatively minor abnormalities, such as mucosal edema, hyperemia, and loss of vascular pattern, to severe pancolitis with diffuse edematous and erythematous mucosa, granularity, friability, and petechial hemorrhages similar to ulcerative colitis (Fig. 11.86).

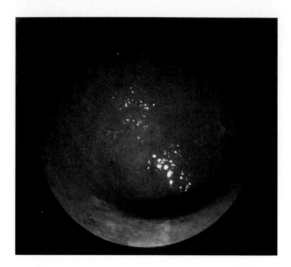

Figure 11.86 *Salmonella colitis can mimic ulcerative colitis.*

Discrete ulcers are usually seen only in the more proximal colon. In severe cases, the markedly edematous mucosa may be covered by a greenish necrotic slough, similar to antibiotic-associated colitis. Occasionally, multiple, regularly distributed, pustular lymph follicles may be present, suggestive of small ulcers seen in Crohn's disease. This finding, together with the predominantly right-sided involvement and the presence of skip areas, may occasionally create an appearance resembling Crohn's disease. Rapid reversal, however, over a 3–4-week period is an important finding that favors the bacterial etiology of the colitis.

Shigellosis may be responsible for severe colitis. In general, the endoscopic appearance may be indistinguishable from idiopathic ulcerative colitis. The severity of the endoscopic abnormalities may vary from intense mucosal erythema and hyperemia with adherent mucus to pronounced hyperemia, minor friability, and superficial ulceration in a background of erythematous mucosa (Fig. 11.87). Although the mucosa may have a magenta hue, the striking friability seen in ulcerative colitis is usually absent. In very severe forms, ulceration may spread and coalesce to involve large segments of the entire circumference. Occasionally, the lesions may be patchy and consist of focal areas of erythema and granularity with some scattered aphthoid erosions or superficial ulcers, usually confined to the rectosigmoid region; this appearance is more suggestive of Crohn's disease.

▼ **A**   ▼ **B**   ▼ **C**

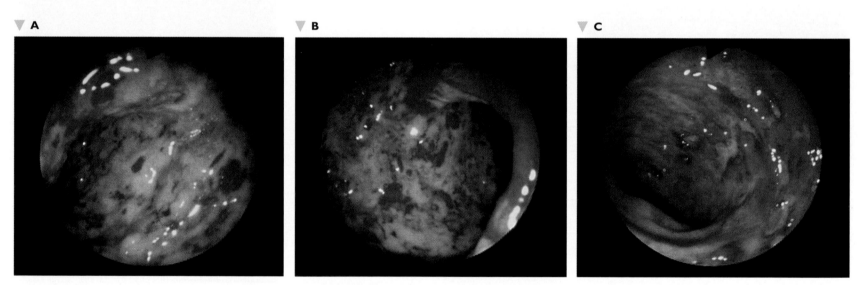

Figure 11.87 *(**A** and **B**) Severe Shigella flexneri colitis with extensive, coalescent, superficial ulceration involves nearly the entire bowel circumference. Increased erythema of the remaining mucosa contrasts with the extensive mucosal necrotic slough. This had the appearance of a pseudomembrane. (**C**) Appearance after 2 weeks of antibiotic therapy shows marked improvement.*

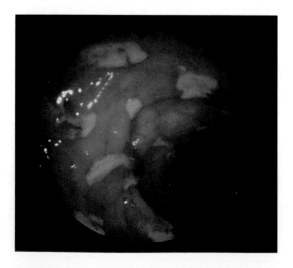

Figure 11.88 *Tuberculosis with ulceration in the cecal area.*

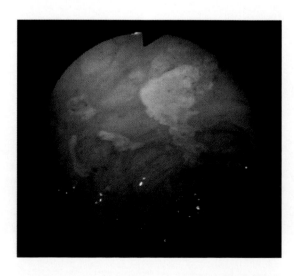

Figure 11.89 *Tuberculous ulcers in the ascending colon.*

Tuberculosis has a predilection for the ileocecal area rich in lymphatic tissue. The overall endoscopic appearance of colonic tuberculosis is indistinguishable from that of Crohn's disease, with ulcers, strictures, and skip lesions (Figs. 11.88 and 11.89). The ileocecal valve may show thickened, nodular, and ulcerated patches (Fig. 11.90). Sometimes the valve is gaping, surrounded by heaped-up and ulcerated folds. The cecum and ascending colon may be narrowed and contracted; focal stenotic areas may be deeply ulcerated. The transverse colon may also be involved with ulceration and, at times, irregular stricturing. Shorter segments of the colon are involved than in Crohn's disease. The mucosa may be focally erythematous and edematous with superficial and deep ulceration, often with raised indurated margins. As in Crohn's disease, ulcers are surrounded by normal-looking mucosa. In addition, cobblestoning, segmental involvement, and linear ulceration are seen. At times, a hypertrophic ulcerated flaky mass resembling a carcinoma may be discernible, especially in the cecal area. A rare presentation is that of a pancolitis with either diffuse or segmental edema, erythema, friability, and ulceration. The rectum is commonly spared. Strictures, mass lesions, and fistulas may also be noted.

Chronic infection with *Mycobacterium avium-intracellulare* may occur in immunocompromised patients and is responsible for pseudo-Whipple's disease of the rectocolon. Large segments of the circumference of the bowel show a whitish hue caused by the massive accumulation of lipid-filled macrophages packed with mycobacteria (Figs. 11.91 and 11.92).

The endoscopic features of gonorrhea are nonspecific and include edema, erythema, friability, and – rarely – ulceration. Usually only the area 3–5 cm immediately above the anus is involved, with abundant purulent material present in the anal canal. Diagnosis is made by Gram's stain and culture of this material. Several pathogens may be cultured simultaneously, further complicating endoscopic interpretation (Fig. 11.93).

The endoscopic presentation of anorectal syphilis includes solitary or multiple anal and rectal ulcers surrounded by friable and slightly edematous mucosa. At times, thickened hyperplastic fibrotic anorectal masses or condylomas may be seen, which are easily mistaken for anal fissures, cryptitis, fistula, or even cancer.

Amebiasis caused by *Entamoeba histolytica* has a predilection for the cecal and rectosigmoid area. The endoscopic features of amebic colitis vary. Especially during acute stages of the disease, the mucosa of the rectum and sigmoid may show diffuse edema, erythema and friability, granularity, and abundant mucopurulent exudate together with scattered ulcerations. This appearance is indistinguishable from that of acute ulcerative colitis. Smears made from the exudate reveal trophozoites, as do biopsies from the ulcerations.

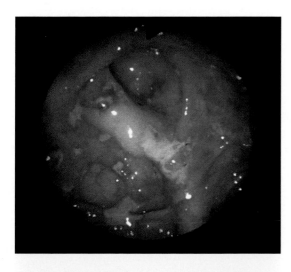

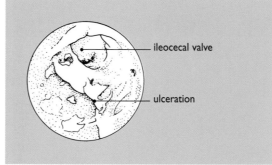

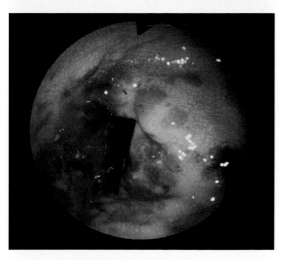

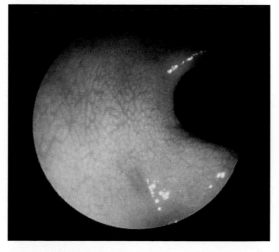

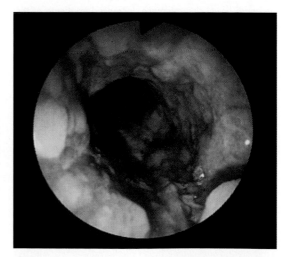

Figure 11.90 *In this case of tuberculosis, the diseased ileocecal valve did not allow intubation of the strictured terminal ileum. Ulcerations of the mucosa are similar to those found in Crohn's disease.*

Figure 11.91 *Pseudo-Whipple's disease due to M. avium-intracellulare in an AIDS patient. Characteristic whitish discoloration contrasts with the reddish zones representing uninvolved mucosa.*

Figure 11.92 *Pseudo-Whipple's disease caused by M. avium-intracellulare in a patient with AIDS. The mucosa has a white hue caused by lipid-filled macrophages.*

Figure 11.93 *Proctitis caused by gonorrhea, Chlamydia, and betahemolytic streptococci. Appearance 7 days after ampicillin therapy still shows erythema and ulcerations.*

Chronic mucosal involvement has a more classic appearance. Ulcerations a few millimeters in diameter with slightly undermined edges are seen in areas where the mucosa is otherwise normal, or minimally abnormal with blurring of the vascular pattern (Fig. 11.94). The ulcers may be covered by a yellow–white exudate and may, at times, resemble aphthoid-type erosions or small ulcers seen in Crohn's disease (Fig. 11.95). Occasionally the ulcers may be deep, punched-out, and surrounded by an intense erythematous halo (Fig. 11.96). Linear ulcers may be seen (Fig. 11.97). Inflammatory pseudopolyps

▼ A ▼ B

▼ C ▼ D

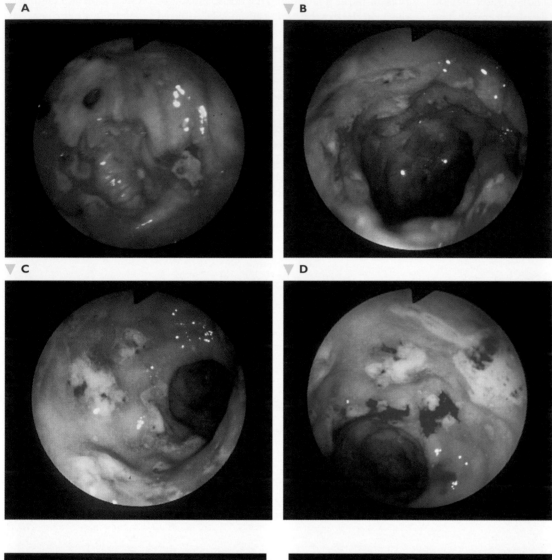

Figure 11.94 (**A–D**) *Discrete ulcers with slightly undermined edges are depicted in these four views of amebiasis. The mucosa surrounding the ulcers is erythematous, edematous and friable. Ulcers may also appear confluent.*

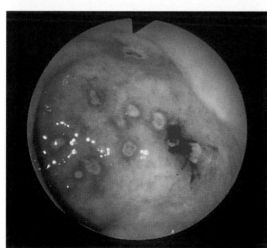

Figure 11.95 *Amebiasis of the rectosigmoid junction. Small superficial ulcerations are covered with whitish exudate and surrounded by an erythematous rim. Mucosa adjacent to the ulcers is unremarkable except for some blurring of the vascular pattern. Smearing of the ulcers may cause mild bleeding because of hyperemia at the edges.*

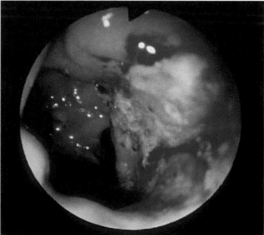

Figure 11.96 *Amebiasis of the colon with a large deep ulcer with an intense red margin.*

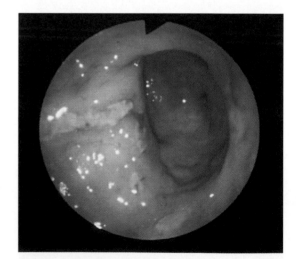

Figure 11.97 *Amebic colitis with linear ulcers.*

may then be seen, often adjacent to ulcers (Fig. 11.98). Rarely, involvement in amebiasis is limited to the cecal area. Endoscopy may reveal cecal erosions, ulcerations, or mass lesions (amebomas) with superficial ulceration.

The colonic complications of schistosomiasis are related to deposition of schistosomal eggs in the terminal venules within the colonic mucosa. *Schistosoma japonicum* involves primarily the cecum and ascending colon, *Schistosoma mansoni* the descending colon, and *Schistosoma haematobium* the bladder and rectum. The colonic features include edema, marked hyperemia, friability, punctate hemorrhages, granularity, and focal shallow ulcerations, closely resembling ulcerative colitis (Fig. 11.99). In addition, there may be mucosal thickening and luminal narrowing. A further similarity with ulcerative colitis is the appearance of multiple inflammatory pseudopolyps largely in the rectum and sigmoid colon (Fig. 11.100). These polypoid lesions are composed of degenerating ova and surrounding granulomatous inflammatory reaction. Their characteristic feature is central ulceration in the presence of abundant amounts of exudate (Fig. 11.101).

Vibrio parahaemolyticus is usually associated with explosive watery diarrhea and shows striking inflammatory changes in the terminal ileum. Usually,

mucoid bloody diarrhea is noted and at endoscopy a patchy erythematous friable mucosa without ulceration may be observed.

Cytomegalovirus (CMV) infection may present as isolated large punched-out ulcers predominantly on the right side in renal transplant patients. In AIDS patients, multiple smaller ulcers may be seen, usually right-sided but occasionally throughout the colon (Fig. 11.102). CMV may also appear as multiple discrete zones of intense erythema (Fig. 11.103). There may be thickening of the folds and the mucosal vascular pattern may be blurred or lost, presenting an appearance similar to ulcerative colitis.

Lymphogranuloma venereum-type (LGV) Chlamydia proctitis is a problem in the homosexual male population. The rectum and sigmoid colon are most often involved, with abnormalities that usually do not extend beyond the sigmoid colon. Endoscopically, there is patchy or diffuse edema. The mucosa is erythematous, friable, and granular; skip lesions may be seen. Ulcerations are noted occasionally, with a predilection for the valves of Houston (Fig. 11.104). In more chronic disease, strictures may occur, usually within a few centimeters of the anus. Also, fistula formation may occur, which may mimic Crohn's disease.

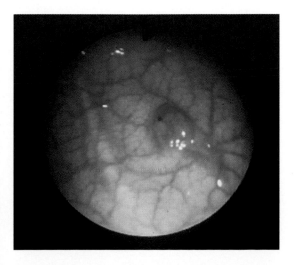

Figure 11.98 *Colonic amebiasis with pseudopolyp-like structures.*

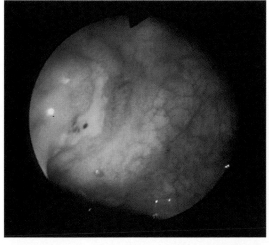

Figure 11.99 *Schistosomiasis at the rectosigmoid junction. A shallow ulceration is surrounded by slightly raised edematous mucosa.*

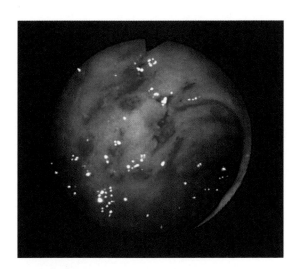

Figure 11.100 *Pseudopolypoid elevations in schistosomiasis contain degenerating ova.*

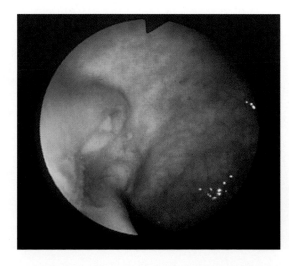

Figure 11.101 *Colonic schistosomiasis. The mucosa is hyperemic, friable and granular.*

▼ **A**

▼ **B**

▼ **C**

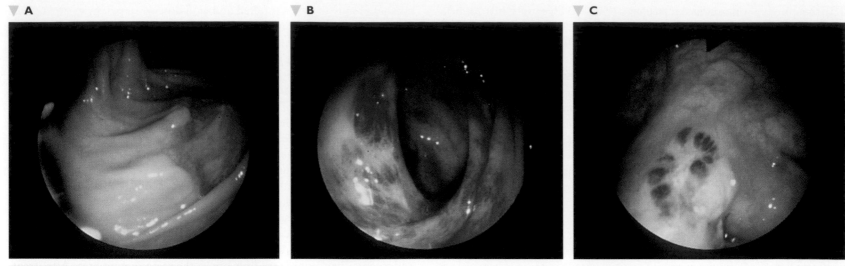

lumen

ulcer

surrounding mucosa

Figure 11.102 (**A**) *Large CMV ulcer in the colon of an AIDS patient.* (**B**) *CMV colitis in an AIDS patient with ulcers and erythema.* (**C**) *Ulcer and erythema in an AIDS patient with CMV colitis.*

▼ **A**

▼ **B**

Figure 11.103 (**A** and **B**) *CMV colitis appearing as intense erythematous mucosa in two AIDS patients.*

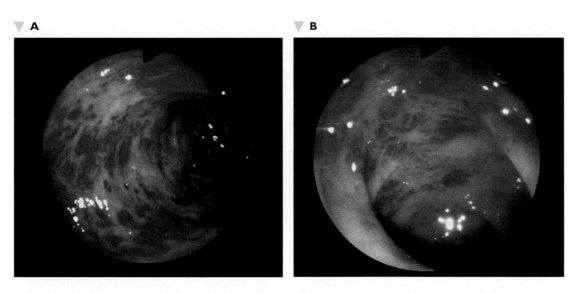

▼ **A**

▼ **B**

Figure 11.104 (**A** and **B**) *Views of LGV-type Chlamydia trachomatis infection show detail of an ulcer across the distal valve of Houston.*

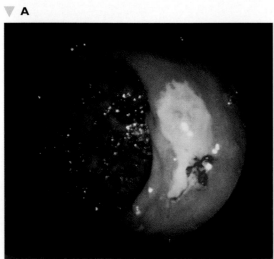

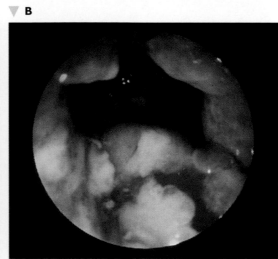

The abnormalities in non-LGV Chlamydia proctitis are usually milder and consist of erythema, edema with minimal friability, and rarely ulceration. In a few patients there may be superficial necrosis of the epithelium (Fig. 11.105).

Herpes simplex virus (HSV) of the anorectal area is an increasingly common diagnosis, especially among homosexual men. At endoscopy, one usually finds patchy or diffuse edema, erythema, and friability, and a variable number of erosions or ulcerations in the anorectal area. Occasionally ulcers coalesce, leading to denudation of nearly the whole circumference of the anorectal canal (Fig. 11.106). Infrequently, small vesicles may be seen in the rectum. HSV intranuclear inclusions and herpes multinucleated cells may be identified in biopsies.

Condylomata acuminata are warts that are caused by the papillomavirus. They occur characteristically in the perineum and over the genitalia; involvement of the anal canal is generally thought to be associated with anal intercourse. The warts may extend into the rectum for 1–2*cm above the pectinate line or columnar squamous junction (Fig. 11.107). They appear as excrescences of varying size that, if left untreated, may extend to form larger confluent lesions. Condylomata may be seen during colonoscopy or flexible sigmoidoscopy when the tip of the endoscope is retroflexed to examine the rectal mucosa just above the anal canal. These human papillomavirus-associated warts are thought to be linked to squamous cell carcinoma of the anus, especially when lesions are large.

ANTIBIOTIC-ASSOCIATED COLITIS

Certain antibiotics predispose to development of diarrhea, most often without evidence of previous inflammation or *Clostridium difficile* infection. Sometimes, however, this organism emerges with antibiotic use, producing a cytotoxin that causes focal necrosis of the epithelium along with an acute inflammatory exudate. If pseudomembranous plaques form over the area of superficial ulceration, the term pseudomembranous colitis is used. This disorder is identified by the presence of sharply demarcated, elevated yellow–white plaques that vary in size from pinhead to several centimeters (Fig. 11.108). The surrounding mucosa may look normal or appear edematous, friable, and covered with mucopurulent exudate. The mucosa may bleed when the plaques are removed. In severe cases the plaques coalesce, and edema, erythema, and friability with punctate hemorrhages may be seen (Fig. 11.109). Rarely, there is extensive sloughing of necrotic mucosa.

Generally, the involvement is distal or left-sided, but it may be universal, especially if plaques are large. In up to one-third of affected patients, the endoscopic changes are seen only above the rectosigmoid area. After treatment with vancomycin, the pseudomembranes usually disappear rapidly.

In up to one-third of cases, only edema and erythema are seen and no obvious pseudomembranes are present. This form of antibiotic-associated colitis has become a major clinical consideration in the differential diagnosis of inflammatory bowel diseases. This is particularly true if the condition occurs without raised whitish plaques attached to the mucosal surface and if the rectum is not involved.

▼ **A**

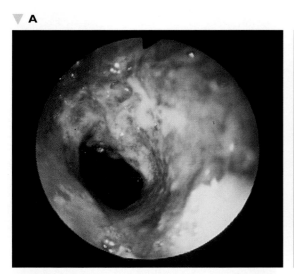

▼ **B**

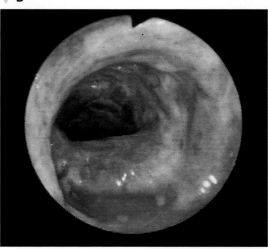

Figure 11.105 (**A** and **B**) Two cases of non-LGV Chlamydia proctitis of unusual severity appearing as superficial necrosis of the mucosa in the anal canal.

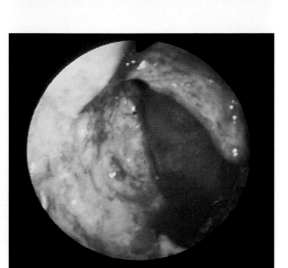

Figure 11.106 This view of herpes proctitis in an AIDS patient shows confluent, nearly circumferential ulceration of the anal canal and distal rectum.

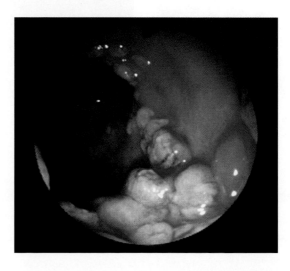

Figure 11.107 Condylomata acuminata in the rectum just above the pectinate line.

A peculiar, transient, right-sided hemorrhagic colitis is occasionally seen after antibiotic therapy, especially after penicillin and ampicillin, and less often after amoxycillin, erythromycin, and clindamycin. The hemorrhagic inflammation is due to overgrowth of toxin-producing *Escherichia coli*. Such patients usually present with bloody diarrhea of acute onset. Edema, friability, and mucosal hemorrhage, sometimes with scattered erosions, are usually located in the hepatic flexure and ascending colon (Fig. 11.110). The affected area may be well demarcated. Follow-up colonoscopies 7–14 days after the initial examination usually demonstrate complete clearing of hemorrhagic mucosal changes.

ISCHEMIC DAMAGE OF THE COLON

Ischemic colitis caused by inadequate tissue perfusion is being diagnosed with increased frequency, especially in elderly patients. Mesenteric ischemia is most often associated with low cardiac output noted with cardiogenic shock or severe intravascular volume depletion. Less often the ischemia may be secondary to occlusion of the superior or inferior mesenteric artery. Primary venous obstruction is rare. In many patients, inadequate tissue perfusion is caused by distal colonic obstruction from carcinoma or diverticular disease.

The pathologic changes evoked by ischemia range from submucosal edema to infarction. Between these two extremes are gradations of tissue damage with resulting diverse clinical courses and endoscopic appearances. In mild ischemia, morphologic changes regress and disappear, whereas severe ischemia may result in irreparable damage with gangrene, perforation, or persistent nonresolving colitis.

The most severe form of ischemic damage is transmural gangrene. Patients with severe abdominal pain, high fever, and evidence of peritoneal irritation are likely have gangrenous infarction and should not undergo endoscopy because of the risk of perforation. In the rare instance when endoscopy is performed, the whitish-gray or purple–black discoloration characteristic of gangrenous mucosa is evident.

Less severe forms of ischemic damage usually correspond to the clinical variant of transient ischemic colitis. Endoscopy may be useful in this less severe form of ischemia. Three stages have been arbitrarily defined. The acute stage is characterized initially by patchy areas (Fig. 11.111). These pale areas are caused by intense vasoconstriction of mucosal blood vessels. Over

▼ **A**   ▼ **B**   ▼ **C**

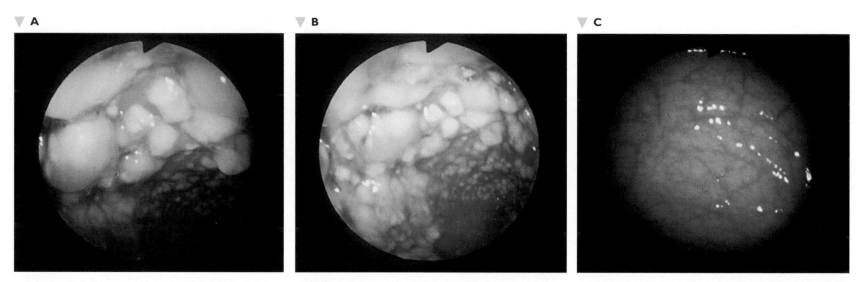

Figure 11.108 (**A** and **B**) After clindamycin therapy, C. difficile overgrowth leads to this severe form of pseudomembranous colitis. Raised, strongly adherent, yellow plaques are characteristic features. (**C**) After 7 days of oral vancomycin the colon appears normal.

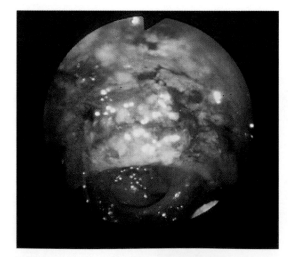

Figure 11.109 C. difficile post antibiotic colitis with pseudomembranes, friability and erythematous mucosa.

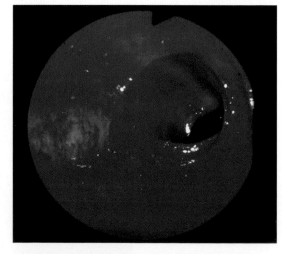

Figure 11.110 Hemorrhagic right-sided colitis after penicillin therapy.

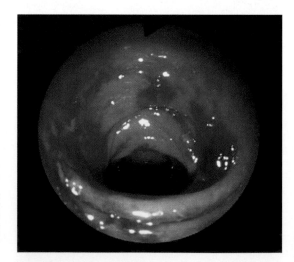

Figure 11.111 Acute phase of ischemic damage involving the sigmoid colon. Patchy erythema contrasts with paler mucosa.

24 hours, the erythematous areas may coalesce. At this point there is usually evidence of submucosal bleeding with petechiae or hemorrhages (Fig. 11.112), or even large submucosal bluish hemorrhagic blebs. In addition, the interhaustral folds may be thickened because of edema and submucosal hemorrhage, creating the characteristic thumb-printing appearance noted radiographically (Fig. 11.113). Spots of superficial mucosal necrosis ranging from 2 to 4 mm in diameter develop. The overall appearance of this acute stage resembles ulcerative colitis and usually lasts about 3 days.

The subacute stage lasts from the third to the seventh day and is characterized by ulceration. The ulcers may be linear, elongated, and serpiginous or trough-like (Fig. 11.114). Sometimes they are longitudinal, resembling those in Crohn's disease (Fig. 11.115). A more extensive superficial form of ulceration may also be found (Fig. 11.116). The necrotic ulcerative lesions are sometimes covered initially by a yellowish-gray, strongly adherent exudate and slough (Fig. 11.117). In some cases, acute inflammatory exudate appears as the predominant lesion, mimicking the pseudomembranous patches in antibiotic-associated diarrhea. The segment involved is usually demarcated at both ends, but occasionally erythema and tiny ulcerations may be separated from the major involment segment by a few centimeters. This ulcerative stage of ischemic damage is similar to idiopathic inflammatory bowel disease, especially Crohn's disease. However, the single-segment distribution of the disease, the predilection for the splenic flexure area or descending colon, the absence of perianal disease, and the histology of biopsies suggest the ischemic nature of the damage.

The chronic stage, lasting between 2 weeks and 3 months, is characterized by gradual resolution and healing. The edema slowly disappears, the ulcer craters become whitish, devoid of all debris and necrotic material, and gradual re-epithelialization of the denuded surfaces occurs. Healing usually takes 6 weeks, but may take as long as 3 months. Colonoscopy at that time may show normal mucosa or residual granularity; sometimes a criss cross pattern of scarring may be visible. A smooth stricture may develop with slight mucosal pinkness, loss of normal vascularity, and scarring as the only visible abnormalities.

The nonresolving form of ischemic damage is most peculiar. After 3 months, extensive superficial ulceration remains, leading to chronic blood loss and excessive intestinal loss of protein (Fig. 11.118).

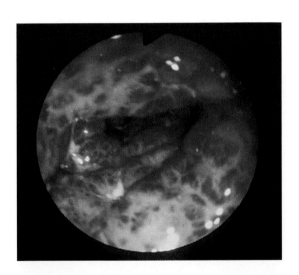

Figure 11.112 *Acute phase of ischemic damage. There is severe luminal narrowing because of marked swelling and muscle contraction. Ecchymotic spots are evidence of submucosal bleeding.*

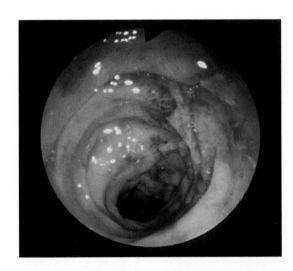

Figure 11.113 *Early ischemic damage. Erythema, swelling, and intramural bleeding are evident. This can result in macropseudopolypoid swelling that corresponds with thumb-printing. Superficial necrosis is also noted.*

▼ **A**   ▼ **B**   ▼ **C**

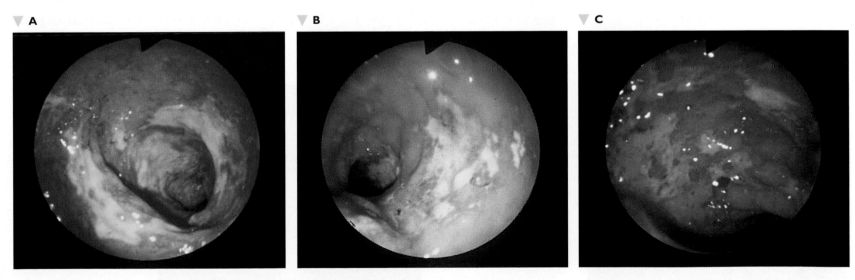

Figure 11.114 *(A–C) Three cases of the subacute or ulcerative stage of ischemic damage after aortic aneurysm surgery. Large serpiginous ulcers are evident. The ischemic segment is clearly demarcated.*

Endoscopic Guidelines

The differential diagnosis of ischemic damage is not simple. It includes carcinoma, inflammatory bowel disease, and diverticulitis. Endoscopy may be helpful in the differential diagnosis and to help determine the extent of mucosa affected. This endoscopic information may be useful because at surgery it may be difficult to assess the extent of the ischemic segment. However, one should note that endoscopy in patients with colonic ischemia may be associated with an increased risk of complications. The wall may be ischemic and potentially weakened, increasing the risk of perforation with the endoscope tip. Distension of the colon with gas during colonoscopy may further compromise the blood supply to the wall, worsen the ischemic injury, and increase the chance of perforation.

The topographical distribution of lesions of ischemic damage is important in diagnosis. In patients who have had abdominal vascular surgery, preferential sites of involvement are the rectosigmoid area or the left colon, especially around the region of the splenic flexure. This corresponds to the watershed area between the vascular territories of the superior and inferior mesenteric arteries. Rectal involvement is unusual, which is a useful differential point. Moreover, ischemic damage always involves a single segment of the gut with sharp demarcations at the proximal and distal borders of the infarcted segment. Therefore, the major endoscopic criteria favoring a diagnosis of ischemia rather than inflammatory bowel disease are:

- Lack of rectal involvement
- Presence of petechiae and ecchymoses, and evidence of submucosal edema and hemorrhage
- Occurrence of unisegmental disease
- Rapid resolution.

Although the outcome of colonic ischemia depends on many factors, the initial response to ischemic damage is the same regardless of the severity. It is therefore impossible to predict the progression and outcome of the ischemic process from the initial clinical or endoscopic evaluation.

RADIATION-RELATED COLITIS

Radiation damage of the rectosigmoid area is common, especially in patients treated for cancer of the cervix. Usually the proximal and distal sigmoid and the intra-and supra-anal areas are involved. These are the intestinal segments in close proximity to the cervix and most affected by the radiation treatment.

Radiation damage may occur in an acute or chronic form. The acute form is seen during radiation treatment and up to 6 weeks thereafter. Endoscopy may reveal edematous dusky mucosa with diffuse erythema similar to ulcerative colitis (Fig. 11.119). Severe damage may lead to friability and mucosal ulceration (Fig. 11.120). Delayed effects are seen 6–12 months after radio therapy. Fibrosis and edema of the submucosa may cause the mucosa to appear opaque or pale. Endarteritis causes fibrosis and neovascularization,

▼ A

▼ B

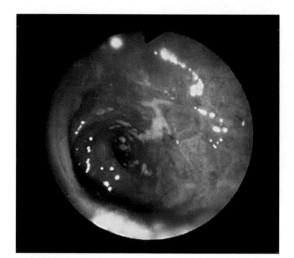

Figure 11.115 Ischemic stricture has a central longitudinal ulceration.

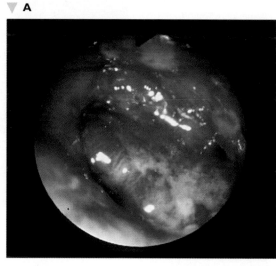

Figure 11.116 (**A** and **B**) Endoscopic findings of ischemic colitis 2 days after onset of sudden hematochezia in a patient with diverticular disease show markedly swollen hemorrhagic mucosa with early patchy superficial epithelial necrosis.

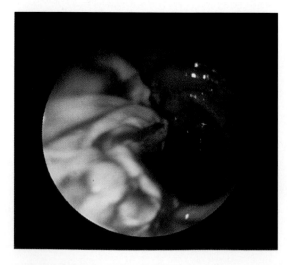

Figure 11.117 Ischemic colitis with adherent mucosal cast. Extensive intramural bleeding was thought to cause mucosa to become necrotic and slough.

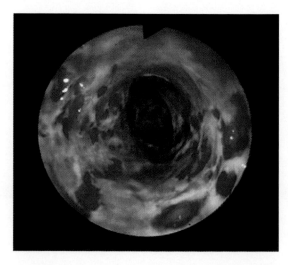

Figure 11.118 Chronic nonresolving ischemic colitis with extensive non-healing necrosis.

seen as telangiectatic mucosal vessels (Fig. 11.121). Such vessels are excessively fragile and may bleed profusely upon slight touch with the endoscope.

In addition to these changes, acute mucosal inflammation may also be noted, with erythema, friability, and granularity. Ulcerations may appear,

especially around the rectosigmoid junction (Fig. 11.122), or into and just proximal to the anal canal (Fig. 11.123). Ulcers from radiation may involve the entire circumference of the rectum (Fig. 11.124). Another common abnormality is the development of a stricture at the rectosigmoid junction

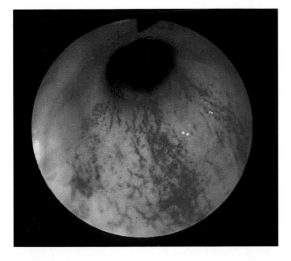

Figure 11.119 Acute radiation damage to rectosigmoid colon. Intense erythema is noted.

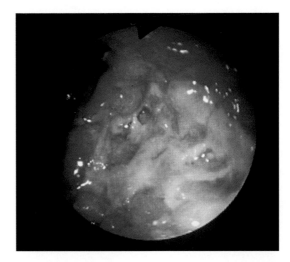

Figure 11.120 Acute radiation injury to the rectosigmoid junction. The mucosa is red and edematous, and an exudate-covered ulcer is seen.

▼ **A**   ▼ **B**

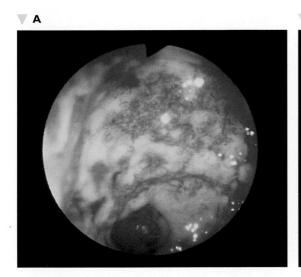
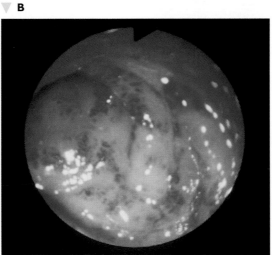

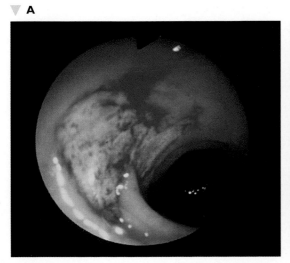

Figure 11.121 (**A** and **B**) Chronic radiation damage at the rectosigmoid junction. Tiny telangiectatic vessels are superimposed on pale and opaque mucosa. The opaque appearance may be caused by fibrosis.

Figure 11.122 Chronic radiation-induced ulcer at the rectosigmoid junction.

▼ **A**   ▼ **B**

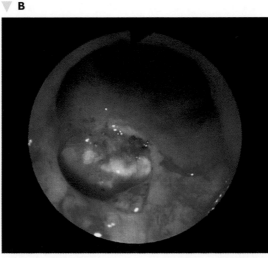

Figure 11.123 (**A** and **B**) Two cases of large radiation-induced ulceration in the rectum; (**B**) is in the anal canal.

(Fig. 11.125). Strictures tend to be associated with pale mucosa or with telangiectasis. Strictures may be relatively short but sometimes extend over a longer distance, especially in the sigmoid colon. This may impede passage of the endoscope.

A dreadful complication is the development of a fistula either in the sigmoid colon (Fig. 11.126), or in the perianal area, resulting in a rectovaginal connection or fistula (Fig. 11.127). Some investigators caution that biopsy should not be obtained from the anterior rectal wall in a female patient with radiation proctitis because of the risk of development of a rectovaginal fistula.

Radiation-related colitis is extremely difficult to treat. Sometimes ulcers remain for a long time or progress to fistulization. Healing may occur with retraction of ulcers (Fig. 11.128).

BYPASS COLITIS

A nonspecific colitis has been observed in colostomy patients with an excluded rectum or rectosigmoid. Termed divergence or disuse colitis, the most characteristic findings are distorted or absent mucosal vascular pattern, erythema and friability, mucosal granularity, and petechial hemorrhages (Fig. 11.129). Occasionally ulcerations and polypoid excrescences may develop. Such changes are almost exclusively in the distal 2–3 cm of the rectum, but may involve the entire excluded segment. Sometimes multiple small lesions

resembling aphthoid erosions, caused by enlarged lymphoid follicles, are seen with red raised margins and central areas of yellow–white exudate with normal intervening mucosa (Fig. 11.130).

Bypass colitis is indistinguishable from ulcerative colitis endoscopically and histologically. Little is known about the pathogenesis of this entity, which may have important diagnostic and therapeutic implications in colostomy patients. This form of colitis resolves upon re-anastomosis.

RARE COLITIS PRESENTATIONS

Behçets Disease

Behçet's disease is a rare illness that may occur with ulceration of the intestinal tract. Other features include ulcers of the genital area and mouth as well as characteristic associations of eye, joint, and cutaneous lesions. The endoscopic finding is discrete, punched-out ulceration on a mucosal background that either appears normal or shows nonspecific erythema or granularity (Fig. 11.131). The location may be predominantly right-sided or involve the colon diffusely, but rectal involvement is variable. The appearance is suggestive of the aphthoid erosions or small ulcers in Crohn's disease. Even histologically, the two diseases are difficult to differentiate.

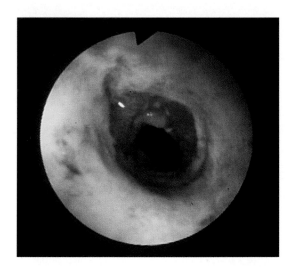

Figure 11.124 *Radiation-induced rectal ulcer involving entire circumference of rectum.*

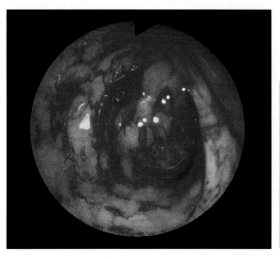

Figure 11.125 *Radiation-induced stricture at the rectosigmoid junction could not be passed with the colonoscope. Telangiectasia is abundant.*

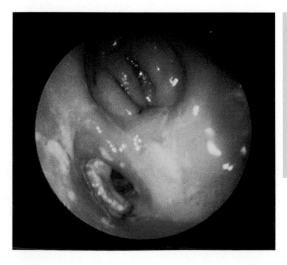

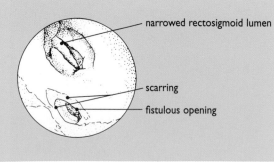

Figure 11.126 *Radiation-induced colonoscopic fistula narrows the sigmoid lumen.*

Neutropenic Colitis

Neutropenic colitis is a rare, poorly understood entity characterized by diffuse inflammatory changes of the colonic mucosa. Neutropenic colitis affects predominantly the right colon. The endoscopic abnormalities are mainly characterized by edema, erythema, and friability.

Collagenous Colitis

Collagenous colitis is a rare abnormality responsible for chronic diarrhea. The endoscopic abnormalities, if any, are usually rather subtle, characterized by mild opalescence and blurring of the vascular pattern (Fig. 11.132).

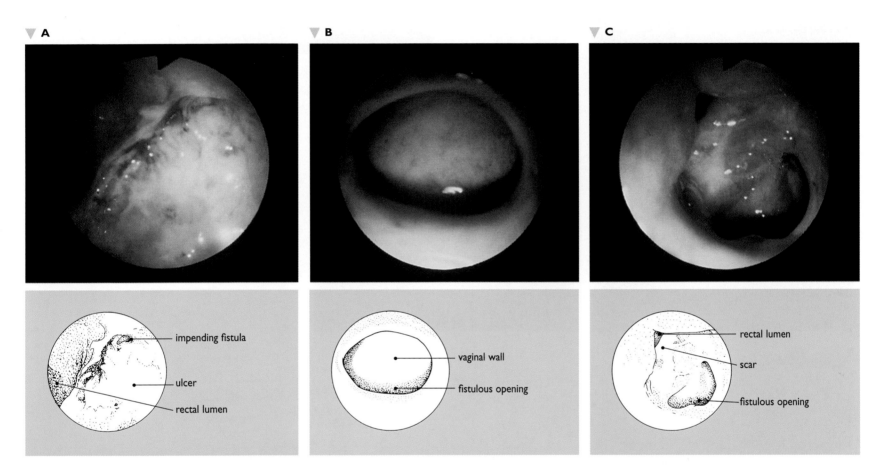

Figure 11.127 *Development of radiation-induced rectovaginal fistula. (**A**) Large radiation-induced ulcer appears near an impending fistula. (**B**) Wide rectovaginal fistula developed a few months later. (**C**) Another rectovaginal fistula.*

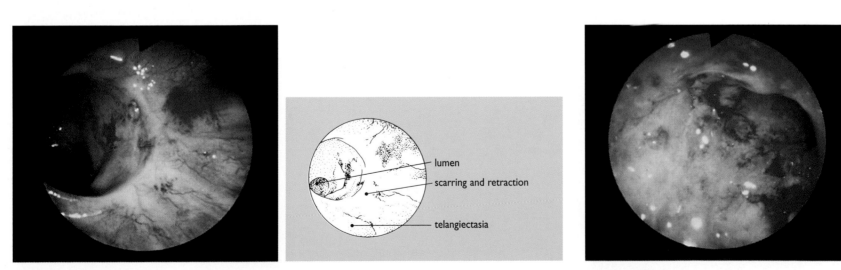

Figure 11.128 *Healing stage of an indolent, radiation-induced supra-anal ulcer.*

Figure 11.129 *Bypass colitis with loss of vascular pattern, erythema, and friability.*

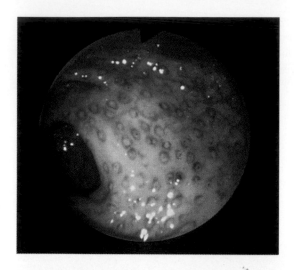

Figure 11.130 *Bypass colitis with enlarged lymphoid follicles mimics aphthoid erosions.*

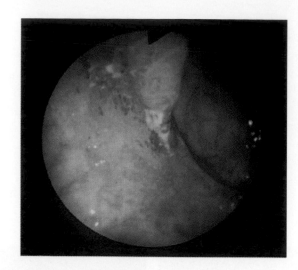

Figure 11.131 *Colonic ulceration in a patient with Behçet's disease.*

▼ **A**

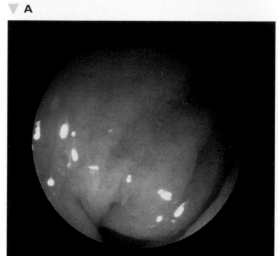

▼ **B**

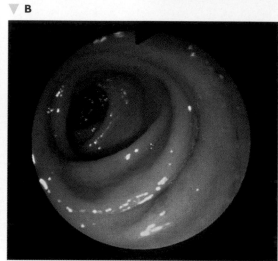

Figure 11.132 (**A** and **B**) *Collagenous colitis. Slight opalescence and blurring of the vascular pattern is seen.*

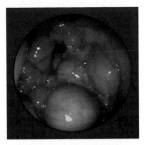

Colon III: Diverticular Disease, Vascular Malformations, and Other Colonic Abnormalities

In this chapter we discuss several common colonic abnormalities, including diverticular disease and its complications, vascular malformations, lower gastrointestinal bleeding, local trauma and a variety of other colonic abnormalities.

DIVERTICULAR DISEASE

Diverticular disease is an increasingly common clinical problem in the aging population of industrialized countries. It ranks with polyps as one of the most common abnormalities seen during colonoscopy. Muscular hypertrophy is the most striking feature. Although some patients have no symptoms, other experience cramping or altered bowel habits. Sometimes symptoms are related to complications of the disease, such as diverticulitis, abscess formation, or fistulization.

Colonoscopy is generally not helpful in the evaluation of patients with acute diverticulitis. However, it may be indicated for diagnosis in diverticular disease in the following settings: ambiguous x-ray findings, especially to exclude carcinoma; colonic bleeding; obstructed flow of barium; and, after a diverting colostomy for obstruction or perforation, to differentiate among polyp, cancer, and inflammation.

Colonoscopy in diverticular disease requires special techniques as the marked muscular hypertrophy causes shortening of the interhaustral segments and marked distortion of the luminal direction. Each fold distorting the lumen must be examined individually. Clues regarding the correct luminal direction may be obtained by observing the arch-like highlights on diverticular folds. However, these may also incorrectly lead the inexperienced endoscopist into a diverticulum.

ENDOSCOPIC APPEARANCE

In general, diverticular orifices are best viewed during the introduction phase of the colonoscopic examination. They represent focal weakness in the wall, usually in the area of penetrating blood vessels (Figs. 12.1 and 12.2). Although the sigmoid colon is the most common site, diverticular outpouchings may occur throughout the colon (Fig. 12.3). They are seen as small circular 2–5 mm widthopenings in the central portion of the interhaustral segment, situated between large thickened folds. Shortening of the teniae leads to the characteristic concertina-like corrugation of the circular muscle. Occasionally there are two or more diverticula per segment (Fig. 12.4) but usually there is only one.

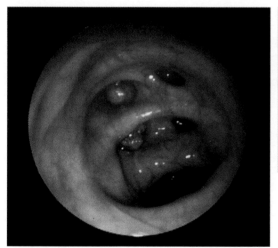

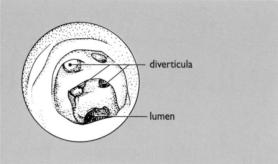

Figure 12.1 *Several diverticular outpouchings are located between thickened haustral folds. The oval-shaped lumen is eccentric.*

▼ **A**　　　　　▼ **B**

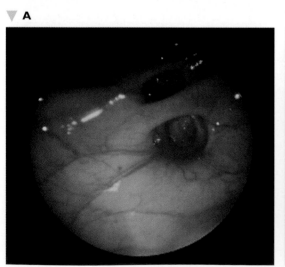

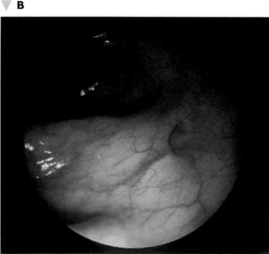

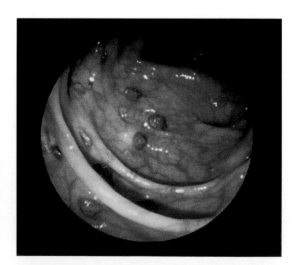

Figure 12.2 *(A and B) The relationship between vessels and diverticular outpouchings are obvious in these views.*

Figure 12.3 *Diverticulosis of the entire colon in a young patient. Numerous diverticula in the ascending colon are shown; fecal impaction is evident.*

Even in a well cleaned colon after gut lavage, diverticular openings may be impacted with stool or barium (Figs. 12.3 and 12.5). Such small fecal pellets within the diverticula may fall into the lumen and obscure endoscopic vision. These diverticular fecaliths can also be confused with a polyp or tumor (Fig. 12.6).

A novice endoscopist may confuse the opening of a diverticulum with the lumen, especially when multiple diverticula are associated with prominent haustral folds. There are some helpful clues to help the colonoscopist find the correct luminal axis. Diverticular openings occur between haustral folds, whereas the lumen is seen at the point where folds converge. The lumen is almost always at an angle to the axis of the colonoscope. A diverticular orifice usually appears round when seen close up, whereas the colonic lumen is usually distorted and slit-like. If there is any doubt, the operator should withdraw and re-establish the general direction of the lumen rather than proceed blindly. The concern is that one might enter and perforate a large diverticulum.

In uncomplicated diverticular disease, the mucosa is smooth and glistening and has a normal vascular pattern. Occasionally, prediverticular disease may be encountered in the form of muscle thickening and retraction, without evidence of diverticular outpouchings (Fig. 12.7). Upon careful inspection of the mucosa, minute outpouchings between the thickened muscle bands are seen occasionally. An inverted diverticulum is a rare finding (Fig. 12.8).

Stretching and compression of redundant mucosal folds is likely to occur in severe diverticular disease because of the underlying motility disorder, excessive cramping, and abnormal contraction (Fig. 12.9). With excessive cramping, patchy areas of markedly hyperemic and even hemorrhagic mucosa may develop (Fig. 12.10), or slightly elevated patches may seem to prolapse and gradually develop into polypoid excrescences (Fig. 12.11). Such polypoid structures are usually bright red hemispheres about 1 cm high, scattered irregularly between diverticula exclusively in the narrow sigmoid segment. These red patches or polypoid lesions may explain minor recurrent bleeding.

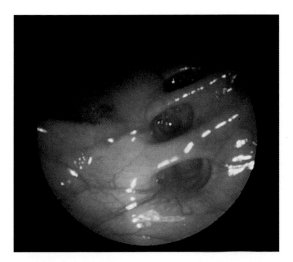

Figure 12.4 *Colonic segment with three diverticula in a row. Vessels are seen at the diverticular orifices.*

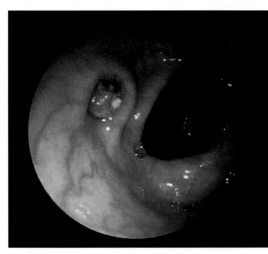

Figure 12.5 *Fecal impaction in a diverticulum.*

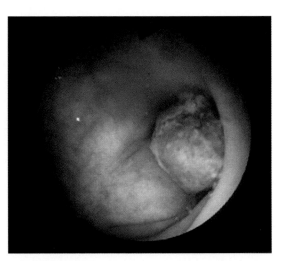

Figure 12.6 *Fecalith from a diverticulum that simulates a polyp or tumor in the colon. With careful observation and manipulation it can be distinguished from a neoplasm.*

▽ **A**

▽ **B**

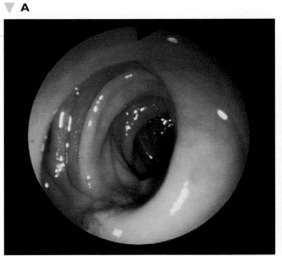

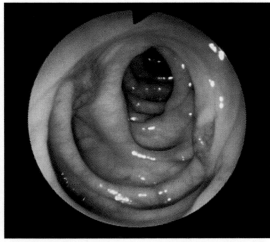

Figure 12.7 *(A and B) Two examples of luminal distortion in diverticular disease due to marked muscle thickening and retraction, and twisting of folds.*

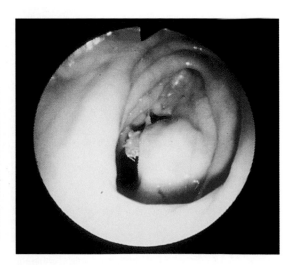

Figure 12.8 *Inverted diverticulum in the sigmoid colon.*

In diverticular disease the colonic mucosa may prolapse back and forth through an area of diverticular narrowing. This erythematous lesion may appear similar to an adenoma (Fig. 12.12), but with careful inspection it will become apparent that the red lesion is pliable, moves easily, and has no pedicle (Fig. 12.13). Furthermore, the absence of any lobulation or nodularity, which are common features in larger adenomas, also points to either a fold or a submucosal polypoid lesion. The gradual decrease in the intensity of the erythema from the top to the wide base, merging into normal mucosa, suggests the correct diagnosis. When inspected in detail, the overall texture of the mucosa covering the polypoid structures is identical to that of the surrounding mucosa. If the patient increases dietary fiber intake, these pseudopolypoid areas of mucosal prolapse may regress (Fig. 12.14).

ACUTE DIVERTICULITIS

The development of acute inflammation in and around the diverticulum-bearing segment is a major complication of diverticular disease. Pressure on the diverticular outpouchings due to fecaliths or other impacted materials leads to necrosis of the mucosal lining. This is followed by intramural invasion of bacteria, producing inflammation and abscess.

The dominant endoscopic features of acute diverticulitis include marked narrowing of the lumen due to excessive spasm, and swelling of the haustral folds (Figs. 12.15 and 12.16). In addition, there is patchy or diffuse erythema of the swollen contracted folds. Occasionally, purulent material exudes from the mouth of the inflamed diverticula or streams along the colonic wall. An intramural abscess may be seen in a narrowed segment (Fig. 12.17). The inflamed segment may narrow to a tiny luminal orifice, which may not be negotiable with a standard or small caliber colonoscope. It should be stressed that endoscopic evidence of acute inflammation does not exclude an underlying carcinoma until the area in question has been intubated and examined. After resolution of the acute episode of inflammation, the erythema, luminal narrowing, and edematous swelling of the folds may disappear entirely and the appearance may return to normal (Fig. 12.18).

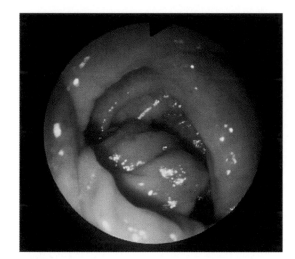

Figure 12.9 *Prolapsing redundant large folds may result from diverticular disease.*

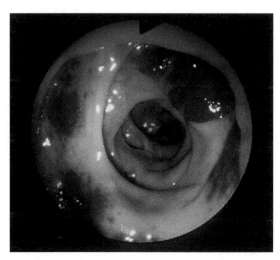

Figure 12.10 *In this patient, severe diverticular disease caused strikingly hyperemic patches as a result of marked congestion.*

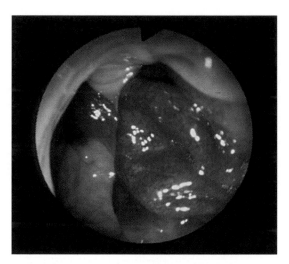

Figure 12.11 *Prolapsing polypoid-appearing folds with erythema in severe diverticular disease.*

▼ **A**

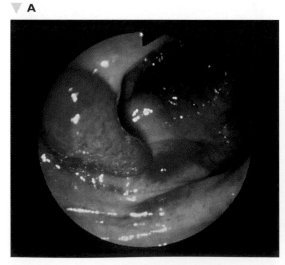

▼ **B**

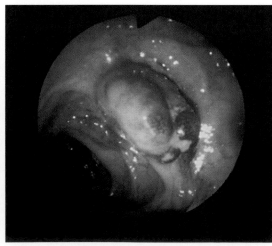

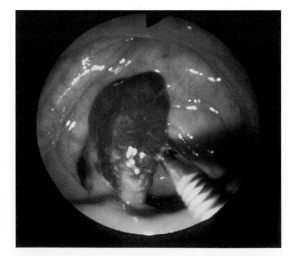

Figure 12.12 (A and **B)** *Examples of polyp-simulating structures due to redundant mucosal invagination in diverticular disease. Note the patches of striking erythema; however, these lesions consist of normal mucosa.*

Figure 12.13 *Markedly congested polyp-simulating structure caused by repetitive intraluminal mucosal invagination shows a pedicle-like base.*

DIVERTICULAR STRICTURE AND MALIGNANCY

The colonic narrowing in diverticular disease is largely caused by thickening of the muscle layers, and is especially apparent in the increased thickness of the haustral folds. Additional compromise of the lumen can result from a superimposed colic–pericolic inflammatory mass or colic and pericolic fibrosis. Because of the tortuosity of the sigmoid colon, it is often not possible to determine radiologically whether obstruction is secondary to inflammation or to carcinoma. If necessary, a small caliber colonoscope can usually be inserted to the point of obstruction.

In diverticulitis, the lumen may narrow abruptly, although the overlying mucosa is still intact and the folds themselves appear symmetrical and regular. By contrast, a malignant stricture usually obliterates and distorts parts of the involved folds. An irregular appearance and a hard consistency of the folds forming the entrance of the narrowed zone are both suggestive of malignancy (Fig. 12.19).

Malignancy is likely when an intraluminal, bulky tumor mass is noted within the narrowed zone. Therefore, all possible effort should be made to pass the obstructed segment with a small caliber colonoscope. If only markedly inflamed but otherwise intact nonsuspicious mucosa is seen, then the chance of underlying malignancy is remote. If, on the other hand, even a small focus of abnormal suspicious tissue is encountered, then there is a strong chance of malignancy. Multiple biopsies should be obtained from any exophytic growth or excessively necrotic-appearing area. Biopsies taken from the concentric folds encircling the narrowed lumen or even from within the strictured area are usually negative.

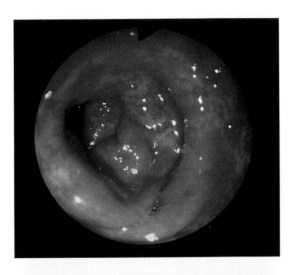

Figure 12.14 *Regression of pseudopolypoid areas of mucosal prolapse in diverticular disease after a year on a high fiber diet. The mucosa is still slightly red, but intense erythema and polyp-like structures have resolved.*

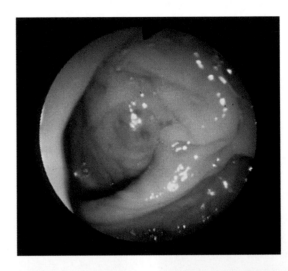

Figure 12.15 *Early diverticulitis. The mucosa is red and swollen, with spasm and swelling of the haustral folds.*

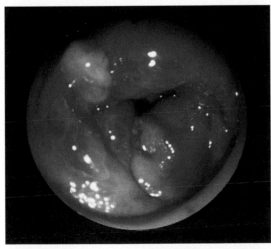

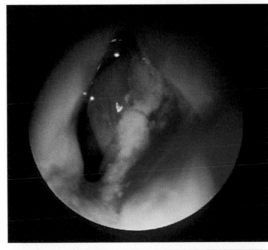

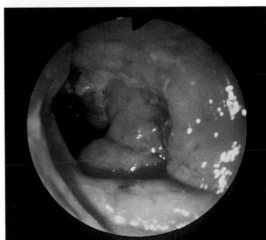

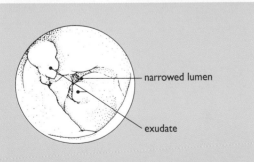

Figure 12.16 *Diffuse swelling obliterates the lumen in full-blown diverticulitis. Erythema and focal purulent exudate are also discernible.*

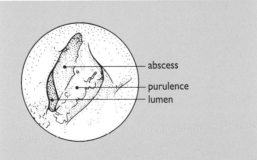

Figure 12.17 *Diverticulitis with intramural abscess. Purulence is noted and the lumen is narrow.*

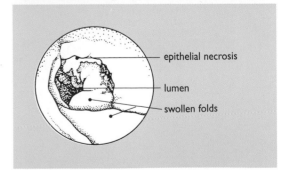

Figure 12.18 *Resolution phase of acute diverticulitis exhibits resolving inflammation and reopening of the lumen. Epithelial destruction is present, and patchy areas of erythema are still visible.*

If the obstructed segment cannot be passed, no conclusion can be reached on the presence or absence of malignancy, and surgical exploration is mandatory. If it cannot be determined at surgery whether the mass is neoplastic or inflammatory, a diversion of the fecal stream is often created with a distal mucous fistula. After several weeks or months, the narrowed area can be re-examined colonoscopically, with biopsies if appropriate, to determine whether the inflammatory changes have resolved (suggesting diverticulitis) or whether malignancy is present. This information will guide decisions about further surgical therapy.

Endoscopic ultrasound will improve the diagnosis and management of diverticulitis by helping the endoscopist to differentiate between diverticulitis and cancer, and by detecting complications such as abscess formation.

VASCULAR MALFORMATIONS

ANGIODYSPLASIA

Angiodysplasia is a microvascular abnormality of the mucosa and submucosa of the colon that may rupture or ulcerate and cause lower intestinal bleeding. It is a common cause of chronic, intermittent, or acute colonic bleeding. The pathophysiology of the formation of angiodysplastic lesions is not known. Speculations have included the relative obstruction, by hypertrophied muscle, of the small veins passing through the muscularis externa. This obstruction gradually backs up until the capillaries are dilated and abnormal arteriovenous connections are formed.

Most angiodysplastic lesions occur in the large diameter cecum and right colon, rarely in the ileum. The greater amount of tension within the bowel wall in these sections contributes to the partial obstruction of the submucosal veins. Angiodysplasia is also encountered in patients with aortic valve disease. Less commonly, angiodysplastic lesions of the colon have been seen in people under 50 years of age, spreading out over the colon and the small bowel (Fig. 12.20). It is possible that congenital abnormalities of the colonic microcirculation lead to the development of this disease in adult life, in conjunction with increased blood pressure and colonic motor disorders.

Angiodysplasia has a variable appearance in the mucosa of the colon. Some of the lesions are large and may seem raised with an irregular border. The smaller lesions appear as bright red spots, often just a few millimeters in diameter (Fig. 12.21). Various shapes are described, including linear, flat, and raised (Figs. 12.22–12.25). The larger lesions may appear superficially eroded and may be responsible for gastrointestinal hemorrhage. The lesions may occur singly or they may appear in groups. Lesions of several variable sizes may

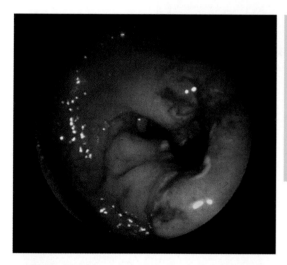

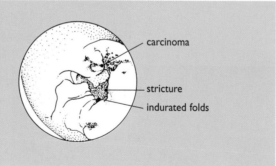

Figure 12.19 *Stenosing sigmoid carcinoma with submucosal spread of tumor. The folds at the entrance to the strictured area were firm and indurated in appearance. An Nd:YAG laser had been used earlier to reopen the stenosis.*

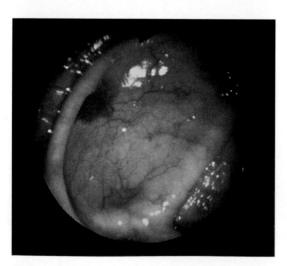

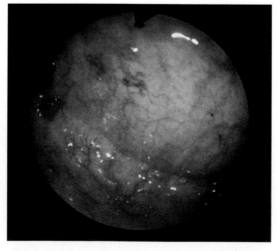

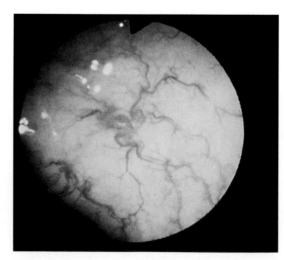

Figure 12.20 *Spectrum of congenital angiodysplastic lesions spread throughout the colon in a young patient.*

Figure 12.21 *Early angiodysplasia with small lesions.*

Figure 12.22 *Early angiodysplastic lesions are seen as slightly dilated tortuous vessels.*

be noted (Fig. 12.26). These lesions can be located anywhere in the gastrointestinal tract and colon. Typically, the right colon and cecum are involved.

The degree of distortion of the adjacent vascular architecture varies with each stage in the evolution of the ectasias. In addition to the reddish vascular clusters or tufts, sometimes bluish draining veins may be seen. The vascular clusters have been compared to the petals of a flower, with the bluish draining veins representing the stem.

Angiodysplastic lesions should not be confused with iatrogenic mucosal injury. The irregular margins of angiodysplastic lesions allow them to be distinguished from colonoscope-induced intramucosal hemorrhage (Fig. 12.27).

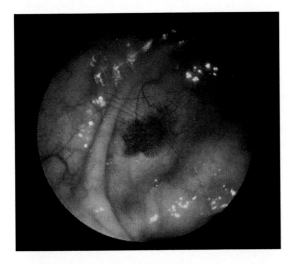

Figure 12.23 *Angiodysplasia. A red capillary tuft has individually recognizable ectatic vessels.*

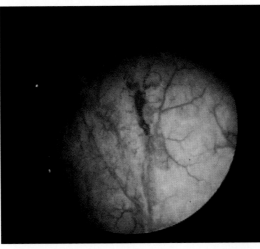

Figure 12.24 *A linear angiodysplasia is connected to a pinhead-sized ectasia by capillaries.*

▼ **A**

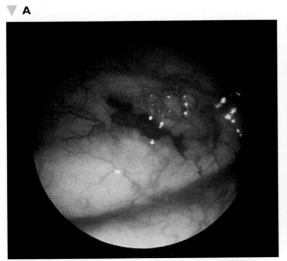

▼ **B**

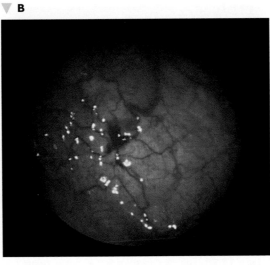

Figure 12.25 *(**A** and **B**) Two cases of angiodysplasia involving the colon. Association with vessels is evident.*

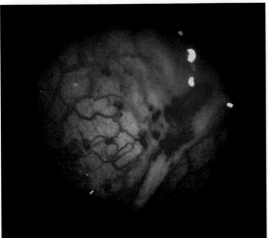

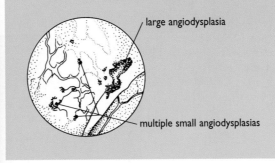

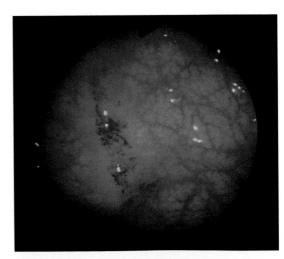

Figure 12.26 *A larger angiodysplasia and multiple small angiodysplasias are apparently interconnected in this view. Draining veins are characteristically bluish.*

Figure 12.27 *Intramucosal bleeding spots in the splenic flexure were induced by the colonoscope.*

The latter areas of mucosal trauma often occur at sharply angulated segments such as the descending–sigmoid junction. Angiodysplasia should not be confused that telangiectasia seen in radiation colitis. A rare cause of vascular malformation that may mimic angiodysplasia is that produced after repetitive trauma of the rectal wall during manual evacuation of feces (Fig. 12.28). The usual therapy for angiodysplastic lesions is eradication with laser energy (Argon or Nd:YAG) or with electrocoagulation using monopolar (hot biopsy forceps) or, more commonly now, bipolar coagulation or a heater probe (Fig. 12.29). In performing a hot biopsy of a vascular ectasia in the cecum, the mucosa should be lifted or 'tented' off the underlying submucosa to avoid transmural burns. Such therapy is especially useful in elderly patients and in patients with complicated medical illnesses who are high operative risks. For younger patients with very extensive lesions, some advocate surgical resection. Studies suggest that therapy of angiodysplastic lesions reduces transfusion requirements over time.

HEMANGIOMA

Hemangiomas of the large bowel arise from submucosal vascular plexuses, usually of the rectum and distal colon. When they create a mass-like deformity, they are usually referred to as cavernous hemangiomas. When they are smaller, they are referred to as the capillary type (Fig. 12.30). They may be responsible for chronic or intermittent bleeding; if so, they may be treated by photocoagulation (Fig. 12.31).

Sizable cavernous hemangiomas are usually recognized endoscopically as ill defined polypoid masses; distinct ulceration is not ordinarily present. These lesions may bleed heavily if biopsied; therefore, most endoscopists do not biopsy a lesion if they think that it is a hemangioma. A dark blue or dark red color is typical of a hemangioma. Some are berry-like lesions with a deep blue to dull red or port-wine coloration (Fig. 12.32).

Hemangiomas may also occur as infiltrating vascular lesions involving large segments of the rectum and sigmoid colon. Such flat or minimally elevated diffuse lesions are often poorly defined and of a bluish color (Fig. 12.33).

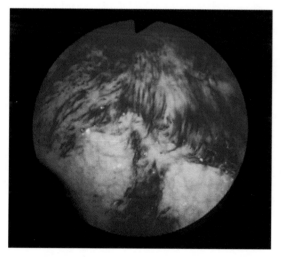

Figure 12.28 *Bizarre vascular malformation of the rectal wall occurred after repetitive trauma caused by manual evacuation of stool.*

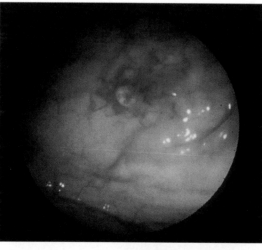

Figure 12.29 *This angiodysplastic lesion was treated with one Nd:YAG laser shot, resulting in blanching.*

Figure 12.30 *Colonic hemangioma of the diffuse capillary type.*

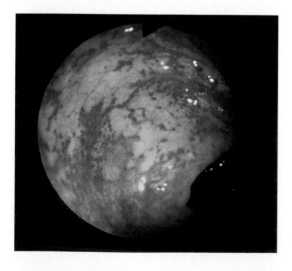

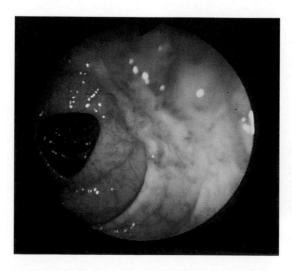

Figure 12.31 *Partial treatment with a single Nd:YAG laser application leaves traces of a large cavernous hemangioma.*

RARE VASCULAR ABNORMALITIES

Other vascular lesions may be encountered in the colon. Varicose veins may occur in patients with portal hypertension. These tend to occur in the rectum and the distal sigmoid colon. The color may appear normal or the varices may have a bluish appearance. These veins tend to run in a longitudinal fashion and are often tortuous, typical of varicose veins elsewhere in the gastrointestinal tract. One must be careful not to mistake these for a polyp. An endoscopic Doppler device might be useful to detect venous flow in what otherwise appears to be a polyp. Endoscopic ultrasound imaging can also assist in the diagnosis of a varix. Careful visual inspection at colonoscopy usually reveals that the varices are part of a venous system (Figs. 12.34 to 12.36).

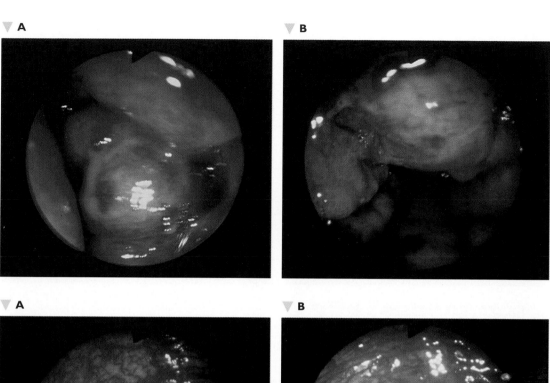

Figure 12.32 (**A** and **B**) Two views of a large rectal hemangioma occurring as a polypoid mass that could be confused with a polyp, malignancy, or internal hemorrhoid.

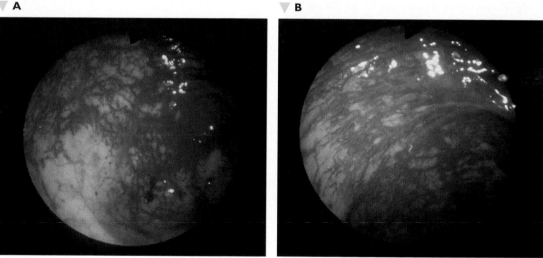

Figure 12.33 (**A** and **B**) Coalescence of diffuse hemangioma involving the rectum and sigmoid colon. Slight protrusion of the vascular anomaly is noted, but the overall pattern is flat.

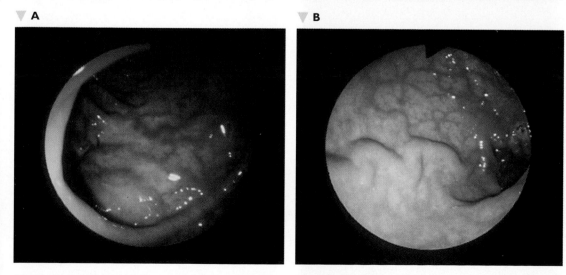

Figure 12.34 (**A** and **B**) Two examples of early varices in the sigmoid colon.

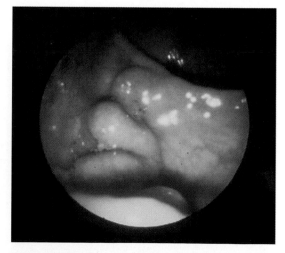

Figure 12.35 Large varix of the sigmoid colon runs perpendicularly to haustral folds.

Evidence of vasculitis may also be found in Henoch-Schönlein syndrome. These patients may present with evidence of gastrointestinal hemorrhage, and at colonoscopy there may be signs of vascular injury of the wall with petechiae (Fig. 12.37). In polyarteritis nodosa and other types of vasculitis the changes may include ulceration and erythema (Fig. 12.38).

Vascular malformations consisting of excessively tortuous protuberant bizarrely developed vascular structures are occasionally encountered in the colon. Such abnormalities, which may be responsible for chronic blood loss, are difficult to classify at present (Fig. 12.39). Abnormalities in vessels may occur at the level of anastomoses (Fig. 12.40).

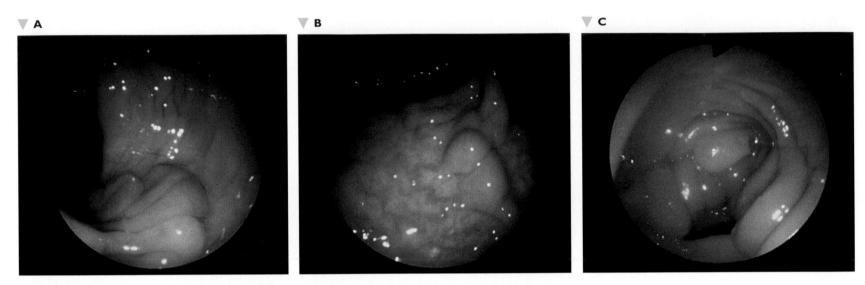

Figure 12.36 (A–C) Three views of varices in the colon. The appearance can vary from polyp-like to a heavy fold. In these examples, the covering mucosa appears normal.

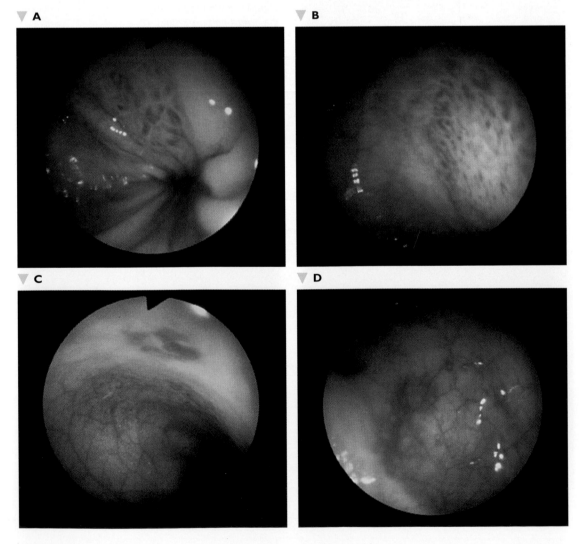

Figure 12.37 (A–D) Henoch-Schönlein vasculitis appears as multiple petechiae (**A** and **B**) or as a central purpura within an area of blanching adjacent to normal vasculature (**C** and **D**).

DIAGNOSIS OF COLONIC BLEEDING

Bleeding from the colon is a frequent problem, especially in the elderly. Colonic bleeding is most often chronic and intermittent, although occasionally bleeding may be massive. A variety of lesions may be responsible for colonic bleeding, as listed in Figure 12.41.

Hemorrhoids and anal fissures can be ruled out easily by appropriate endoscopic examination.

Diverticular disease can cause acute or chronic intermittent colonic bleeding. Stretching and distortion of the vessel walls through increased intraluminal pressure is thought to weaken the vessels and to predispose them to rupture into the diverticulum. Localization of the bleeding site to the left colon in a patient with diverticular disease and no other distinguishable lesions strongly suggests that the bleeding has a diverticular origin. However, one must remember that right-sided diverticula can also bleed. The diagnosis is often one of exclusion, as an actively bleeding diverticulum is only

▼ A

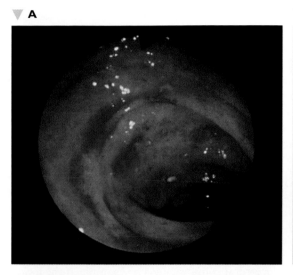

▼ B

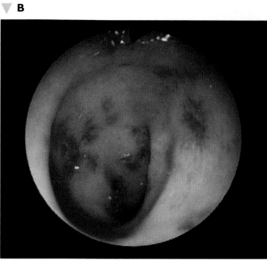

Figure 12.38 *Vasculitic changes involving the colon are mainly characterized by focal erythema and, occasionally, by discrete intramural bleeding.*

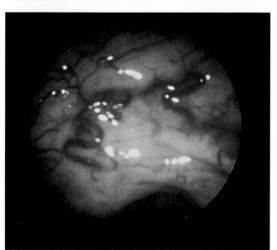

Figure 12.39 *Bizarre vascular malformation.*

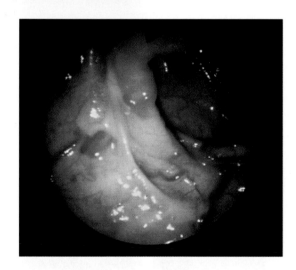

Figure 12.40 *Abnormal vessels at colonic anastomosis.*

Figure 12.41 *Causes of rectal bleeding.*

Causes of Rectal Bleeding

Hemorrhoids
Anal fissures
Diverticular disease
Idiopathic inflammatory bowel disease
      Ulcerative colitis
      Crohn's disease
Radiation colitis
Ischemic colitis
Infectious colitis
Vascular malformations (angiodysplasia/varices)
Colonic polyps
Colorectal cancer
Small bowel lesions (especially distal)
Upper gastrointestinal lesions
Idiopathic ulcerations

rarely identified during colonoscopy. If there is any doubt, colonoscopy should be repeated soon after the bleeding ceases. Diverticular bleeding may be so brisk that the lumen is obscured. Occasionally, blood may be seen welling up from the bleeding diverticulum, resulting in copious amounts of blood filling the distal colon.

Inflammatory bowel disease is occasionally detected during colonoscopy performed for chronic or intermittent bleeding. Ulcerative colitis is usually associated with severe inflammation and diffuse continuous bleeding from the inflamed mucosal surface. In Crohn's disease, deep focal ulceration involving major vessels causes the brisk bleeding. Infectious colitis and radiation damage rarely cause major bleeding.

Occasionally, ischemic damage of the colon may produce bleeding, typically in the splenic flexure area, descending colon, and sigmoid colon. Marked mucosal friability with spontaneous bleeding is seen in conjunction with extensive intramural hemorrhage, as evidenced by the presence of petechiae and ecchymoses.

Vascular malformations, especially angiodysplasia, are increasingly recognized as a cause of intermittent brisk or chronic low-grade bleeding. The visible angiodysplasia is only a manifestation of a diffusely deranged mucosal and submucosal vascular network.

Neoplasms in the form of adenomatous polyps or colorectal cancer are the most common lesions identified at colonoscopy in patients with colonic bleeding. The adenomatous polyps that bleed tend to be large causing the polyps to be repeatedly traumatized. Twisting and bending leads to fracture of the stalk and vascular obstruction, resulting in congestion and hemorrhage. In addition, the surface of a polyp that has bled becomes fragile. Bleeding also occurs after autoamputation.

When a patient notes red blood streaking the stool, a polypoid carcinoma of the sigmoid colon may be the cause. Other cancers detected because of bleeding, especially in the right colon, are usually large centrally ulcerated masses. Distal small bowel lesions may be a cause of lower gastrointestinal tract bleeding, especially in patients whose detectable angiodysplastic lesions of the colon have been adequately treated endoscopically.

The possibility of an upper gastrointestinal bleeding site should always be considered in patients passing large amounts of red blood through the rectum. If an upper gastrointestinal site is suspected, it is worthwhile to pass an endoscope into the stomach and duodenum first to see whether there is evidence of active bleeding and to determine the bleeding site. It is essential in all patients presenting with gastrointestinal bleeding to consider the possibility of an upper gastrointestinal bleed being misdiagnosed as lower gastrointestinal hemorrhage. A brief screening endoscopy can be performed to rule out an upper gastrointestinal source rapidly. Alternatively, one can pass an orogastric tube into the stomach to see whether blood is present.

A careful history usually offers considerable information about the source of the bleeding. Red blood on toilet tissue or bleeding unrelated to defecation is often due to hemorrhoids or fissures external to the sphincter muscles. Dripping red blood after defecation is also usually hemorrhoidal. When a stripe of blood is seen on the stool, or flecks of blood are mixed with the stool, the lesion usually lies above the rectum in the area of the sigmoid colon. Blood from sites proximal to the descending colon is mixed with the stool and may not be grossly visible, but can be detected by fecal occult blood testing.

For any patient with hematochezia, an anorectal sigmoidoscopic examination should be performed first to look for anal or rectal pathology. Blood attributed to hemorrhoids may be related to a low-lying carcinoma or polyp. Although a rigid anoscope is the standard technique, the flexible sigmoidoscope can be retroflexed in the rectal ampulla to examine the hemorrhoidal ring (Fig. 12.42). If no lesion is obvious, it may be necessary to perform a total colonoscopy. If certain lesions are found in the sigmoid colon, it still may be necessary to perform a total colonoscopy. For example, if the lesion detected is an adenomatous polyp, colonoscopy is indicated to detect a synchronous polyp or carcinoma above the low-lying lesion.

To identify a bleeding site, blood must be seen actively trickling or spurting. Presence of blood in the vicinity of an apparent vascular ectasia or diverticulum is not convincing evidence. On the other hand, rapid bleeding usually overwhelms the cleaning capability of the colonoscope.

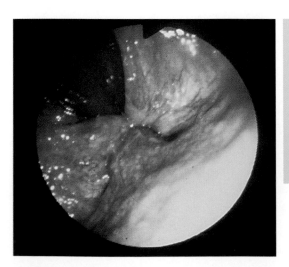

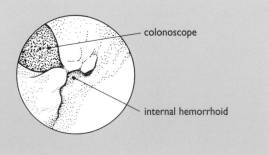

Figure 12.42 *An internal hemorrhoid is seen after retroflexing the colonoscope.*

Colonoscopy is assuming an increasing role in cases of massive dramatic bleeding. Large amounts of blood and clots may make it difficult to examine the colon. Nevertheless, for some patients with massive bleeding, colonoscopy has been reported as having a high diagnostic yield.

Colonoscopy is most valuable for patients with intermittent or moderate bleeding. With the latter, the blood acts as a cathartic to clean the bowel and minimal preparation is necessary. However, blood clots should be evacuated from the rectum by enema before starting the examination, to prevent

blockage of the instrument suction channel during colonoscopy. If there is a pool of blood, the patient can be repositioned so that the blood forms a layer at the bottom of the endoscopic field of vision, and the instrument can then be advanced over it. By maintaining an almost constant spray of water, the image can be kept clear as the insertion proceeds.

The goal of colonoscopy in chronic, more occult bleeding is to define accurately the bleeding source, to provide effective therapy whenever possible, and to help guide the surgical approach. In patients with rectal bleeding it is wise to study the entire length of the colon unless a known source is positively identified. It is a mistake to presume hemorrhoidal bleeding when a polyp or cancer may be present above the level inspected. Flexible sigmoidoscopy is inadequate for this because only a portion of the colon is inspected. Several studies have shown that in a patient who has chronic rectal bleeding with a negative sigmoidoscopy and negative barium enema, colonoscopy is very effective to diagnose causes, for example polyps or cancer, not identified by prior tests.

Some of the causes of colonic bleeding are amenable to endoscopic treatment. Polyps may be removed easily and safely. Telangiectasis may be treated with laser coagulation, heater probe or electrocoagulation. Rebleeding, however, is not uncommon with angiodysplasias because of the widespread nature of the vascular abnormality.

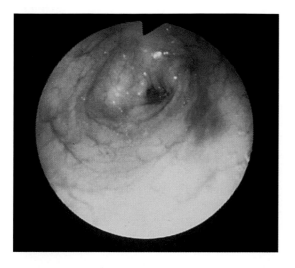

Figure 12.43
Endometriosis of the sigmoid colon causes luminal narrowing. A reddish area is evident.

OTHER COLONIC ABNORMALITIES

ABNORMALITIES OF GENITAL ORIGIN

Because of its proximity to the uterus, the sigmoid colon may become involved with endometriosis. Abrupt severe narrowing is the characteristic finding. The mucosa at the mouth of the narrowed zone appears intact except for some swelling and a glassy appearance (Figs. 12.43 and 12.44). The

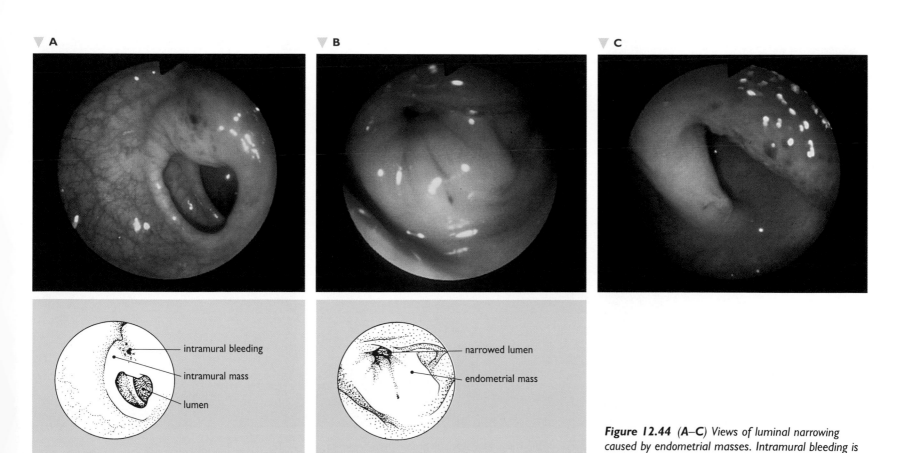

Figure 12.44 (A–C) Views of luminal narrowing caused by endometrial masses. Intramural bleeding is often seen.

obstructing mass is of firm consistency. When examined at the time of the menstrual period, reddish spots or reddish flecks may be observed surrounded by somewhat irregular granular mucosa (Fig. 12.45).

Extrinsic compression of the sigmoid colon by an enlarged fibroid uterus or enlarged ovary may distort the lumen and create an asymmetrical stricture-like appearance. If the fold pattern remains intact and there is no evidence of significant diverticular disease, the examiner should suspect extrinsic compression.

Other suppurative inflammation of the adnexa may occasionally lead to fistulization into the sigmoid colon and the formation of a granulation polyp (Fig. 12.46). Usually the sigmoid colon is markedly fixed to the adnexal mass, which makes polypectomy difficult. The histologic nature of the polyp suggests the correct pathology.

PSEUDOMELANOSIS COLI AND CATHARTIC COLON

Pseudomelanosis coli is caused by the accumulation of a brownish-black lipofuscin pigment in the lysosomes of the subepithelial macrophages, resulting from the ingestion of anthraquinone laxatives. Depending upon the mode of administration of anthraquinone-containing laxatives, the lesions may be distinguished throughout the colon or limited to the rectosigmoid area.

The striking feature at endoscopy is the mucosal coloration, which varies from slightly gray to anthracite or completely black. This discoloration may be seen in patches or streaks (Fig. 12.47). Characteristically, there is a sharp demarcation at the ileocecal valve between the normal-colored small intestine and the pigmented colonic mucosa. When adenomatous polyps are present in pseudomelanosis coli, they characteristically lack the blackish pigment and stand out as whitish excrescences against the dark background (Fig. 12.48). Lymph follicles may also appear as white dots on a pigmented

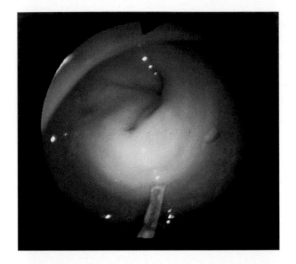

Figure 12.45
Endometriosis of the rectum occurring as an obstruction.

▽ **A**

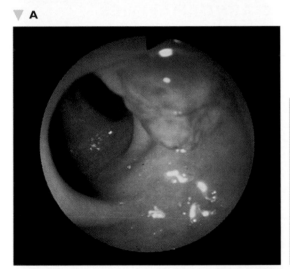

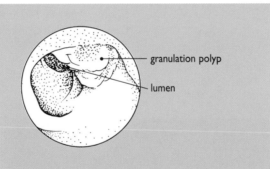

granulation polyp

lumen

▽ **B**

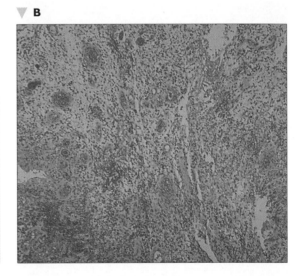

Figure 12.46 (**A**) *Polypoid lesion consisting of granulation tissue at the rectosigmoid junctionis caused by chronic suppurative inflammation of the left adnexa.* (**B**) *Histology of the granulation polyp.*

▽ **A**

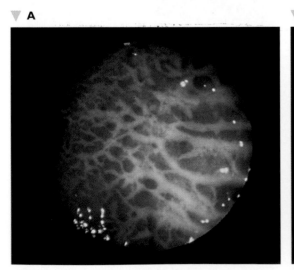

▽ **B**

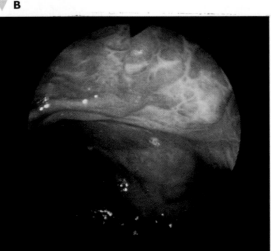

▽ **C**

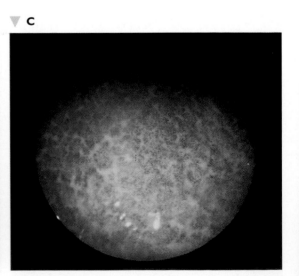

Figure 12.47 (**A–C**) *Different appearances of pseudomelanosis of the colon. Discoloration ranges from brown to black.*

background (Fig. 12.49). On cessation of the anthraquinone laxative, the coloration disappears gradually over several months. Inflammatory changes of the mucosa, such as erythema or granularity, are usually not present in a pseudomelanotic colon.

COLONIC ULCERS
Solitary Rectal Ulcer
The solitary rectal ulcer syndrome is thought to be a consequence of excessive straining, which may cause internal prolapse of the mucosa, with stretching and compression eventually leading to ischemia, inflammation, and an anterior rectal wall ulcer (Fig. 12.50). A solitary rectal ulcer must be distinguished

from traumatic ulceration, as seen in homosexual men. In some patients, the trauma to the rectal wall is self-induced by digital extraction of fecal material to assist defecation or by repeated manual manipulation with foreign objects (Figs. 12.51 and 12.52). Traumatic ulceration may also occur after inadvertent intramucosal injection of hypertonic topical laxative solutions or laceration by instruments such as an enema tip (Fig. 12.53). The ulcers themselves are large, with a well defined edge. Despite the name, solitary ulcers are quite often multiple. Injury can be caused by foreign bodies (Fig. 12.54). Lacerations can be the result of acute trauma (Fig. 12.55). A solitary ulcer can also be seen in association with ulcerative colitis (Fig. 12.56).

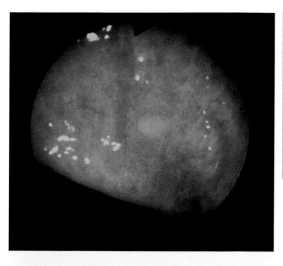

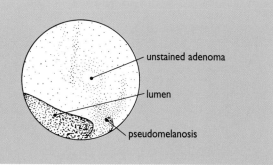

Figure 12.48 *Small unstained adenoma stands out in pseudomelanosis.*

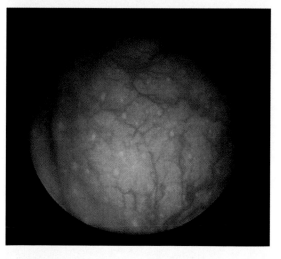

Figure 12.49 *Pseudomelanosis of the colon with lymph follicles, which stand out as white dots.*

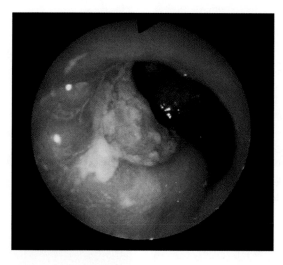

Figure 12.50 *A solitary ulcer of the rectum may be caused by repetitive injury to a small area.*

▼ **A**

▼ **B**

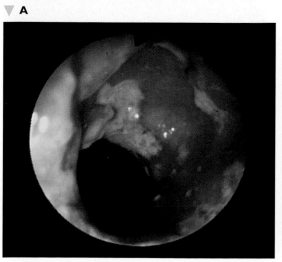

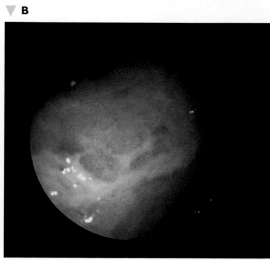

Figure 12.51 *(A and B) Two cases of rectal ulcers caused by encopresis and manual manipulation.*

COLITIS CYSTICA PROFUNDA

Colitis cystica profunda is not well understood. It refers to the finding of mucus retention cysts in the submucosa of the colonic wall. This occurs in the distal colon and rectum, and may be related to the solitary rectal ulcer syndrome. Endoscopically these lesions appear as slightly raised mucosa that may feel firm and be superficially eroded. The firm consistency and abnormally deep cysts may simulate carcinoma but this can be differentiated by histologic interpretation of biopsies (Fig. 12.57).

PNEUMATOSIS COLI

Pneumatosis coli is characterized by the presence of gas-filled cysts within the mucosa and submucosa of the colon. Usually only one segment of the colon is involved, especially the sigmoid or descending colon. At endoscopy, clusters of broad-based smooth polypoid bulges are seen that may have a

peculiar transparency (Fig. 12.58). Quite often there is erythema at the tip of these bulges, presumably secondary to friction. When they are multiple, the cysts may appear to obstruct the lumen, but the endoscope can usually be passed. Some bleeding may occur as a result of breakdown of the hemorrhagic mucosa on the surface of the cysts. When punctured, gas may escape. Such lesions should not be removed with electrocautery snares because the gas within the cysts may be explosive. Upon treatment with pure or hyperbaric oxygen, the cysts may gradually disappear, leaving behind a somewhat thickened brownish discolored granular mucosa (Fig. 12.59).

HIRSCHSPRUNG'S DISEASE AND STERCORAL ULCERATION

Hirschsprung's disease is a rare indication for colonoscopy. Proper cleansing of the colon in such circumstances is usually extremely difficult. The distal

▼ A ▼ B

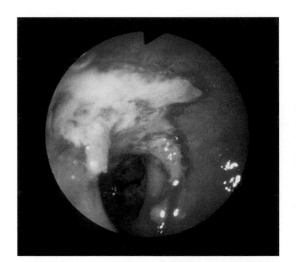 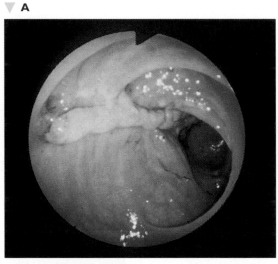 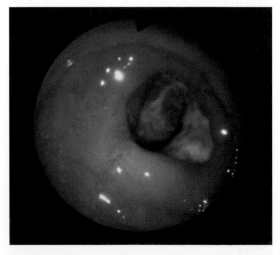

Figure 12.52 *Healing stage of ulcer caused by automanipulation.*

Figure 12.53 *(A and B) Two views of longitudinal laceration of the upper rectum caused by the forceful insertion of an enema cannula.*

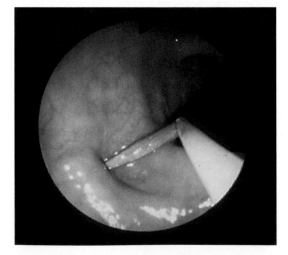 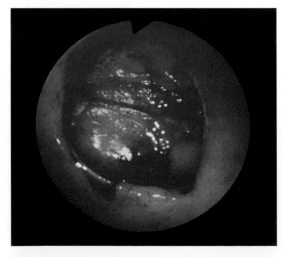

Figure 12.54 *Colonoscopic removal of sharp wooden stick from the colon.*

Figure 12.55 *Laceration of sigmoid colon. The mucosa is torn and submucosal or serosal vessels are seen.*

Figure 12.56 *Solitary rectal ulcer in a patient with ulcerative colitis.*

denervated segment typically has a normal caliber and an unremarkable mucosa (Fig. 12.60). Above the denervated segment is a tremendously dilated colon. Not uncommonly, bizarre-shaped stercoral ulcers are present in the area where the widely dilated colon joins the denervated segment (Fig. 12.61).

Stercoral ulcers may develop whenever there is a colonic stasis with fecalith or fecaloma formation. (Fecaliths are stone-like formations of fecal matter. When they reach a size of 2 cm in diameter or more they are termed fecalomas.) These firm masses of feces may injure and necrose the mucosal lining.

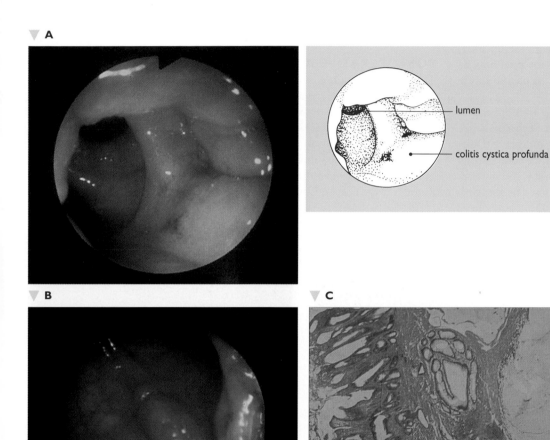

Figure 12.57 (*A–C*) Colitis cystica profunda. (*A*) The thickened area in the distal rectum characterizes the disorder. (*B*) Here the lesion simulates a tumor. (*C*) Corresponding biopsy shows mucin-filled submucosal cysts.

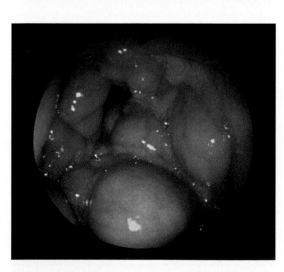

Figure 12.58 Pneumatosis coli. Gas-filled cysts seem to occlude the lumen.

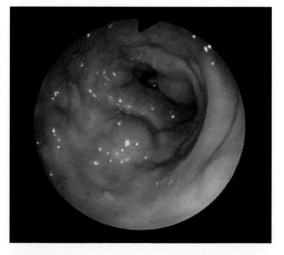

Figure 12.59 Hyperbaric oxygen therapy can cause regression of cysts.

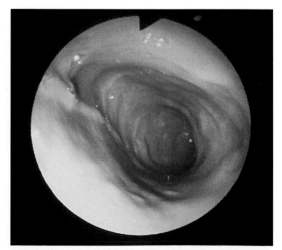

Figure 12.60 Adult Hirschsprung's disease. The distal denervated segment has normal caliber and mucosal appearance.

DEROTATION OF COLONIC VOLVULUS

Colonoscopy is used in the diagnosis and therapy of intermittent volvulus of the sigmoid colon. Usually at the point of obstruction, twisted mucosal folds can be seen (Fig. 12.62). The mucosa usually looks normal, but may have an appearance suggesting a compromised vascular supply with cyanosis. Derotation of the volvulus may occur if the twisted area can be gently entered and liquid stool and gas can be removed through the suction channel of the endoscope.

APPENDIX AND APPENDICEAL LESIONS

The normal appendiceal orifice is a slit-like, semilunar pocket on the posterior medial wall of the cecum. The root may protrude from the opening, especially when the appendix contracts (Fig. 12.63). Fecal material may be present in the appendiceal opening and can be the cause of partial intussusception of the appendiceal structure (Fig. 12.64).

A common abnormality is an inverted appendiceal stump after appendectomy, which may appear as a smooth oblong mass (Fig. 12.65). Such a mass-like deformity can easily be mistaken for an adenomatous polyp, especially if adenomatous polyps are present in the cecal area or if surveillance colonoscopy is performed after previous removal of adenomatous polyps. It is usually covered by normal-appearing mucosa. When in doubt, biopsies should be obtained.

Such a lesion should not be removed with a polypectomy snare if there is the slightest suspicion that it might be an inverted appendiceal stump.

It is most unusual to see purulent material exuding from the appendiceal orifice (Fig. 12.66). More often, an appendiceal inflammatory mass compresses the medial or posterior cecal wall, with edema of the mucosa and stretching of the folds (Fig. 12.67).

The appendiceal region and bottom of the cecum have a unique appearance after intussusception of the ileocecal area. This is a very rarely noted lesion. Because of marked venous congestion, there may be impressive petechial or ecchymotic discoloration of the mucosa.

POSTOPERATIVE APPEARANCES

The colonoscopist needs to be aware of the range of appearances after colonic resection and colonic anastomosis.

An anastomosis between the small intestine and colon may be either side-to-end or end-to-end (Fig. 12.68). The overall color and texture of the two segments are usually sufficiently different to determine the anastomotic line. This line can also be indicated by differences in the vascular pattern. The anastomosis between the ileum and colon may be regular and smooth or nodular (Fig. 12.69). Ring-like Kerckring's folds are often seen just beyond

▼ A   ▼ B

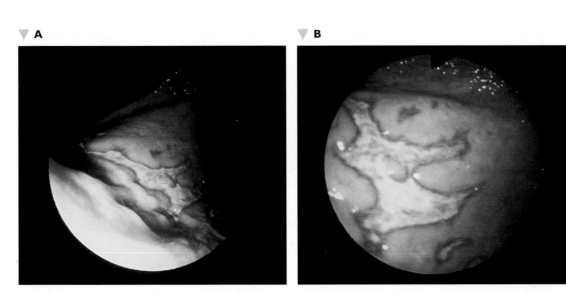

▼ C

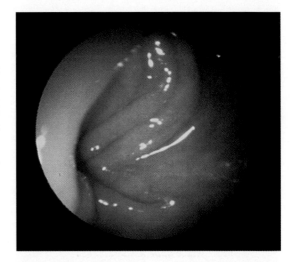

Figure 12.61 (**A** and **B**) Two views of Hirschsprung's disease. Widely dilated segment of the colon often shows bizarre stercoral ulceration caused by fecal stasis.

Figure 12.62 Colonic volvulus. The twisting mucosal fold pattern is characteristic.

▼ A   ▼ B   ▼ C

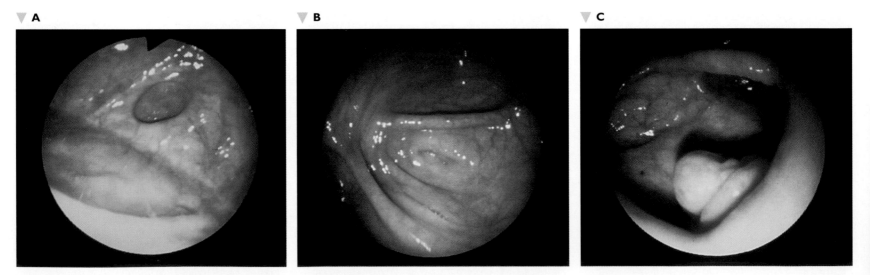

Figure 12.63 (**A–C**) Appendix. (**A** and **B**) Two examples of normal appearance of opening. (**C**) In a different patient, the root of the appendix protrudes upon the appendiceal contraction.

the anastomosis. Features such as erythema and nodularity of the anastomotic line are not specific and should not be interpreted as evidence of recurrent inflammatory disease by itself.

A colocolonic anastomosis is usually fashioned end-to-end. The anastomotic line may be a thin perfectly smooth scar (Fig. 12.70). When interrupted sutures are used, the anastomotic site may be nodular. Sometimes the

▼ **A**

▼ **B**

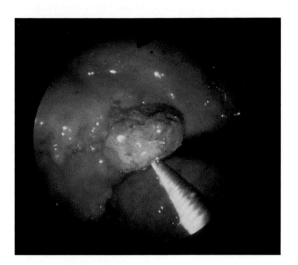

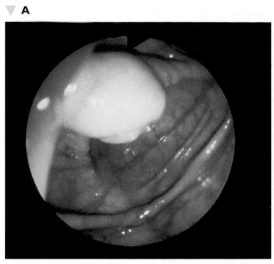

Figure 12.64 *Partial spontaneous intussusception of the appendix encrusted with fecal material.*

Figure 12.65 *(A and B) Two examples of an inverted appendiceal stump. This is common after appendectomy.*

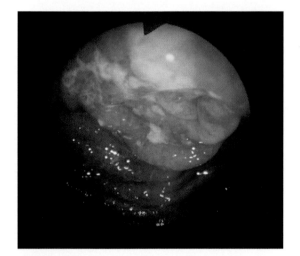

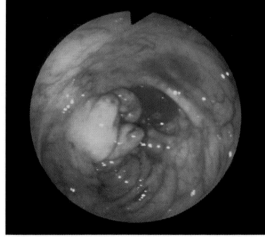

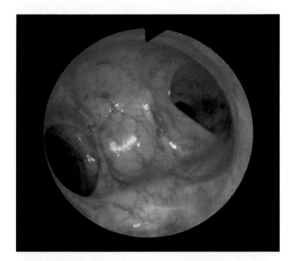

Figure 12.66 *Acute appendicitis is presumably responsible for exudate surrounding the appendiceal opening.*

Figure 12.67 *Appendiceal inflammation with swollen folds.*

Figure 12.68 *Normal side-to-end ileocolonic anastomosis.*

▼ **A**

▼ **B**

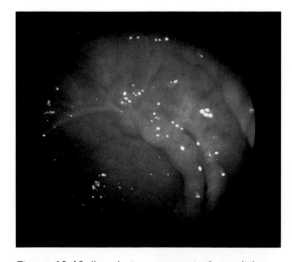

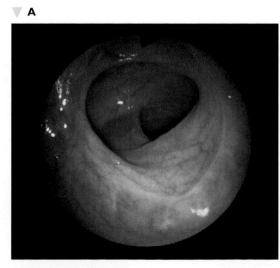

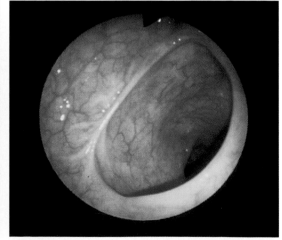

Figure 12.69 *Ileocolonic anastomosis shows slight nodularity at the anastomotic line.*

Figure 12.70 *(A and B) Perfectly smooth colocolonic anastomosis appearing (A) as a fine line of scarring or (B) as a very thin scar fold.*

nodular folds may exceed 5 mm in depth, and the overlying mucosa appears erythematous. However, the mucosa is soft and pliant, and tents easily upon biopsy. In the case of side-to-end colocolonic anastomosis, the closed end of the anastomosed segment may be inverted, creating a polyp-simulating configuration that may fool the endoscopist and lead to inappropriate removal (Fig. 12.71). When in doubt, the polypoid protuberance should be biopsied to prove its non-neoplastic composition.

If a suture granuloma occurs at the anastomosis, the area is usually erythematous and may be eroded or ulcerated (Fig. 12.72). A pseudopolyp caused by a suture granuloma may simulate a polyp (Fig. 12.73).

A peculiar and poorly understood abnormality is the development of chronic ulceration after ileorectal anastomosis, especially on the ileal side (Fig. 12.74). Such ulcers appear resistant to any form of therapy.

Narrowing of a colonic anastomosis to the point where a colonoscope cannot pass suggests disease at the anastomosis, such as inflammation, cancer, or concomitant diverticular disease. The presence of a symmetrical stricture without rigidity, masses, or ulcerations favors the diagnosis of a benign anastomotic stricture rather than recurrent malignancy. Malignancy can never be excluded with certainty, even if biopsy and brush cytology are negative. Endoscopic ultrasound may prove useful to evaluate anastomotic strictures and detect cancer or inflammation.

Endoscopy can also be useful in the evaluation of a Kock pouch or an ileoanal anastomosis with creation of a pelvic pouch. These types of surgery are usually carried out for ulcerative colitis or familial polyposis coli. During the healing stage after creation of a pouch, superficial ulceration and exudate

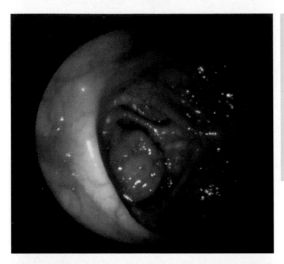
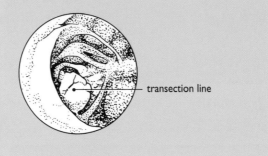

Figure 12.71 Inverted anastomotic line after side-to-end anastomosis, in the closed end of the proximal part of the anastomosis. If uncertain, a biopsy will establish that this is not an adenomatous polyp.

transection line

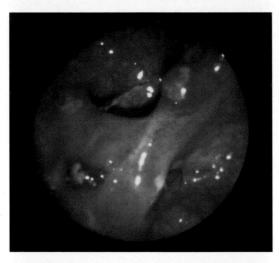
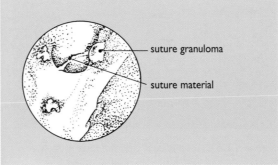

Figure 12.72 Suture granulomas at the anastomotic line; there is some evidence of inflammation.

suture granuloma

suture material

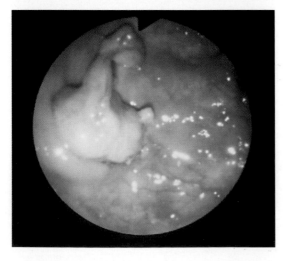

Figure 12.73 Pseudopolyp from a suture granuloma 1 year after colon resection simulates a polyp.

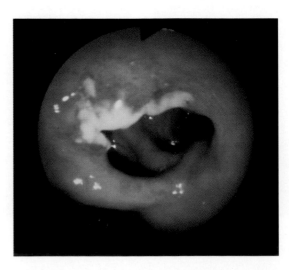

Figure 12.74 Chronic ulceration after ileorectal anastomosis for polyposis coli.

*Numbers in **Bold** refer to Figure numbers*

*Numbers in **Bold** refer to Figure numbers*